FATTY ACIDS

SYNTHESIS AND APPLICATIONS

FATTY ACIDS
SYNTHESIS AND APPLICATIONS

N.E. Bednarcyk
W.L. Erickson

NOYES DATA CORPORATION
Park Ridge, New Jersey   London, England
1973

Copyright © 1973 by Noyes Data Corporation
   No part of this book may be reproduced in any form
   without permission in writing from the Publisher.
Library of Congress Catalog Card Number: 76-188405
ISBN: 0-8155-0485-3
Printed in the United States

Published in the United States of America by
Noyes Data Corporation
Noyes Building, Park Ridge, New Jersey 07656

FOREWORD

The detailed, descriptive information in this book is based on U.S. patents since 1962 relating to fatty acids technology.

This book serves a double purpose in that it supplies detailed chemical information and can be used as a guide to the U.S. patent literature in this field. By indicating all the information that is significant and eliminating legal jargon and juristic phraseology, this book presents an advanced, commercially oriented review of fatty acids preparation and applications.

The U.S. patent literature is the largest and most comprehensive collection of technical information in the world. There is more practical, commercial, timely process information assembled here than is available from any other source. The technical information obtained from a patent is extremely reliable and comprehensive; sufficient information must be included to avoid rejection for "insufficient disclosure."

The patent literature covers a substantial amount of information not available in the journal literature. The patent literature is a prime source of basic commercially useful information. This information is overlooked by those who rely primarily on the periodical journal literature. It is realized that there is a lag between a patent application on a new process development and the granting of a patent, but it is felt that this may roughly parallel or even anticipate the lag in putting that development into commercial practice.

Many of these patents are being utilized commercially. Whether used or not, they offer opportunities for technological transfer. Also, a major purpose of this book is to describe the number of technical possibilities available, which may open up profitable areas of research and development. One should have to go no further than this condensed information to establish a sound background before launching into research in this field.

Advanced composition and production methods developed by Noyes Data are employed to bring these durably bound books to you in a minimum of time. Specialized techniques are used to close the gap between "manuscript" and "completed book." Industrial technology is progressing so rapidly that time-honored, conventional typesetting, printing, binding and shipping methods can render a technical or scientific book quite obsolete before the potential user gets to see it.

The Table of Contents is organized in such a way as to serve as a subject index. Other indexes by company, inventor and patent number help in providing easy access to the information contained in this book.

15 Reasons Why the U.S. Patent Office Literature Is Important to You—

(1) The U.S. patent literature is the largest and most comprehensive collection of technical information in the world. There is more practical commercial process information assembled here than is available from any other source.

(2) The technical information obtained from the patent literature is extremely comprehensive; sufficient information must be included to avoid rejection for "insufficient disclosure."

(3) The patent literature is a prime source of basic commercially utilizable information. This information is overlooked by those who rely primarily on the periodical journal literature.

(4) An important feature of the patent literature is that it can serve to avoid duplication of research and development.

(5) Patents, unlike periodical literature, are bound by definition to contain new information, data and ideas.

(6) It can serve as a source of new ideas in a different but related field, and may be outside the patent protection offered the original invention.

(7) Since claims are narrowly defined, much valuable information is included that may be outside the legal protection afforded by the claims.

(8) Patents discuss the difficulties associated with previous research, development or production techniques, and offer a specific method of overcoming problems. This gives clues to current process information that has not been published in periodicals or books.

(9) Can aid in process design by providing a selection of alternate techniques. A powerful research and engineering tool.

(10) Obtain licenses — many U.S. chemical patents have not been developed commercially.

(11) Patents provide an excellent starting point for the next investigator.

(12) Frequently, innovations derived from research are first disclosed in the patent literature, prior to coverage in the periodical literature.

(13) Patents offer a most valuable method of keeping abreast of latest technologies, serving an individual's own "current awareness" program.

(14) Copies of U.S. patents are easily obtained from the U.S. Patent Office at 50¢ a copy.

(15) It is a creative source of ideas for those with imagination.

CONTENTS AND SUBJECT INDEX

INTRODUCTION	1
PREPARATION BY OXO SYNTHESIS	2
Sulfuric Acid Catalyst	2
High Sulfuric Acid Concentration	2
Spent Alkylation Acid Containing 80 to 90% Sulfuric Acid	5
Use of Isoolefins	9
Use of Long Chain Olefin	12
Boron Trifluoride-Phosphoric Acid Catalyst	15
Continuous Single Stage Process	15
Reconstituting and Recycling Catalyst Internally	21
Anhydrous Reaction Mixture	23
Boron Trifluoride-Phosphoric Acid-Water Mixture	26
Hydrated Boron Trifluoride Catalyst	29
Low Olefin Concentration	29
Multistaged Hydrolysis	32
Group VIII Metal Catalysts	35
Treatment of Residue from Carbonylation Process	35
Oxidation with Cobalt Oxonation Catalyst	37
Complex Palladium Salt	41
Use of Halogenated Olefin	42
High Partial Pressure of Carbon Monoxide	45
Pt or Pd, Aromatic Phosphine and Surface Active Agent	50
Removal of Cobalt Catalyst	54
Iridium Compound with an Iodide Promoter	57
Rhodium Compounds	61
Other Catalysts	62
Hydrogen Fluoride	62
Oxidation of Oxo Synthesis Product Without Catalyst	65
Phosphoric Acid	68
Organic Sulfonic Acid	70
Oxonium Tetraborate	73
PREPARATION FROM OLEFINS BY OTHER METHODS	75
Oxidation of Olefins with Gaseous Oxygen	75
Bromine and Heavy Metal Catalyst	75
Cerium Salt-Nitric Acid Mixture as Catalyst	80
Use of Dinitrogen Tetroxide	83
Selective Oxidation	86
Continuous Atomization	88
Ozonolysis of Olefins	91

Formic Acid Solvent	91
Alkoxyalkanol Solvent	94
Phosphoric Acid Promoting Agent	97
Pyridine Solvent	99
Lower Alkanol Reaction Medium	102
Use of Oxidizing Agents	106
Metal Salt of Oxyhalide Acid	106
Periodic Acid or Potassium Permanganate	109
Reaction with Formic Acid	112
Sulfuric Acid Catalyst	112
Free Radical Initiator	116
Transaddition Reaction with Saturated Carboxylic Acids	120
Alkali Metal Catalyst	120
Water-Soluble Initiator	123
PREPARATION FROM OTHER SOURCES	129
From Hydrocarbons	129
Step-Wise Process	129
Continuous Withdrawal of Formed Acid	131
ω-Aryl Saturated Acids	135
From Alcohols and Ketones	139
Oxidation Using Platinum Catalyst	139
Oxidation Using Cobalt-Bromine-Carboxylic Acid Catalyst	141
Cyclic Secondary Alcohols and Caustic	144
Dicarboxylic Acid from Cyclic Alcohols and Ketones	146
Oxidation of Ketene-Ketone Polymers	148
From Derivatives	151
Decomposition and Isomerization of Anhydrides	151
3,3-Disubstituted Acids from Lactones	153
Hydrolysis of Nitriles	155
From Sulfates and Sulfonates	158
Oxidation of Alkyl Sulfuric Acids	158
Hydroxyalkane- and Alkenesulfonates	161
From Natural Sources	163
Seed Oils	163
Steam Hydrolysis of Fats	165
Hydrolysis and Acidification of Cocoa Butter	168
Miscellaneous Starting Materials	169
Nitroalkane and Sulfuric Acid	169
Magnesium Dialkyls and Carbon Dioxide	173
Preparation of Unsaturated Acids	175
C_{18} Cyclic Acid	175
Hydrolysis of 2-Substituted-2-Oxazolines	177
Acetylenic Acids by Grignard Synthesis	179
Reduction of Polyacetylenes	181
Preparation of Queen Substance	183
α-Substituted Unsaturated Acids	189
Trienoic Acids	190
BIOLOGICAL SYNTHESES	193
Conjugated Unsaturated Acids	193

Octadecatrienoic Acid Using Tung Nut Enzymes	193
Isolinoleic Acid Using Bacteria	194
Dibasic Acid	196
Using Yeast Fermentation	196
Acids and Esters	199
Microbial Production	199

SYNTHESIS OF HYDROXY ACIDS — 205

Catalytic Processes	205
Cation Exchange Resin Catalyst	205
Lewis Acid Catalyst	208
Cobalt Catalyst	212
Neo-Acids Using Acid Catalyst	215
Noncatalytic Processes	218
From Haloalkanols	218
From Alpha-Nitratocarboxylic Acids	221
Use of Alkanol Reaction Medium	223
Lesquerolic Acid from Seed Oil	226
Omega-Hydroxypelargonic Acid Using Polymeric Aluminum Alkyls	227

SYNTHESIS OF SALTS AND SOAPS — 231

Reactions with Acids	231
Calcium and Magnesium Soaps Using Liquefied Acids	231
Metal Soaps by Catalytic Grinding Process	233
Steam Distillation Process for DMOA	234
Divalent Metal-Zirconium Compounds by Water Removal Process	238
Basic Cadmium Salts as Vinyl Resin Stabilizers	241
Water Removal Process for Molybdenum Salts	245
Molybdenum and Vanadium Salts Using Oxalate	246
Silver Salts from Silver Complexes	248
Reactions with Alcohols	250
Alkali Salts by Oxidation in Presence of Cu(II) and Noble Metal	250
Selective Process for Straight Chain Soaps	251
Monounsaturated Soaps by Selective Hydrogenation	254
Caustic Fusion Improvement by Pretreatment	257
Oxidative Dehydrogenation in Presence of Carbon	260
Oxidative Dehydrogenation in Presence of Water	262
Other Starting Materials	265
Phenyl Mercuric Salts Using Branched Chain Acid Salts	265
Aluminum Salts from Aluminum Trialkyls	267
Lead, Cadmium and Divalent Tin Salts Using Acid Anhydrides	271
Alkali Metal Salts from Aldehydes	273
Salts from Tetravalent Alkoxides and Divalent Metal Carboxylates	274
Diorganoantimony Compounds Using Carboxylic Acid Salts	278

PREPARATION OF OTHER DERIVATIVES — 281

Esters	281
Neoalkylpolyol Esters	281
Dehydrogenation of Alcohols	284
Polymeric Esters	286
Lactones	288

Oxidation of Ketones	288
Anhydrides	291
Symmetrical Anhydrides of Hydroxy Acids	291
Keto Acids	294
From Dicarboxylic Dihalides and Organic Aluminum Halides	294
Halo Acids	296
Halooxidation of Aldehydes	296
Metal-Containing Derivatives	297
Magnesium Oxide Adducts	297
Werner Complexes of Chromium and Fatty Acids	301
PURIFICATION AND SEPARATION	303
Purification Processes	303
Using Acid Activated Crystalline Clay	303
Using Organic Aldehyde and Acidic Crystalline Clay	304
Stilbene Removal with Boron Trifluoride Etherate	306
Stilbene Removal with Boron Trifluoride Etherate and Activated Carbon	309
Using Amino Compounds	310
Using a Solvent Mixture	311
Neocarboxylic Acid in Two Stages with H_2SO_4	312
Using Alkyl Ester of Titanic Acid	314
Using Alkyl Ester of Silicic Acid	316
Using Alkali Metal Borohydride	317
Separation Processes	319
Using Aliphatic Hydrocarbon and Furfural	319
10-Hydroxydecanoic Acid by Acetylation	320
Using a Fatty Acid Distillation Residue	323
Using a Halofluoroalkane	326
Using 2-Nitropropane	327
Using Column Chromatography	328
Using Aryl Sulfonates	330
Using Reactive Extraction with Amines	331
Using Selective Crystallization	333
Using Detergent Fractionation	336
Using Crystal Modifiers	339
Simultaneous Separation and Purification	344
Countercurrent Process Using NH_4OH	344
Using Acidic Clay and Boron Trifluoride Etherate	346
COMPANY INDEX	349
INVENTOR INDEX	350
U.S. PATENT NUMBER INDEX	352

INTRODUCTION

This book describes practical syntheses and applications of those fatty acids that are used by the rubber and synthetic resin industries, and to some lesser extent by manufacturers of paints, printing inks, adhesives, and allied products.

All patents with edible applications have been excluded here, but will be used in a forthcoming new edition of the Noyes Data book on edible oils and fats.

Since the term "fatty acids" means many things to many people, we have tried to adhere to the definitions set forth by Klare S. Markley in his monumental five volume standard work entitled "Fatty Acids, Their Chemistry and Physical Properties" and published during the last decade by Wiley and Sons.

Naturally occurring fatty acids are higher straight chain unsubstituted carboxylic acids containing an even number of carbon atoms. They may be saturated or unsaturated, i.e., they may contain double bonds. Since synthetic modifications are countless, the definition is broadened to include odd- and even-numbered compounds containing six or more carbon atoms in the carbon chain and resembling the natural fatty acids. They may have various substituents along the chain; they may be branched and even contain certain additional short side chains. They may be oxidized to yield dicarboxylic acids and/or aldehyde acids.

Short chain, water-soluble acids, such as maleic acid, do not fall into this definition. Such acids will be covered in separate monographs to be published shortly by Noyes Data Corporation.

PREPARATION BY OXO SYNTHESIS

It has been known for some time that fatty acids can be produced by high pressure synthesis from olefins, carbon monoxide and water in the presence of a variety of catalysts. The patents in this chapter are grouped according to the type of catalyst used.

SULFURIC ACID CATALYST

High Sulfuric Acid Concentration

In a process described by G.A. Kurhajec, D.L. Johnston and K.E. Furman; U.S. Patent 3,047,622; July 31, 1962; assigned to Shell Oil Company an olefinic compound is combined with relatively dilute polybasic inorganic acid, thereby obtaining an olefinic compound-dilute acid admixture, reacting the olefinic compound-dilute acid admixture, while in liquid phase, with carbon monoxide, in the presence of sufficient concentrated sulfuric acid to result in a reaction mixture having a sulfuric acid strength above about 90%, in the absence of any substantial amount of water addition, at a temperature of from -10° to 100°C. and a pressure of from about atmospheric to 1,500 psig.

Thereafter water is added to the resulting reaction mixture in the substantial absence of carbon monoxide addition, and organic acid is separated from the resulting reaction mixture after the water addition. Olefinic compounds employed as charge to the process comprise organic compounds containing an olefinic unsaturation, such as, for example, the monoolefinic hydrocarbons having at least 3 carbon atoms to the molecule. Examples of suitable olefins comprise propylene, butene-1, butene-2, isobutene, the pentenes, hexenes, etc., and their homologues; olefinic polymers, such as propylene tetramer; the cyclic olefins, such as cyclopentene, cyclohexene, 4-vinylcyclohexene-1, and the like; etc. Olefinic compounds having a carbinol group in addition to olefinic unsaturation, as well as olefinic compounds having substituents, such as halogen, which do not adversely affect the course of the reaction, for example, 4-methyl-4-pentene-2-ol, ricinoleic acid, soya fat acid, methallyl chloride, and the like, are comprised in the suitable unsaturated olefinic compounds which may be reacted in accordance with the process. The olefinic charge to the process may comprise a single one, or a plurality of two or more, of the suitable olefinic compounds; hydrocarbon fractions comprising them; and the like.

Preferred olefinic charge material comprises the monoolefins having up to 20 carbon atoms to the molecule. A particularly preferred charge comprises the tertiary base olefins (that is, those yielding a tertiary alcohol upon hydrolysis). The olefinic charge to the process need not necessarily be in a state of high purity. Impurities generally encountered in the olefinic materials as commercially available do not adversely affect the efficiency of the process to any substantial extent.

Essential to the process is the initial combining of the olefinic charge to the process with a relatively dilute polybasic acid, such as, for example, aqueous sulfuric acid, or aqueous phosphoric acid, etc., aqueous sulfuric acid being preferred. The relatively dilute, or weak, acid thus initially combined with the olefinic charge is preferably of an acid strength not substantially in excess of about 80%. Preferred is the use of aqueous sulfuric acid containing from about 60 to 75%, and still more preferably from about 65 to 70%, by weight of sulfuric acid.

The specific strength of the dilute acid preferably employed will depend to some extent upon the specific olefinic material charged and specific operating conditions employed. Admixture of the relatively dilute acid with the olefinic charge is generally effected at a temperature at which no substantial polymerization of the olefins is encountered. Thus, the dilute acid may be combined with olefinic charge at a temperature in the range of from about 0° to 40°C. The specific temperature employed will depend upon the specific olefinic charge and degree of acid strength used. Higher temperatures may however be employed.

Thus, at times it is desirable to produce reaction mixtures comprising higher boiling organic acids, corresponding approximately to the polymeric compounds of the olefinic charge. In such case initial admixing of dilute acid with olefinic charge may be carried out at a higher temperature, for example, as high as about 100°C., to obtain polymerization of at least a substantial part of the olefinic compounds charged while in contact with the dilute acid during the initial phase of the process. The resulting admixture obtained by combining dilute acid and olefinic charge in the initial phase of the process is thereupon reacted with carbon monoxide in the presence of sufficient added concentrated sulfuric acid to obtain a reaction mixture having an acid strength of at least 90%. The dilute acid-olefinic charge mixture thus initially formed may comprise at least a part or all of the olefinic constituents in the form of suspension, solution, or reaction product with the acid.

The method of combining the preformed admixture of dilute acid and olefinic charge with the concentrated sulfuric acid may vary. Thus, the admixture of dilute acid and olefinic charge may be introduced into a large body of concentrated sulfuric acid. In such case, the body of concentrated sulfuric acid is preferably under carbon monoxide pressure. In continuous operation it is generally preferred to effect the addition of a continuous stream of the preformed dilute acid-olefinic compound admixture to a body of concentrated sulfuric acid in a reaction zone maintained under a substantial carbon monoxide pressure.

Contact of the fortified acid-olefinic compound admixture with carbon monoxide is carried out at relatively mild conditions. Temperatures of from -10° to 100°C., and preferably in the range of 20° to 60°C. are employed. Carbon monoxide pressures ranging from atmospheric to 1,500 psig and higher may be used. However, pressures higher than 700 psig need generally not be used. A constant carbon monoxide pressure in the range of from 100 to 650 psig is generally preferred. A particularly suitable pressure range is that from 450 to 550 psig. Conditions are controlled so that at least the greater part of the olefinic charge is in the liquid phase throughout the course of the reaction.

Essential to the process is the avoidance of introduction of any substantial amount of water into the reaction zone from an outside source during the course of the reaction with carbon monoxide. Upon completion of the reaction the reaction mixture is brought to substantially atmospheric pressure, and contacted with water. The water so added may be in the form of ice, liquid water or steam. Organic acid is thereupon separated from the reaction mixture resulting from the reaction with the water, by conventional means comprising one or more such steps as, for example, decantation, distillation, extractive distillation, adsorption, solvent extraction, etc.

Example 1: Isobutylene is dissolved in aqueous 65% H_2SO_4 at 30°C. and a pressure of 150 psig. The resulting solution contains a ratio of isobutylene to 65% H_2SO_4 of 1:2 by weight. The solution of isobutylene in 65% H_2SO_4 so obtained is then added to concentrated (92%) H_2SO_4 under a carbon monoxide pressure of 500 psig with vigorous stirring at 20°C. The mol ratio of isobutylene to total sulfuric acid in the resulting fortified mixture is 3.3:10. The resulting fortified solution is subjected to a constant carbon monoxide pressure of 500 psig at a temperature of 20°C. until no further absorption of carbon monoxide is evident. Pressuring with carbon monoxide is then terminated, and the pressure reduced to substantially atmospheric by venting.

Water is added to the resulting reaction mixture in an amount equal to 400% by volume at a temperature of 0°C. while at atmospheric pressure. Reaction is rapid with the formation of two separate liquid layers; an upper organic layer and a lower aqueous sulfuric acid layer. Analysis of the products thus obtained indicates that substantially all butylene has reacted with the production of 0.9 mol organic acid product per mol isobutylene charged with a yield of trimethylacetic acid of 83%; the rest of the organic acid obtained being polymeric in character.

Example 2: For the purpose of comparison isobutylene is added directly to concentrated sulfuric acid (92%) under a carbon monoxide pressure of 500 psig. The mol ratio of isobutylene to sulfuric acid in the resulting admixture is 3.3:10. The resulting solution is maintained at a constant carbon monoxide pressure of 500 psig at a temperature of 20°C. until no further absorption of carbon monoxide is apparent. Pressuring with carbon monoxide is then stopped and the pressure brought to atmospheric by venting. Water is then added to the resulting reaction mixture in an amount equal to 400% by volume at 0°C.

Reaction is rapid with the formation of two separate liquid layers; an upper organic layer and a lower aqueous sulfuric acid layer. Analysis of the products thus obtained indicates that substantially all isobutylene has undergone reaction with the formation of 0.59 mol of organic acid product per mol of isobutylene charged with a yield of 47% of trimethylacetic acid; the rest of the organic acid obtained being polymeric in character.

Spent Alkylation Acid Containing 80 to 90% Sulfuric Acid

C.G. McAlister, R.J. Lee and H.M. Knight; U.S. Patent 3,053,869; September 11, 1962; assigned to Standard Oil Company describe a process for the preparation of fatty acids from carbon monoxide and an olefin of 3 to 20 carbon atoms under mild reaction conditions; i.e., temperatures not exceeding 100°C. and pressures no higher than 100 atmospheres, using as the catalyst spent alkylation acid. Spent alkylation acid is essentially a petroleum refinery waste stream whose principal use is a feed to a system for recovery of sulfuric acid values therefrom by a thermal decomposition process such as heating in admixture with fine coke particles to liberate SO_2 which is dried and charged to a catalytic sulfuric acid process.

Spent alkylation acid is obtained as the result of alkylating olefins with isoparaffins in the presence of concentrated sulfuric acid of no less than 89% H_2SO_4. Such a process is well-known to those skilled in the art. The acid withdrawn from such an alkylation process may have an H_2SO_4 content of from 80 to 95% total titratable acidity as H_2SO_4, more usually it contains not more than about 90% H_2SO_4 on the same basis, and is unsuitable for further use as an alkylation catalyst. Hence, it is known as spent alkylation acid. Although spent alkylation acid may contain 80 to 90% H_2SO_4 on the basis of total titratable acidity, it is recognized by those skilled in the art as being quite different from 80 to 90% fresh sulfuric acid, for such a fresh sulfuric acid contains water as the only other principal ingredient in an amount of from 10 to 20%.

Spent alkylation acid on the other hand, while containing 80 to 90% H_2SO_4 on the above basis, contains only from 1 to 5% water with the remainder being "red oils" which are complex mixtures of polyolefins, organic sulfates and sulfonates. The free H_2SO_4 content of spent alkylation acid as determined by the aniline method will be 5 to 7% below the total titratable acidity concentration. The process is applicable for the preparation of carboxylic acids from such olefins as simple alkenes; i.e., straight and branched chain, terminal and internal unsaturated alkenes, cyclic olefins, diolefins, and unsaturated difunctional compounds such as unsaturated carboxylic acids from which dicarboxylic acids are prepared among others.

The olefin reactant employed may be a single normal olefin, or such branched chain olefins as the liquid polymers of propylene containing 5 to 20 carbon atoms and copolymers of propylene and butylene containing 5 to 20 carbon atoms a mixture of the foregoing olefins, or mixtures of olefins with saturated hydrocarbons or other inert solvents such as in a catalytic gasoline containing 50% olefins. In general, olefins containing 3 to 20 carbon atoms and especially branched chain olefins of 5 to 20 carbon atoms are preferred.

More specifically, the process comprises adding the olefin to stirred, spent alkylation acid at reaction temperature pressurized with CO. The mol ratio of spent alkylation acid employed is at least 1 mol H_2SO_4 per mol of olefin. The reaction mixture is maintained at a temperature in the range of -10° to 100°C. The reaction pressure employed is 10 to 100 atmospheres of carbon monoxide. The mixture resulting is held for 5 to 30 minutes after all the olefin has been added. The resulting mixture is depressurized, and water is added until the titratable acidity of the aqueous layer is between 65 to 75% and preferably 70 to 72% by weight, calculated as H_2SO_4. The temperature during dilution is controlled to not exceed about 60°C. The organic phase is separated from the aqueous phase and the fatty acid is recovered from the organic phase. Recovery of the fatty acid product may be

Preparation by Oxo Synthesis

accomplished by extraction, distillation, converting the fatty acid to a soap and extracting the soap with water or other solvent and springing the acid from its soap, and other methods understood by those skilled in the art. While mol ratios of up to 100 mols of H_2SO_4 per mol of olefin can be employed, little advantage is gained by employing more than 10 mols per mol. Satisfactory yields of fatty acids can be obtained for commercial operation by employing less than 10 mols H_2SO_4 per mol of olefin, and preferably the mol ratio is in the range of 1.5 to 5 mols per mol of olefin.

The reaction temperature need not exceed 100°C., so temperatures in the range of from -10° to 100°C. will be useful with temperatures in the range of 20° to 45°C. being preferred. As hereinbefore stated, the CO pressure need not exceed 100 atmospheres and pressures in the range of 10 to 50 atmospheres are advantageously employed. To illustrate the mode of operating according to the process, the following example is given. In this example a 316 stainless steel autoclave equipped with an internal cooling coil, baffles, an efficient stirrer and a dip-tube for introducing olefin below the spent alkylation acid surface is employed. Olefin from a weighed reservoir is pumped into the autoclave.

Example 1: Spent alkylation acid containing 83.1 weight percent free H_2SO_4, 4% water, 5% red oil, and having a total titratable acidity of 89.5 weight percent and a specific gravity of 1.7170 at 20°C. is charged to the autoclave in an amount (2,954 g.) to provide 25 gram mols H_2SO_4. The autoclave is closed. The spent alkylation acid is stirred and maintained at a temperature of 20° to 21°C. and pressured with carbon monoxide to 400 psig (about 27 to 28 atmospheres). Pentene-1 is pumped into the autoclave over a 6-hour period until 9.1 mols (635 g.) are added, which is equivalent to a mol ratio of "free H_2SO_4"/pentene-1 of 2.75.

The reaction temperature is maintained in the range of 20° to 21°C. during the olefin addition while the reaction mixture is stirred. Stirring is continued for 15 minutes after all the olefin is added. The recovered reaction mixture weighed 3,589 g. which indicates that approximately 130 g. of CO (plus the amount of handling losses) is taken up by the olefin. The stirred depressurized reaction mixture is cooled to 10°C. and there is added 2,700 grams of water to provide an aqueous phase of about 45% titratable acidity. The mixture is maintained at 30°C. during the addition of water. Heptane in an amount equal to about 1/2 the volume of the olefin charged is added and thoroughly mixed with the diluted reaction mixture.

Stirring is stopped. Two phases form. The lower aqueous phase is withdrawn. The heptane phase, containing the organic acids, is washed with 5 volume percent of water and then 3 times with 5 volume percent of a 10% sodium bicarbonate solution in order to remove the sulfuric acid, sulfur dioxide, and the like which are present in this phase. The organic acids in the heptane phase are taken up in 3,220 ml. of aqueous sodium hydroxide (7 weight percent NaOH concentration). The sodium hydroxide solution is then extracted several times with 200 ml. quantities of benzene to remove nonacidic organic polymers. The sodium soap solution is next acidified with hydrochloric acid to spring the free aliphatic carboxylic acids. The aqueous phase is extracted with a small amount (5%) of benzene, and the benzene washings are combined with the aliphatic acid phase.

Benzene and a water azeotrope are distilled off. The remaining aliphatic acids weighed 598 g. These are fractionated at atmospheric pressure through a 12" Vigreux column yielding 571 g. of C_6 acid boiling between 180° to 200°C. (largely 185° to 190°C.), and 27 g. of higher boiling acids. The C_6 acid product contained 85 to 90% of 2,2-dimethylbutyric acid as determined by gas chromatographic analysis. The yield of total C_6 acid is 54.3 mol percent or 90.0 weight percent, based on the pentene-1 charged. The yeild of polymer, after correction for the "red oils" present in the spent alkylation acid, amounted to 8.5 weight percent based on the olefin charged.

A similar run was made at a 2.32 mol ratio of "free H_2SO_4"/pentene-1. In this run, 2,490 g. of spent alkylation acid (83 weight percent free H_2SO_4) was charged to the autoclave, and 634 g. of pentene-1 was added over a 6-hour period. A carbon monoxide pressure of 400 psi and a temperature of 20°C. were maintained in identical fashion to the previous run. The total aliphatic acid product amounted to 503 g., of which 473 g. was C_6 acid. The yield of C_6 acid was 45.0 mol percent and the yield of polymer (corrected) was 16 weight percent based on pentene-1 charged.

In a third run in this series, the mol ratio of "free H_2SO_4"/pentene-1 was reduced to 1.85. In this run, 1,985 g. of spent alkylation acid was charged to the autoclave, and 638 g. of pentene-1 was added over a 6-hour period while maintaining 400 psi carbon monoxide pressure in the autoclave. The product was worked up in the same manner as the 2 previous runs, yielding 370 g. of aliphatic acids of which 359 g. was C_6 acid. The yield of C_6 acid was 34.0 mol percent and the yield of polymer (corrected) was 23.5 weight percent based on the olefin charged. Results are summarized below.

Production of Aliphatic Acids from Pentene-1 and CO Using Spent Alkylation Acid as the Condensing Agent

Temperature: 20°C. CO pressure: 400 psi

Mol Ratio "Free H_2SO_4":Olefin	Total Yield of Aliphatic Acids*	Yield of C_6 Acid*	Mol % Yield of C_6 Acid	Weight % Yield of Polymer**
2.75	94.3	90.0	54.3	8.5
2.32	79.4	74.8	45.0	16.0
1.85	58.0	56.3	34.0	23.5

*Weight percent based on pentene-1 charge
**Polymer yield corrected for the polymer (red oil) present in the spent alkylation acid used in the runs.

Use of Isoolefins

J.E. Anderson and N.W. Franke; U.S. Patent 3,167,585; January 26, 1965; assigned to Gulf Research & Development Company have found that optimum amounts of organic acids are formed in the process wherein an olefin which gives tertiary carbonium ions upon proton addition is reacted with carbon monoxide and water when the olefin and carbon monoxide are reacted in the liquid phase in the presence of sulfuric acid having a concentration of about 82 to 88% and the reaction product so produced is thereafter taken up with water. Olefins which give tertiary carbonium ions upon proton addition and which can be employed in this process can be defined by the following structural formula:

$$R_1-\underset{\underset{R_2}{|}}{C}=\underset{\underset{R_4}{|}}{C}-R_3$$

wherein R_1 and R_2, the same or different, can be alkyl radicals having from 1 to 20 carbon atoms, preferably from 1 to 15 carbon atoms, such as methyl, ethyl, propyl, n-butyl, isobutyl, tert-butyl, pentyl, neopentyl, methylbutyl, decyl, eicosyl, ethylmethylpentadecyl, etc.; and R_3 and R_4 can be hydrogen or similar to R_1 or R_2 above. Examples of olefins which can thus be employed are isobutylene, 2-methylbutene-1, 2-methylbutene-2, 2,4-dimethylpentene-2, 2,4,4-trimethylpentene-1, 2,2,4-trimethylpentene-2, 2-methylpentadecene-2, etc.

The reaction requires approximately equal molar amounts of each of the reactants, carbon monoxide, water and olefin, and sulfuric acid. Desirably, it is preferred that the molar ratio of sulfuric acid to olefin be at least 3 to 1. Using the preferred ratios we obtain less polymerization of olefin under the reaction conditions. The sequence in which the reactants and catalyst are brought together is of utmost importance. Sulfuric acid and carbon monoxide, separately or together, are introduced into the reaction zone. Only after the catalyst and reaction zone have been saturated with carbon monoxide is the addition of the defined olefin made. This is done primarily to reduce or inhibit olefin polymerization in the presence of sulfuric acid.

Water is then added to the reaction product obtained from the reaction of carbon monoxide and sulfuric acid with olefin. The desired organic acid is thereafter recovered from the final reaction product. It has been found that in order to obtain optimum yields of organic acids in the above process when the olefin employed is one which will give tertiary carbonium ions upon proton addition it is absolutely imperative that the concentration of the sulfuric acid be between about 82 to 88%, preferably between about 83 to 86%. Carbon monoxide is added to the reaction zone at the beginning of the reaction and by periodic addition or any other suitable means as required during the course of the reaction to maintain the desired concentration of the same as well as the desired reaction pressure. The reaction of carbon monoxide and sulfuric acid with olefin is extremely fast. Thus, it was found that when 1.5 mols of olefin were added at the rate of 1 ml. per minute to an autoclave containing 4.5 mols of H_2SO_4 having a concentration of 85% under a carbon monoxide pressure of 1,000 pounds per square inch gauge, the reaction was completed in 4 hours without undue polymerization. Under reaction conditions employed, care must be exercised to have only sufficient olefin present to facilitate the desired reaction and not such an excess that will promote the polymerization thereof. The amount of olefin introduced therein must, therefore, correspond approximately to the amount of olefin reacted.

The temperature and pressure required for the reaction of carbon monoxide and sulfuric acic with olefin are moderate. Thus the temperature can be about -20° to 70°C., preferably about 0° to 50°C. and the pressure in excess of about 100, preferably about 800 to 2,000 pounds per square inch gauge. At least one mol of water must be added to the reaction product for each mol of olefin which has reacted in the desired reaction. The temperature employed in this phase of the reaction can be about -10° to 60°C. and the pressure about 1/2 to 10 atmospheres.

The reaction product obtained upon the addition of water contains the desired organic acid along with some minor amounts of alcohol, esters and polyolefins. If the organic acid has 4 to 6 carbon atoms it will be completely soluble in the sulfuric acid associated therewith. One having 7 to 10 carbon atoms will be extremely soluble in the sulfuric acid. If the organic acid has from 11 to 15 carbon atoms it will be slightly soluble in the sulfuric acid, while one having 16 or more carbon atoms will be insoluble therein.

Thus, the separation of the desired organic acid from the sulfuric acid and other constituents associated therewith will depend upon its solubility in the sulfuric acid. With an organic acid having 4 to 6 carbon atoms, the mixture is diluted further with water. The solubility of the organic acid in dilute sulfuric acid being small, ordinary decantation is satisfactory. Organic acids having from 7 to 10 carbon atoms can be extracted with a saturated hydrocarbon such as hexanes, pure or mixed pentanes, heptanes, etc.

The organic acid is then separated from the saturated hydrocarbon by distillation. Since organic acids having 11 or more carbon atoms are slightly soluble or insoluble in sulfuric acid, ordinary separation such as decantation is satisfactory. The sulfuric acid can be recovered and reused. The mechanism of the reaction is believed to be as follows, using isobutylene as the representative olefin.

Preparation by Oxo Synthesis

(1) $CH_3-\underset{\underset{CH_3}{|}}{C}=CH_2 + H_2SO_4 \longrightarrow CH_3-\underset{\underset{CH_3}{|}}{\overset{+}{C}}-CH_3 + HSO_4^-$

(2) $CH_3-\underset{\underset{CH_3}{|}}{\overset{+}{C}}-CH_3 + {}^-C\equiv\overset{+}{O} \longrightarrow CH_3-\underset{\underset{\overset{+}{C}=O}{|}}{\overset{\overset{CH_3}{|}}{C}}-CH_3$

(3) $CH_3-\underset{\underset{\overset{+}{C}=O}{|}}{\overset{\overset{CH_3}{|}}{C}}-CH_3 + HSO_4^- \longrightarrow CH_3-\underset{\underset{\underset{OSO_3H}{|}}{C=O}}{\overset{\overset{CH_3}{|}}{C}}-CH_3$

(4) $CH_3-\underset{\underset{\underset{OSO_3H}{|}}{C=O}}{\overset{\overset{CH_3}{|}}{C}}-CH_3 + H_2O \longrightarrow CH_3-\underset{\underset{COOH}{|}}{\overset{\overset{CH_3}{|}}{C}}-CH_3 + H_2SO_4$

The process is illustrated using sulfuric acid of various concentrations and diisobutylene feed (about 80% by weight of which was 2,4,4-trimethyl pentene-1 and 20% by weight 2,4,4-trimethyl pentene-2).

Example 1: In each run 4 1/2 mols of the sulfuric acid was placed in a container and sufficient carbon monoxide (about 100% carbon monoxide) was introduced therein to saturate the sulfuric acid, obtain a carbon monoxide atmosphere and a pressure of 1,000 pounds per square inch gauge. Periodically during the reaction carbon monoxide was introduced therein to maintain a constant pressure of 1,000 pounds per square inch gauge. In each run after the desired pressure was obtained the olefin was introduced therein at the rate of 1 ml. per minute until 1.5 mols of olefin had been introduced. The temperature during the reaction was maintained at 20°C.

When the reaction was complete the container was depressured and drained. Sufficient water was then added to the container to dilute the acid to a concentration of 75%. This resulted in an almost complete separation of organic product from the sulfuric acid. The sulfuric acid layer, after decantation, was extracted with 500 ml. of n-hexane to recover contained organic acids. The organic product was stirred into 600 g. of a 10% by weight of sodium hydroxide solution, and this basic mixture was shaken in a separatory funnel with the aforementioned hexane extract to recover any organic acid in the extract. The organic acids are more soluble in a basic solution and, consequently, were removed from the n-hexane phase. The basic layer containing the organic acids was separated from the n-hexane layer by decantation. Then the basic layer was placed into a vessel provided with means for cooling. Sufficient amount of hydrochloric acid (about 20% by weight hydrochloric acid) was added with cooling until the pH of the solution was about 2 and the organic acid layered out from the basic solution.

To improve this separation, the entire organic layer was placed into another separatory funnel and 250 ml. of n-hexane was added. In this acidic medium and with proper shaking, the organic acid dissolved into the n-hexane layer. About 300 ml. of water was added to wash out any traces of the mineral acid (hydrochloric acid). The hexane layer was then recovered by decantation. It was passed over Drierite (anhydrous calcium sulfate) to remove any absorbed water and distilled at atmospheric pressure to recover the n-hexane which could be reused. The remaining bottom from this distillation was vacuum distilled at 10 mm. of mercury to recover the carboxylic acid.

Run No.	Sulfuric Acid Concentration % by Wt.	Weight of CO Absorbed, grams	Isononanoic Acid Recovered % by Wt.
1	78.2	14.5	49
2	80.0	24.9	75
3	82.8	34.3	92
4	85.0	38.7	96
5	87.0	38.4	97
6	88.7	36.2	93
7	90.0	38.7	93
8	96.9	26.9	40

Use of Long Chain Olefin

E.T. Roe and D. Swern; U.S. Patent 3,170,939; February 23, 1965; assigned to the U.S. Secretary of Agriculture describe the carboxylation of long carbon chain olefinic compounds with carbon monoxide at atmosphere pressure. Direct carboxylation of long chain olefinic compounds with carbon monoxide can be achieved at atmospheric pressure by employing a narrow range of operating conditions in which the concentration of the sulfuric acid and also the molar ratio of sulfuric acid to the long chain olefinic compound must be regulated.

According to the process carbon monoxide at atmospheric pressure is (a) dispersed in aqueous sulfuric acid having a concentration in the range of about

93 to 98% H_2SO_4, (b) the olefinic compound is combined with this sulfuric acid at about 10° to 20°C. in such proportions that the resulting mixture contains at least about 3 mols water to each mol of olefinic compound, and (c) during the mixing of olefinic compound and sulfuric acid additional carbon monoxide is dispersed in the mixture. The entire operation is conducted at substantially atmospheric pressure, and the new carboxylic acid derivative is recovered from the sulfuric acid by dilution with water and solvent extraction or mechanical separation.

The product is typically recovered from the reaction mixture by pouring the sulfuric acid solution into a mixture of ice and water, followed by extraction of the product with a suitable solvent such as ether. Alternatively, procedures for extracting the product directly from the reaction mixture may be employed. A critical variable in the high yield atmospheric carboxylation of the less reactive, long carbon chain nonterminally unsaturated compounds is the concentration and quality of water. The importance of water is quite evident as shown in the table in which the results of the carboxylation of oleic acid are tabulated. In all of these examples the amount of water does not change during carboxylation, since the carbon monoxide is generated externally. The following equation summarizes the chemistry involved:

$$CH_3-(CH_2)_7-CH=CH-(CH_2)_7-CO_2H + CO + H_2O \longrightarrow$$

$$CH_3-(CH_2)_x-\underset{\underset{COOH}{|}}{CH}-(CH_2)_{15-x}-COOH$$

(wherein x may be 6 to 9)

Commercial oleic acid was purified by crystallization at low temperature followed by fractional distillation to give the oleic acid employed as the starting material in these examples. The process is illustrated with particular reference to Example 6 in the table. Carbon monoxide was passed through 80.4 g. (0.795 mol) of 97.2% sulfuric acid contained in a 500 ml. 3-necked flask, vented to the atmosphere, using a gas dispersion tube with a coarse fritted cylinder. With stirring, 7.1 g. (0.025 mol) of oleic acid was added dropwise in 16 minutes to the sulfuric acid solution which was saturated with carbon monoxide. Carbon monoxide was allowed to pass through the stirred mixture for a total of 2 hours, while the temperature was maintained between 9° and 13°C. with external cooling.

At the end of this time the mixture was poured into approximately 300 ml. of a mixture of ice and water. The product was extracted with ether and washed free of sulfuric acid. The ether solution was dried over anhydrous sodium sulfate, filtered, and the ether was then evaporated, yielding

6.4 g. of pale yellow syrupy material having an iodine number of 12.9, acid number, 300, and saponification number, 300. The reaction conditions for the other examples were the same as described for Example 6 with the exceptions listed in the table, specifically, mol ratio of sulfuric acid to oleic acid, concentration of sulfuric acid, and time of stirring the mixture.

Reaction of Oleic Acid with Gaseous Carbon Monoxide

Example No.	Mol Ratio			Sulfuric Acid, %	Time, Hours	Acid No.[2]	Iodine No.
	Oleic Acid	Sulfuric Acid	Water[1]				
1	1	5.5	3.0	91	2	150[3]	18
2	1	9.6	1.5	97	2	222	--
3	1	9.6	1.5	97	6	226	--
4	1	18.0	2.8	97	1	252	34
5	1	19.1	3.0	97	2	287	20
6	1	31.8	5.0	97	2	300	13
7	1	63.6	10.0	97	2	297	16
8	1	24.0	0	100	2	215[4]	63

[1]Water present in sulfuric acid.
[2]Saponification number essentially the same as acid number, except where given below.
[3]Saponification number 201.
[4]Saponification number 251.

Referring to Examples 1 through 8, the extent of carboxylation is indicated by an increase in acid number and a decrease in iodine number. With 91% sulfuric acid (Example 1) no carboxylation takes place. The acid number actually indicates a loss of carboxyl group. Since the same mol ratio of water, 3 mols of water to 1 mol of oleic acid, when contained in a more concentrated sulfuric acid (Example 5) is adequate, one must conclude that 91% sulfuric acid is too dilute for this process.

However, 1.5 mol of water per mol of oleic acid is insufficient for carboxylation to proceed in a satisfactory manner (Examples 2 and 3) even though the concentration of sulfuric acid is 97% and the reaction time is extended to 6 hours. With 100% sulfuric acid (Example 8) carboxylation, if occurring, is negligible, showing conclusively that water must be present during the reaction. The greatest increase in acid number and decrease in iodine number, indicating maximum carboxylation is obtained when 5 mols of water per mol of oleic acid is employed (Example 6). Increasing the amount of water above 5 mols per mol of oleic acid (Example 7) or increasing the reaction time beyond 2 hours does not increase the amount of carboxylation.

The product obtained by the carboxylation of oleic acid, the pale yellow viscous liquid described in Example 6, could not be purified by low temperature solvent crystallization, but distilled readily at about 200°C. and 0.45 mm. mercury pressure to give a product having an acid number of 341, carbon and hydrogen analyses of 69.4 and 11.7%, respectively, and molecular refractivity of 92.8. Infrared spectra and gas chromatographic analyses of the product were also obtained. All the data substantiate the conclusion that the product is carboxystearic acid of the formula:

$$CH_3-(CH_2)_x-\underset{COOH}{CH}-(CH_2)(15-x)-COOH$$

In a major portion of the product, the carboxyl group in probably in the 9 or 10 position ($x = 7$ or 8). However, in view of the nature of strong acid-catalyzed double bond addition reactions, the 8 and 11 isomers ($x = 6$ or 9) are also formed. The source of carbon monoxide may be other than that already illustrated. For example, it may be generated in situ by the decomposition of formic acid in the sulfuric acid reaction medium, but the composition of the reaction mixture must still adhere to the concentration of sulfuric acid and mol ratio of water to compound to be carboxylated must be approximately as defined by Examples 5 and 6.

Highly purified oleyl alcohol (98 to 99%), methyl ricinoleate and linoleic acid were also carboxylated by the process. After pouring the reaction product obtained by carboxylation of oleyl alcohol into an ice and water mixture, it was necessary to hydrolyze the sulfate ester by boiling. Otherwise the procedure was substantially that employed in Example 6.

BORON TRIFLUORIDE-PHOSPHORIC ACID CATALYST

Continuous Single Stage Process

In a process by M.J. Waale and J.M. Vos; U.S. Patent 3,059,004; October 16, 1962; assigned to Shell Oil Company carboxylic acids are produced by continuously introducing charge materials consisting essentially of carbon monoxide, an olefinic compound having at least 3 carbon atoms, an amount of water in at least the stoichiometrical equivalent of the olefinic compound, and a catalyst consisting essentially of a boron trifluoride-inorganic acid complex into a reaction zone, maintaining a substantially homogeneous liquid phase of relatively constant composition at a substantially constant temperature in the range of from -10° to 150°C. in the reaction zone throughout the course of the reaction, continuously withdrawing a portion of the liquid phase from the reaction zone, and separating carboxylic acid from the portion of liquid phase withdrawn from the reaction zone. Olefinic compounds employed as charge to the process comprise the monoolefinically unsaturated organic compounds having at least 3 carbon atoms to the molecule. Examples of such suitable olefinic compounds are the monoolefinic hydrocarbons, polymers and copolymers of alkenes, cyclic alkenes, as well as unsaturated fatty acids or hydroxy fatty acids which may form unsaturated fatty acids under the reaction conditions, etc. Commercially available mixtures comprising these alkenes may also be used, for example, olefin-containing hydrocarbon fractions such as obtained by thermal vapor phase cracking or paraffin wax in the presence of steam.

These fractions not only contain alkenes but generally also paraffins, naphthenes and aromatics, which usually do not take part in the synthesis. Their presence promotes the separation into layers of the reactor effluence, the same also being true of the alkenes unconverted during the reaction. The carbon monoxide reactant need not necessarily be pure. Suitable carbon monoxide charge material comprise the commercially available carbon monoxide and carbon monoxide-containing gases. The presence therein of fixed gases and minor amounts of saturated hydrocarbons does not adversely affect the efficiency of the process.

The process is executed in the presence of a liquid, highly acidic, inorganic compound as catalyst. Suitable catalysts comprise the liquid complex mixtures obtained by combining boron trifluoride, water and a polybasic inorganic acid, such as for example, phosphoric acid, sulfuric acid and the like. Preferred catalysts comprise the complex mixtures of boron trifluoride-phosphoric acid-water containing a mol ratio of phosphoric acid to boron trifluoride in the range of from about 0.8:1.3 to 1.3:0.8 having a water content of from about 7 to 12% by weight (based upon total boron trifluoride and phosphoric acid). A particularly preferred catalyst comprises the complex mixtures containing about 1 1/2 molar amount of boron trifluoride for 1 molar amount of phosphoric acid and approximately 10% by weight of water (based upon the total weight of boron trifluoride plus phosphoric acid).

In accordance with the process the olefinic reactant, carbon monoxide, catalyst and water are continuously introduced into the reaction zone throughout the course of the operation. The molar ratio of the amount of water to the amount of alkenes charged is generally maintained in the range of from about 1:1 to 30:1, preferably from about 2:1 to 6:1. The greater this ratio the greater should be the weight ratio of catalyst supplied to alkenes supplied. The water supplied usually is in the range from about 2 to 15% by weight of the total quantity of liquid inorganic material (mainly the catalyst) supplied during the same period of time. The catalyst decreases in activity at excessive and too low water to catalyst ratios.

Preparation by Oxo Synthesis

Essential to the process is the maintaining of the liquid contents of the reaction zone in the form of a substantially homogeneous liquid phase of substantially constant composition throughout the course of the reaction. Essentially constant composition of the reaction zone contents is obtained by controlling and correlating the rate at which materials are charged to the reaction zone and withdrawn therefrom.

Conventional means are employed to maintain the desired state of homogeneity in the liquid contents of the reaction zone. Thus one or more means such as stirring, passage of normally gaseous material therethrough, and the like may be employed. The temperature at which the reaction is carried out is generally in the range of from about -10° to 150°C. In many cases excellent results are obtained at temperatures in the range of 40° to 100°C. The carbon monoxide pressure generally is maintained in excess of about 20 atmospheres gauge. Suitable values of this pressure are usually in the range of from about 50 to 150 atmospheres gauge. The average residence time of the reaction mixture in the reaction space is often in the range of from 1 to 4 hours. The gas phase is preferably vented separately from the reaction zone.

The reaction conditions may be varied according to the type of the alkenes to be converted and the specific catalyst selected for this purpose. With the use of liquid complex mixtures of phosphoric acid, boron trifluoride and water, in which the $H_3PO_4:BF_3$ mol ratio is in the range of from about 0.8 to 1.3 to about 1.3:0.8, preference is given to: a water content of from 7 to 12% by weight (based on the mixture of H_3PO_4, BF_3 and H_2O at the inlet), temperatures in the range of from about 40° to 80°C. and CO pressures of from about 50 to 150 atmospheres gauge. Lower or higher water contents may be used in accordance with increase or decrease in the $H_3PO_4:BF_3$ ratio. With the use of sulfuric acid containing 4 to 10% by weight of water the reaction will be preferably executed at about room temperature and at the higher pressures within the specified range.

A particular advantage of the process resides in the ability to carry out the desired reaction therein at optimum conditions for the reaction mixture as a whole throughout the entire reaction zone; i.e., conditions under which alkenes are converted at a relatively high reaction rate to carboxylic acids and at a relatively low reaction rate to such undesirable by-products as polymers. Composition of the reaction mixture in the reaction space is obtained at a constant rate of supply of the reactants and of the catalyst, as well as of the materials which may be supplied together with the components and the catalyst, provided the temperature and pressure are also kept constant and the reaction mixture is kept substantially homogeneous. Small deviations from the constant conditions envisaged may occur during operation, for example, as a result of irregularities or inaccuracies in the working of the apparatus used for the supply of materials. These deviations are, however, readily compensated for by taking appropriate conventional measures to regulate the process. When the composition of the reaction mixture is constant the concentration of each component remains constant. For each of the components to be reacted therefore the supply per unit of time and per unit of volume should be equal to the sum of consumption and withdrawal. In the case of the product the production per unit of time and per unit of volume should be equal to the withdrawal.

Conventional means are employed to maintain the desired state of homogeneity in the liquid contents of the reaction zone. Thus one or more means such as stirring, passage of normally gaseous material therethrough, and the like may be employed within the scope of the process. As a consequence of the maintaining of the above defined catalytic reaction conditions, comprising the maintaining of liquid contents of the reaction zone in the form of a homogeneous, liquid phase of substantially constant composition, water can now be added in an amount sufficient to form the desired acid directly to the single reaction zone, and the carboxylic acids produced efficiently at moderate conditions of temperature and pressure in a continuous single stage operation.

Reactor effluence in the process may be worked up in the conventional manner. After releasing the pressure and degassing, it may, if it has not already separated into two layers of its own accord, be separated by the addition of a suitable organic diluent. Suitable diluents comprise the normally liquid hydrocarbons, for example, a gasoline fraction having a boiling range of from about 60° to 80°C. The addition of the diluent facilitates the separation of the reactor effluence into two layers, viz an organic phase containing the carboxylic acid product and an inorganic catalyst containing phase. The latter may be recycled to the reaction zone after the addition of sufficient water thereto to replace that consumed in the reaction. The water may optionally be introduced, in part or entirety, as a separate stream into the system.

Fatty acid products are recovered from the organic phase by conventional methods, preferably after the removal of the last traces of catalyst therefrom. Removal of residual catalyst may comprise such steps as washing with water and the like. Recovery of the product carboxylic acids may comprise such steps as, for example, ester or salt formation, extraction, crystallization, decantation, distillation with or without steam, etc.

Example: The starting alkenes were a fraction of a product obtained by thermal vapor phase cracking of a paraffinic feedstock in the presence of steam. This fraction contained chiefly alkenes having from 8 to 10 carbon atoms. The original diene content had disappeared as a result of partial

Preparation by Oxo Synthesis

hydrogenation. In percentages by weight the monoalkene content was 76% in addition to which 17% of saturated hydrocarbons and 7% of aromatics were present. Of the 76% of monoalkenes, 38.5% were unbranched, 20% branched and 17.5% cyclic alkenes. The monoalkenes mainly had a cis- or trans-configuration, only 2% were alpha-alkenes, while 1% had a $CH_2=CR_1R_2$ structure (in which R_1 and R_2 are alkyl groups). The catalyst used contained equimolar amounts of H_3PO_4 and BF_3, and also water. When the catalyst was introduced into the reaction space, the water content, based on the sum of H_3PO_4, BF_3 was about 10% by weight.

The reaction was carried out in a cylindrical, stainless steel 5 liter reaction vessel which had a spherical bottom. The reactor was provided with a mechanically driven stirrer, a steam or water jacket for raising the reaction mixture to the desired temperature, supply lines for alkenes, carbon monoxide and catalyst, and discharge lines for liquid reaction mixture and the gas phase. The volume of liquid reaction mixture in the reaction vessel was kept at 3 liters.

The molar ratio of water to alkenes supplied to the reaction vessel was varied between 3 and 25. The carbon monoxide pressure was varied between 36 and 100 atmospheres gauge. The temperature in the reaction vessel was kept at 60°C. The contents of the reaction vessel were stirred at a speed of 750 rpm. In each experiment the reaction vessel remained in continuous operation for 1,500 hours. The results shown in the table relate to the period between the 600th and 1,500th hour.

The reactor effluence was led to a separator in which two layers formed. The bottom layer (the catalyst layer) was passed from the separator to a buffer vessel to which sufficient water was added for the water content to be about 10% by weight, based on the total amount of the inorganic material present. The catalyst layer also contained organic material in an amount which during the reaction was able to increase to an average of 16% by weight, based on the sum of inorganic and organic material. In some experiments the organic material content in the catalyst was lower owing to the supply of fresh catalyst, but this fact had little effect on the results. The catalyst with the organic material present therein was returned from the buffer vessel to the reaction vessel.

The top layer was removed from the separator and freed from inorganic acid compounds by water-washing. The washing water was then used in order to bring the catalyst to the desired water content. The fatty acids were then converted into their sodium salts by adding a 25% solution of aqueous NaOH in 5% excess. The solution of the soaps was separated from unconverted alkenes and by-products; extracted with a light, aromatic-free gasoline; acidified with HCl; and again extracted with an aromatic-free gasoline.

The gasoline was distilled from the last extract obtained, after which the remaining fatty acid mixture was fractionated in vacuo; a column having 7 theoretical plates and a 4:1 reflux ratio being employed. At a pressure of 3 mm. mercury temperatures in the range of 101° to 125°C. were measured at the top of the column. Fourteen fractions were obtained, of which the average molecular weight, determined from the acid numbers, rose from 157 to 182 (theory: $C_8H_{17}COOH = 158$, $C_{10}H_{21}COOH = 186$).

The conditions, in so far as they differed in the various experiments, are listed in the following table which also shows the conversions and yields. The figures under the heading "alkene" are grams per hour of the hydrocarbon mixture supplied which, as stated above, contained 76% by weight of alkenes. In the molar ratio of H_2O to alkene no other hydrocarbons are included except alkenes. Under the heading "catalyst" is given the number of grams per hour of the catalyst including the organic material present therein and after the water content had been made up. The percentage of total converted alkene is based on the alkene content of the feed.

A comparison of experiments 2, 3 and 4 shows the favorable effect which an increasing ratio of water-containing catalyst to alkene has on conversion (last column) and selectivity (last column but one). A comparison of experiments 1, 5 and 6 shows the favorable effect of increasing the CO pressure. Experiment 1 is considered the most favorable, since a high production capacity of the reactor (see first column) is retained therein with a reasonable conversion and selectivity.

No.	Feed g./hour		Organic Material in Catalyst Supplied, percent by Weight	Water to Inorganic Material in Catalyst, percent by Weight	Mol Ratio of H_2O to Alkene in Feed	CO-Pressure Atm. Gauge	Residence Time, hours	Fatty Acid, mol percent to Converted Alkene	Total of Converted Alkene percent
	"Alkene"	"Catalyst"							
1	275	1,175	11.7	9.9	3.4	100	2.7	67	80
2	264	2,475	15.8	10.2	7.4	100	1.6	63	85
3	134	2,400	12.3	9.7	14.0	100	1.8	83	93
4	77	2,425	9.0	9.6	25.0	100	1.9	90	96
5	264	1,155	10.2	10.2	3.7	71	2.8	60	84
6	268	1,170	11.4	9.7	3.5	36	2.8	52	68

A separation process, entirely consisting of distillations, was also applied to samples of the crude products still containing the unconverted alkenes, but from which the catalyst had already been removed by washing. The alkenes were distilled off at atmospheric pressure, after which the fatty acids were distilled in vacuo. The resulting fatty acid fractions were less pure than those resulting from the method discussed above in the example, this being offset by a simpler process. The fatty acids separated in such simple manner were, however, found to be sufficiently pure for satisfactory use in various practical scale applications.

Modifications of this low temperature, liquid phase carboxylic acid process are described in the following patents. J.G. Van de Vusse and L. Alders; U.S. Patent 3,059,005; October 16, 1962; assigned to Shell Oil Company provide a method for separating and purifying the catalyst within the system in the absence of agents from an outside source.

A process by J.G. Van de Vusse; U.S. Patent 3,059,006; October 16, 1962; assigned to Shell Oil Company concerns a method of regulating the carbon monoxide partial pressure in the reactor.

J.M. Vos and R. de Vries; U.S. Patent 3,059,007; October 16, 1962; assigned to Shell Oil Company produced increased yields and better quality product by eliminating polyolefins from the olefin charge to the reactor.

Reconstituting and Recycling Catalyst Internally

In order to avoid the excessive temperatures and pressures and relatively low yields of the one-step processes for producing carboxylic acids from olefins, carbon monoxide and water with mineral acid catalysts, it has been found necessary to carry out the reaction in two steps. In the first step, the olefin and carbon monoxide are reacted in the presence of an acidic catalyst, essentially in the absence of water, to form an intermediate, hydrolyzable, reaction product. This intermediate product is thereafter hydrolyzed in the second step to liberate the desired carboxylic acid product in good yield and the acidic catalyst.

C. Roming, Jr.; U.S. Patent 3,068,256; December 11, 1962; assigned to Esso Research and Engineering Company describes a process for producing carboxylic acids from olefins, carbon monoxide and water which surprisingly combines the advantages of the two-step process with those inherent in the one-step process. This desirable result is accomplished by conducting the reaction in a manner such that the acid catalyst is continuously reconstituted and recycled internally to catalyze the reaction of freshly introduced olefin and carbon monoxide feed. The recycling of the acid catalyst internally is accomplished by utilizing the relatively large difference in density between the acid catalyst and the carboxylic acid reaction products and unreacted feed olefin.

Internal recycling of the catalyst in this way affords a considerable advantage over the two-step process because of reduced equipment costs and reduced acid catalyst requirements, as will be shown more fully hereinafter. At the same time, the improved yields and ability to operate at mild reaction conditions, heretofore possible pnly with a two-step operation, are not sacrificed. Generally speaking, the process comprises passing carbon monoxide and a C_2 to C_{24} olefin into a reaction zone in the presence of a liquid mineral acid catalyst having a specific gravity in the range of 1.25 to 1.90. The reaction mixture is maintained in the reaction zone for a sufficient time to form an intermediate, hydrolyzable reaction product which is then passed into a hydrolysis zone. Water is countercurrently flowed into the hydrolysis zone, whereby intimate contact between the water and intermediate reaction product occurs and the product is hydrolyzed to yield the desired carboxylic acid product and reconstituted mineral acid catalyst. The carboxylic acid product is removed from the hydrolysis zone for further processing, and the reconstituted mineral acid is internally recycled through the hydrolysis and reaction zones to catalyze the reaction of fresh olefin and carbon monoxide feed.

The pressures under which the reaction is conducted are given in terms of carbon monoxide pressures; however, it is not meant to imply that pure carbon monoxide gas is required. Carbon monoxide in the form of synthesis gas, for example, is suitable. Other forms of carbon monoxide may also be utilized as long as the indicated carbon monoxide partial pressures are attained in the reaction vessel. It is, of course, preferable that objectionable acidic components of impure carbon monoxide gases, such as sulfur compounds, carbon dioxide, oxygen or metal carbonyls, be removed from the carbon monoxide feed; however, inert gases such as hydrogen, methane and nitrogen may be present as impurities or diluents, since they do not adversely affect the desired reaction.

Regardless of whether pure gas or a diluted mixture is used, the amount of carbon monoxide supplied to the reactor is, of course, in excess of that required to stoichiometrically react with the olefin feed. To provide an adequate excess, at least 1,000 scf carbon monoxide/bbl. olefin feed should be provided and preferably, between 1,500 and 2,500 scf/bbl. of feed.

The olefin feed to the reactor can be any olefin which normally is in the liquid state under the conditions of reaction. That is to say, olefins having from 2 to 24 carbon atoms and mixtures thereof are suitable. For example, aliphatic olefins such as ethylene, propylene, butylene, isobutylene, pentylenes, decenes, hexadecenes, octadecenes, etc., and mixtures of these olefins may be used. However, olefins having 4 to 15 carbon atoms are preferred. The C_6 to C_{15} branched olefins produced by the polymerization of propylene, are an especially desirable feedstock for they give rise to sterically-hindered acids, which in turn yield very stable esters. Such esters are valuable in the production of synthetic lubricants.

The acidic catalysts utilized in the process are liquid mineral acids having specific gravities greater than about 1.25. It is essential that the specific gravity of the acid not be lower than this value in order that the proper degree of recycling be attained in the reactor. Preferred acids are those having specific gravities of at least 1.35 and especially preferred are acids of 1.5 to 1.85 specific gravity. With the latter acids, not only is improved recycling realized, but the yields of product produced in the presence of such catalysts are greater. Suitable mineral acids having specific gravities in the proper range include sulfuric acid, boron trifluoride dihydrate, and mixtures of boron trifluoride with sulfuric or phosphoric acids. The boron trifluoride comprising catalysts are especially preferred, with boron trifluoride dihydrate being most preferred because of its superior activity in producing high yields of the desired carboxylic acid products, particularly those derived from branched chain, higher molecular weight olefins.

Example: To demonstrate the advantage of the one-step process in which the acid catalyst is internally recycled over the two-step process of the prior art, wherein the catalyst is externally separated from the carboxylic acid product, the following series of experiments were conducted.

Tripropylene, derived from the phosphoric acid catalyzed polymerization of propylene, was reacted in a stainless steel autoclave at a pressure of 1,000 psig CO pressure and at ambient temperature (about 23°C.). The catalyst used was produced by saturating 85% phosphoric acid with boron trifluoride (1.5/1/1 mol ratio of $BF_3/H_3PO_4/H_2O$, specific gravity about 1.75). During the reaction, which varied from 2 to 6 hours, the temperature rose to about 40°C. and the pressure to 1,200 to 1,500 psig.

At the completion of the reaction, the autoclave was vented to the atmosphere, and the products transferred to a separatory funnel. A stoichiometric amount of water, based on olefin, was added. The mixture was then extracted with an equal volume of petroleum ether in order to separate as completely as practicable the carboxylic product layer from the acid catalyst layer. Even by this stringent separation procedure, however, only 94 to 97% of the original amount of acid catalyst utilized could be recovered. In contrast to the catalyst losses of at least 3%, obtained even under the careful separation of this example of the two-step process, catalyst losses are reduced by employing the internal recycling to the order of 1% and certainly less than 2%.

Anhydrous Reaction Mixture

A process by H. Chafetz and J.A. Patterson; U.S. Patent 3,282,993; November 1, 1966; assigned to Texaco Inc. comprises a reaction of an olefin, carbon monoxide and essentially a stoichiometric amount of water in the presence of an inorganic acid carbonylation catalyst under an elevated carbon monoxide pressure, advantageously between about 400 and 50,000 psi, and at a temperature between about -40° and 60°C., to form an essentially anhydrous final reaction mixture of fatty acid and the catalyst.

The process then involves contacting with agitation the final reaction mixture under essentially anhydrous conditions with an organic solvent selective for the fatty acid but not for the catalyst at a temperature between about $-40°$ and $75°C.$, separating the fatty acid-containing solvent layer from the acid catalyst layer, recycling the acid catalyst layer to the initial reaction of the carbon monoxide and the olefin and separating the fatty acid product from the solvent layer. By essentially anhydrous is meant less than about 10% stoichiometric excess of water.

Under advantageous conditions the essentially stoichiometric amount of water expressed in terms of mol ratio of olefin reactant to water is between about 1:0.9 and 1:1.1. In addition, in the extraction of the fatty acid product from the final reaction mixture the volume ratio of selective solvent to final reaction mixture is desirably between about 1:1 and 20:1. The olefins which may be employed in the procedure may be any of the alkenes having from 3 to 40 carbons such as butylene, diisobutylene, 2-methylhexene-3, and pentadecene-1. The branch chain olefins such as diisobutylene are particularly suitable for the production of highly branched chain fatty acid which in turn when reacted with alcohols produce synthetic ester lubricating oils of good thermal stability.

The inorganic acid carbonylation catalyst which may be employed are any of the standard Koch reaction catalysts such as sulfuric acid, hydrochloric acid, phosphoric acid, hydrofluoric acid, monohydroxy fluoroboric acid and boron trifluoride complexes resulting from the reaction of boron trifluoride with mineral acids. Under the advantageous conditions the catalyst is present in the reaction in a mol ratio of olefin to catalyst of between about 1:1 and 1:20. Suitable organic solvents for fatty acid product extraction are, for example, liquid alkanes which have a boiling point different and advantageously lower than the carbonylation product and are essentially immiscible in water. Specific examples of the liquid alkanes contemplated herein are the C_3 to C_{20} alkanes such as hexane, isooctane, decane and tetradecane.

In the extraction step of the process any of the standard solvent extraction procedures can be employed. For example, in one procedure the extraction solvent and final reaction product are contacted with one another under mixing conditions. Then upon cessation of mixing the extraction mixture is allowed to form two layers followed by the separation of the fatty acid enriched solvent layer from the acid layer by decantation. This procedure is particularly adaptable to a batch type operation. Alternatively, a procedure particularly adaptable in a continuous process is where the final reaction mixture is introduced at the top of an elongated extraction column and the selective extraction solvent is introduced at the bottom of the column. The extractant and product are passed in countercurrent flow to one another thereby accomplishing the transfer of the fatty acid product to extractant. The fatty acid enriched solvent is then withdrawn from the top of the extraction column and the acid catalyst withdrawn from the bottom. Whether a batch or continuous extraction procedure is employed, the recovered catalyst and solvent may be sent to storage for eventual reuse or may be immediately recycled to the initial carbon monoxide-olefin reaction.

Example: A 1,530 cc stainless steel autoclave equipped with a motor driven stirrer and capable of operating up to 10,000 psig was purged with carbon monoxide and then pressured with carbon monoxide to about 3,000 psi. Following the carbon monoxide pressuring, liquid $BF_3 \cdot H_3PO_4$ catalyst was introduced into the reactor. Then while holding the reactor at an autogenous temperature, diisobutylene was pumped into the reactor at a rate of about 2 cc/min. After each addition of approximately 1 mol of diisobutylene, 15 to 20 cc of water was pumped into the reactor. The cycle of diisobutylene and water addition was repeated until the amounts recited in the following table were charged. During the addition, the reaction temperature averaged out to that given in the table. Usually at the end of the run the temperature was higher than at the beginning.

In each run and after the last addition of water the reaction mixture was stirred for approximately 1/2 hour and then was degassed and the product removed from the reactor. The removed liquid product was a homogeneous solution and was contacted in a stirred container with isooctane for 5 minutes at 20° to 30°C. Upon cessation of the stirring two layers were formed and the upper isooctane layer was decanted and distilled to a 140° to 160°C. pot temperature. The distillation residue was further fractionated under reduced pressure of 20 mm. Hg and fraction collected at 128° to 133°C. was identified as 2,2,4,4-tetramethylpentanoic acid. Further analysis of the remaining fractions determined the presence of C_5 to C_{13} monobasic fatty acids. The foregoing procedure was repeated 3 additional times with the catalyst in Run 1 being consecutively reused in Runs 2, 3 and 4.

The acid catalyst employed in the foregoing procedure was prepared by placing concentrated phosphoric acid in a 3-neck flask (equipped with a condenser, thermometer and gas inlet tube) heated to a temperature of 100°C. Gaseous boron trifluoride was introduced in excess for a period of about 4 hours while maintaining the reaction temperature at between about 100° to 130°C. The reactants, catalyst, product and reaction data in which the catalyst is reused are reported in the table shown on the following page.

One feature of the process can be seen from the data tabulated in the table. It appears the catalyst increases its activity when recovered by solvent extraction in the process. For example, the fatty acid yields in Runs 3 and 4 are substantially above the yields of Runs 1 and 2.

Description	Run 1	Run 2	Run 3	Run 4
Reactants, gms.:				
Diisobutylene	518	460	468	518
CO	125	152	161	115
Water	90	72	70	88
Catalyst:				
Name	$H_3PO_4 \cdot BF_3$	Cat. Run 1	Cat. Run 2	Cat. Run 3
Amt., gms	935	854	787	715
Reaction Conditions:				
Avg. Temp., °C	32	27	31	23
Avg. Pres., p.s.i.g	3,360	3,240	2,410	3,370
React. Time, Hrs	6	8½	6	9½
Extraction Conditions:				
Gms. React. Mixt./Gms. Isooctane	1.1	1.1	1.1	1.1
Temp., °C	30	30	30	30
Product [1]:				
Amt., gms	623	580	729	776
Neut. No	286	292	291	315
Yield, wt. percent [2]	120	126	156	150

[1] C_5 to C_{13} monobasic fatty acid residue after stripping isooctane extracts to pot temperature of 140–160° C.
[2] Based on weight of olefin reactant.

Boron Trifluoride–Phosphoric Acid–Water Mixture

B. Paulis, H.G. Merkus and J.P. Campen; U.S. Patent 3,527,779; September 8, 1970; assigned to Shell Oil Company outline a process for the preparation of carboxylic acids which comprises contacting, at a temperature in the range of from about 60° to 150°C., a monoolefinically unsaturated organic compound and carbon monoxide with a catalyst consisting of a mixture of H_3PO_4, BF_3 and H_2O, the molar ratio of H_2O to BF_3 in the mixture having a value between about 1 to 1 and about 2.3 to 1 and the molar ratio of BF_3 to H_3PO_4 having a value between about 2 to 1 and about 20 to 1.

Use of this catalyst mixture and special temperature range makes it possible to react olefinically unsaturated organic compounds with CO and H_2O to give high yields of carboxylic acid, good separation between the carboxylic acid formed and the catalyst being obtained after reaction, the heat set free being easily removed, the catalyst not decomposing to an undesired extent owing to hydrolysis, and commercial materials being used for the equipment without these materials being heavily corroded.

Preferred olefins have from 3 to about 18 carbons, such as, for example, propene, butene-1, butene-2, isobutene, branched or nonbranched pentenes, hexenes, octenes, nonenes, decenes; oligomers of lower olefins such as trimers or tetramers of propene, dimers or trimers of isobutene; cyclic alkenes such as cyclopentene and cyclohexene. Isobutene and oligomers thereof, in particular diisobutene, are especially preferred. Mixtures of olefins also can be used as starting materials for the preparation of carboxylic acids according to the process. The volume ratio of catalyst (i.e., H_3PO_4, BF_3, and water) to olefin may vary between wide limits. Volume ratios between about 6 to 1 and about 0.5 to 1 are very suitable with volume ratios between about 4 to 1 and about 1 to 1 being preferred.

The CO pressure during the process can be varied between wide limits. Pressures above 250 kg./cm.^{2} can be used, but make high demands on the construction of the reactor. It is very convenient for the preparation of carboxylic acids to be carried out at a CO pressure between 10 and 250 kilograms per square centimeter, particularly suitable are CO pressures between 30 and 150 kg./cm.^{2}. The presence of an inert diluent during the reaction is advantageous in that it minimizes the formation of undesired by-products. Very favorable results are obtained when liquid saturated hydrocarbons are used as inert diluent.

Preferred hydrocarbons are lower acyclic or alicyclic alkanes, e.g., pentane, hexane, heptane and octane and mixtures thereof. An especially preferred diluent is n-heptane or a mixture consisting substantially of n-heptane. The process may be carried out batchwise or continuously. Batchwise operation may be conveniently effected by introduction of the olefin, CO and, if desired, inert diluent into a reactor which contains the catalyst. If the acid derived from the olefin introduced by addition of 1 mol CO and 1 mol H_2O to 1 mol of that olefin is the desired product it is advantageous to keep the contents of the reactor in vigorous motion (e.g., by stirring), in order that the olefin introduced is contacted with CO as soon as possible.

If the reaction is carried out in batch, the H_2O content of the catalyst mixture of BF_3, H_3PO_4 and H_2O decreases, as H_2O is built in the carboxylic acids formed. For that reason in most cases it will be necessary to add water during the reaction in order to keep the molar ratio of H_2O to BF_3 of the catalyst between the limits set.

At the end of the reaction the addition of CO and olefin and diluent is stopped and the reaction mixture, which is no longer kept in vigorous motion, settles to form a catalyst layer and an organic layer which contains the carboxylic acids, and from which the carboxylic acids can be isolated by conventional means, e.g., by distillation, by crystallization of via esters or salts. It is also possible to separate the organic layer and the catalyst layer with the aid of devices such as a centrifuge. The catalyst layer can be reused.

Example 1: In each experiment in a stirred 1-liter autoclave provided with a 4-blade peddle stirrer which contained 200 ml. of a mixture of H_3PO_4, BF_3 and H_2O, isobutene and water were simultaneously introduced, by pumping, at a rate of, respectively, 240 and 60 g. per hour. The CO pressure was kept constant at 100 kg./cm.^{2} by adding gaseous CO. After 30 minutes the addition of isobutene and water was discontinued, and when CO absorption ceased the pressure was released. In a separatory funnel the reactor contents separated into 2 layers, the upper-organic-layer containing the carboxylic acids formed. The lower-catalyst-layer was extracted three times with pentane, and the combined organic layers were washed with saturated sodium chloride and dried. The bulk of the solvent was distilled off. The composition of the remaining reaction product was determined with the aid of gas chromatography. In all cases the conversion of the isobutene was above 99.9%. In Table 1 the results are given of several experiments in which the ratios between H_3PO_4, BF_3 and H_2O, and the temperature were varied.

TABLE 1

Exp. No.	Reaction conditions				Selectivity (percent m. on isobutene intake)			
	Temp., °C.	Molar ratio of catalyst components			C_5 acids	C_9 acids	C_{13} acids	Neutral compounds
		H_3PO_4	BF_3	H_2O				
1	41	1	2.37	6.72	5			95
2	40	1	2.51	4.96	37	10		53
3	61	1	2.51	4.96	75	25		
4	60	1	2.50	4.99	74	22	4	
5	40	1	2.68	5.12	59	13		28
6	60	1	2.68	5.12	81	18	1	
7	41	1	3.00	5.62	56	14	1	29
8	61	1	3.00	5.62	70	22	4	4
9	40	1	3.50	6.34	75	19	6	
10	60	1	3.50	6.34	80	17	3	
11	40	1	4.00	6.80	76	17	7	
12	60	1	4.00	6.50	82	15	3	
13	61	1	4.00	6.80	88	12		

Example 2: All experiments, in which the ratio between H_3PO_4, BF_3 and H_2O and the temperature were varied, were carried out as described in Example 1, the difference being that diisobutene was used as the starting olefin instead of isobutene. The results are given in Table 2.

TABLE 2

Exp. No.	Reaction conditions				Selectivity (percent m. on isobutene intake)			
	Temp., °C.	Molar ratio of catalyst components			C_5 acids	C_9 acids	C_{33} acids	Neutral Compounds
		H_3PO_4	BF_3	H_2O				
14	60	1	3.00	5.00	39	55	1	5
15	60	1	3.50	6.30	47	53		
16	8	1	4.00	6.50	7	86	6	1
17	20	1	4.00	6.50	12	84	4	
18	40	1	4.00	6.50	29	70		1
19	60	1	4.00	6.50	42	56	1	1
20	63	1	4.00	6.50	63	35		2
21	80	1	4.00	6.50	73	27		

Example 3: A continuous experiment was carried out by separately introducing into a vigorously stirred reactor a catalyst consisting of H_3PO_4, BF_3 and H_2O in the molar ratio of 1 to 4 to 6.78, and a mixture of isobutene and CO, the latter mixture being introduced near the tips of the stirrer blades. The contents of the reactor were continuously withdrawn from it.

In the reactor the CO pressure was maintained at 100 kg./cm.^{2}, the temperature at 100°C. 143.5 kg. isobutene per m.^{3} reactor volume was fed per hour, the volume ratio between catalyst and isobutene fed being kept at 2 to 1. The residence time of the materials in the reactor was 1.5 hours. The ratio between H_3PO_4, BF_3 and H_2O present in the reactor at equilibrium was 1 to 4 to 5.32. From the reaction product obtained the pressure was released; the reaction product separated into an upper organic layer, and a lower inorganic layer comprising H_3PO_4, BF_3 and H_2O.

The organic layer which contained the carboxylic acids formed was washed with water, and analyzed with the aid of gas chromatography. It contained 93.5% α,α-dimethylpropionic acid, 1.4% carboxylic acids with 6, 7 or 8 carbon atoms, 2.7% carboxylic acids with 9 carbon atoms and 2.4% carboxylic acids with 13 carbon atoms. Less than 0.1% of neutral compounds was found. All percentages given refer to the amount of isobutene fed into the reactor having been converted to the compound in question. The conversion of isobutene was quantitative. So much water was added to the inorganic layer that the ratio between H_3PO_4, BF_3 and H_2O contained in that layer was 1 to 4 to 6.78; this layer was recycled to the reactor.

HYDRATED BORON TRIFLUORIDE CATALYST

Low Olefin Concentration

It has been known that carboxylic acids may be synthesized by the reaction of water, carbon monoxide and olefins using an inorganic acid catalyst such as hydrated boron fluoride. One of the practical problems encountered in conducting this synthesis is the unavoidable formation of undesired by-products and particularly the production of olefin polymers. This results from the circumstance that the highly acidic catalyst employed is a very active polymerization catalyst.

S.D. Sumerford, H.G. Ellert and R.C. Lohman; U.S. Patent 3,205,244; September 7, 1965; assigned to Esso Research and Engineering Company provide an improvement of this acid synthesis process in which undesired by-products are minimized by maintaining low olefin concentrations in the reactant mixture, preferably below 2 weight percent, and by avoiding any localized concentration of the olefins. This is accomplished by introducing the olefinic feed material into a carbon monoxide rich vapor space above the liquid inorganic acid catalyst while maintaining the rate of olefin introduction at or below the rate of olefin conversion.

The introduction of the olefin in the carbon monoxide vapor space in this manner enables the olefin to be well mixed with carbon monoxide prior to contact with the acid catalyst and permits the carboxylic acid synthesis to initiate at the top surface of the acid catalyst in a manner avoiding any localized concentration of olefins, thereby minimizing by-product formation. The acidic catalyst employed in the process is any of the liquid, highly acidic catalysts which are known to promote the reaction of carbon monoxide, olefins and water. Such catalysts include concentrated sulfuric acid, phosphoric acid and hydrofluoric acid. However, the catalyst which is preferably employed is boron fluoride combined with water in molar ratios of at least 1:1 and preferably about 2 to 2.5:1. Boron fluoride combines or complexes with water so as to form definite chemical compounds corresponding to the empirical formula of boron fluoride monohydrate and boron fluoride dihydrate, both of which may include additional quantities of water which may be present as a solvent or may, in fact, complex with the boron fluoride in other ratios.

Such catalysts are referred to herein as "hydrated boron fluoride catalysts". While greater quantities of water may be employed, if desired, it is particularly preferred in the practice of this process to use a boron fluoride catalyst containing about 1 to 2.5 mols of water per mol of boron fluoride, and particularly, a catalyst containing about 2 mols of water per mol of boron fluoride. Optionally, the hydrated boron fluoride catalyst may be used in combination with other of the inorganic acid catalysts. Sulfuric acid or phosphoric acid, in particular, may usefully be employed with the hydrated boron fluoride catalyst.

The relative proportions of the acids employed may be varied, although use of approximately equal molar amounts of boron fluoride and phosphoric acid or sulfuric acid is preferred. The process may be used for the preparation of carboxylic acids from any monoolefinic compound containing 3 to 20 carbon atoms. The olefin feed stock can comprise straight or branched chain alkenes including propylene, butylene, pentene and the higher homologues and isomers of these alkenes. The olefins of this class can constitute either terminal or internal unsaturated alkenes. Similarly, cyclic olefins having up to 20 carbon atoms may be employed as the feed stock, including cyclopentene, cyclohexene, and the higher homologues.

Any desired mixtures of these compounds such as the C_4 fraction recovered in petroleum refining operations may be used if desired. All of these monoolefinic compounds can include functional groups such as carboxylic acid (carboxyl) or alcohol (hydroxyl) groups. Thus the C_3 to C_{20} monoolefinic compound can be one selected from the group consisting of unsubstituted C_3 to C_{20} monoolefinic hydrocarbons and substituted C_3 to C_{20} monoolefinic hydrocarbons wherein the substituent is a functional group selected from the group consisting of carboxylic acid and alcohol groups. The acid synthesis process may be conducted at temperatures within the range of about

−20° up to 150°C., although the preferred temperature is in the range of 20° to 100°C. Elevated pressures are required in order to maintain a high carbon monoxide partial pressure. Pressures of 10 to 600 atmospheres or more can be employed, although it is preferred to use a pressure of about 40 to 100 atmospheres.

The process may be conducted in either a semibatch or continuous fashion. In a semibatch process the liquid, inorganic acid catalyst is first introduced to a suitable reactor or autoclave and thereafter carbon monoxide and olefin are introduced to the reactor continuously until the catalyst is exhausted. In continuous processing, a similar reactor and procedure can be employed, but with the continuous withdrawal of reactant products and the continuous introduction of fresh or recycle catalyst. However conducted, it is the particular feature of this process that the reaction is carried out in such a manner that the olefin concentration in the reactant mixture is maintained below at least 5 weight percent and preferably below 2 weight percent at all times.

In order to accomplish this, it is necessary to add the olefinic feed to the reactant mixture at a rate no greater than the rate of olefin conversion. The reaction of the olefin, carbon monoxide and catalyst occurs readily to form a complex of these reactants so that 90% olefin conversion can be obtained in about 20 minutes. However, extended reaction periods of at least 1 hour and preferably 2 to 4 hours are required to attain the maximum practicable olefin conversion. In a lined-out continuous reaction, unreacted olefin content of the reactor effluent may be analytically determined by gas chromatography. The feed introduction rate, temperature and the holding time may be controlled to maintain the unreacted olefin concentration below about 5 weight percent and preferably less than 2 weight percent based on crude acid product.

The reaction of the carbon monoxide in this manner results in the formation of a complex which can be decomposed by hydrolysis to release the carboxylic acid product. The carboxylic acid will correspond to an acid produced by removing an olefinic linkage of the olefinic feedstock and attaching a carboxylic group directly to one, and a hydrogen atom to the other, of the two olefinic carbon atoms. Thereby olefins are converted to a carboxylic acid having one additional carbon atom. Similarly, application of the process to an olefinically unsaturated acid results in production of dicarboxylic acid having one more carbon atom in the molecule.

Example: In order to illustrate this process and to demonstrate its advantages, a series of carboxylic acid syntheses were carried out in which varied levels of olefin concentration were maintained in the reactants. The olefin feedstock constituted a C_9 olefin stream, a propylene trimer, having the composition: C_9 olefins, 90%; C_8 olefins, 6%; and C_{10} olefins, 4%.

The acid catalyst employed was a hydrated boron fluoride catalyst corresponding to the dihydrate of boron fluoride. The reaction was carried out in a continuous flow reactor by continuous introduction of catalyst, carbon monoxide and olefin to a well mixed reactor which was partially filled with the liquid catalyst and products. Product was continuously withdrawn from the reactor. At all times the carbon monoxide pressure was maintained at about 800 to 900 psi, and the temperature within the reactor was maintained at about 125°F. In each run the rate of introduction of the propylene trimer was varied from a level somewhat below the reaction rate of the olefin to a rate of introduction greater than the rate at which the olefin was reacting.

The unreacted olefin concentration was analyzed in the reactor effluent during the course of the reaction. The reaction products were then hydrolyzed at about 100°F. with a molar excess of water based on the olefin-carbon monoxide-acid catalyst complex, and the liberated carboxylic acid product was distilled in a 1-inch Oldershaw column. The following results were obtained:

C_9 Olefin Concentration Remaining, Percent of Crude Acid	Distilled C_{10} Acid Product Purity, Percent of Theoretical
0.8	100
2.0	99.9
5.2	97.7
7.4	96.5

It will be noted from this data that when the olefin feed was introduced at a rate such that substantially complete olefin reaction was obtained, high purity carboxylic acid product was produced. Thus, the final acid product was found to have a purity of substantially 100% of theoretical in the runs in which the olefin feed introduction was sufficiently slow so that less than about 2 weight percent of unreacted olefins remained in the reactant mixture. On the other hand, at higher olefin feed rates, resulting in higher concentration of unreacted olefins in the reactant mixture, by-product impurities resulted which could not be separated from the carboxylic acid product by fractionation. This results from the circumstance that such by-products may have approximately the same boiling point as the desired carboxylic acid product.

Multistaged Hydrolysis

In related work A.H. Wehe, Jr., H.G. Ellert, R.C. Lohman and W.T. Boyd; U.S. Patent 3,262,954; July 26, 1966; assigned to Esso Research and Engineering Company and A.H. Wehe, Jr., H.G. Ellert,

Preparation by Oxo Synthesis

R.C. Lohman and W.T. Boyd; U.S. Patent 3,296,286; January 3, 1967; assigned to Esso Research and Engineering Company describe a process for synthesizing the carboxylic acid by a first step formation of a complex of carbon monoxide, an olefinic compound, and a hydrated boron fluoride catalyst and by a second step hydrolysis of the complex, the improvement residing in the technique of hydrolyzing the complex in a continuous multistaged hydrolysis step. According to the process, this multistage hydrolysis step comprises at least three, but preferably more than three, discrete stages.

In a first of these stages, the complex is hydrolyzed with aqueous hydrolysis medium into a mixture of crude carboxylic acid product and dilute boron catalyst having a water to BF_3 mol ratio of less than about 3.0 to 1. In another of the discrete stages, other than the first stage and the last stage, it is critical that the mixture of crude carboxylic acid product and boron catalyst be diluted with BF_3-containing aqueous medium having a water to BF_3 mol ratio of greater than 15 to 1 into a crude carboxylic acid product and a reconstituted boron catalyst having a maximum water to BF_3 mol ratio of about 3.0 to 1. In the latter stage, or stages, the crude carboxylic acid product is washed with the BF_3-containing aqueous medium and the stage, or stages, are maintained at a water to BF_3 mol ratio of greater than 15 to 1.

The process may be used for the preparation of carboxylic acids from any monoolefinic compound containing 3 to 20 carbon atoms. The olefin feedstock can comprise straight or branched chain alkenes including propylene, butylene, pentene, and the higher homologues and isomers of these alkenes. The olefins of this class can constitute either terminal or internal unsaturated alkenes. Similarly, cyclic olefins having up to 20 carbon atoms may be employed as the feed stock, including cyclopentene, cyclohexene, and the higher homologues. Any desired mixtures of these compounds such as the C_4 fraction recovered in petroleum refining operations may be used if desired. All of these monoolefinic compounds can include functional groups such as carboxylic acid, ester, or alcohol groups.

The preferred catalyst for use in the process is a hydrated boron fluoride catalyst having the empirical formula: $BF_3 \cdot xH_2O$, where x equals about 2 to 2.5. Such catalysts involve the combination or complexing of boron fluoride with water so as to form definite chemical compounds including those corresponding to the empirical formula of boron fluoride monohydrate and boron fluoride dihydrate, and which may include additional quantities of water which may be present as a solvent, or may complex or otherwise react with the boron fluoride in other ratios. Optionally, the hydrated boron fluoride catalyst may be used in combination with other inorganic acid catalysts. Sulfuric acid or phosphoric acid in particular may usefully be employed with the hydrated boron fluoride catalyst. The relative proportions of the acids employed may be varied, although use of approximately equal molar amounts of boron fluoride and phosphoric scid or sulfuric acid is preferred. The acid synthesis step may be conducted at temperatures within the range of about -20° up to 150°C., although the preferred temperature is in the range of 20° to 100°C. Elevated pressures are required in order to maintain a high carbon monoxide partial pressure. Pressures of 10 to 600 atmospheres or more can be employed, although it is preferred to use a pressure of about 40 to 100 atmospheres.

The process may be conducted in either a semibatch or continuous fashion. In a semibatch process, the liquid, inorganic acid catalyst is first introduced to a suitable reactor or autoclave and thereafter carbon monoxide and olefin are introduced to the reactor continuously until the catalyst is exhausted. In continuous processing, a similar reactor and procedure can be employed, but with the continuous withdrawal of reactant products and the continuous introduction of fresh or recycle catalyst.

Broadly, the hydrolysis step consists of hydrolyzing the complex in a hydrolysis zone so as to form the crude carboxylic acid product and subsequently washing the crude carboxylic acid product in an acid washing zone wherein both of the zones comprise a plurality of continuous countercurrent mixing-settling stages. In these stages BF_3-H_2O concentrations are maintained to avoid those where solid boric acid precipitates. The hydrolysis step may be conducted at temperatures of 30° up to 100°C., preferably from 45° to 80°C. Elevated pressures may be employed although such use is not required.

Example: In an experiment conducted to demonstrate the operability of the hydrolysis system a complex was formed with propylene trimer, carbon monoxide and $BF_3 \cdot 2H_2O$ catalyst. The reactor effluent of the complex formation step was then diluted with about 15 volume percent of normal hexane, and unreacted excess $BF_3 \cdot 2H_2O$ catalyst was settled and removed. The remaining complex was then hydrolyzed in stages at a tower temperature of about 75°C. using water that had been used to wash an equivalent amount of crude acid resulting from such hydrolysis.

Thus the water of hydrolysis used had been obtained by contacting crude carboxylic acid in equilibrium stages. Small amounts of solid boric acid were carried over with the C_{10} organic acid product. There was no evidence of solid boric acid formation in the column itself.

The washed organic acid had a pH of 4 indicating good washing. The regenerated catalyst had a density of 1.61 at 27°C. The recovered acid was found suitable for recycle to the synthesis stage with apparently the same activity and selectivity as fresh $BF_3 \cdot 2H_2O$ catalyst.

GROUP VIII METAL CATALYSTS

Treatment of Residue from Carbonylation Process

It is well-known to synthesize oxygen-containing compounds by reacting olefins with carbon monoxide and hydrogen in the presence of a catalyst comprising cobalt. The product, which consists largely of aldehydes, is then hydrogenated, whereby a mixture consisting largely of primary alcohols is obtained. This mixture is normally subjected to separation by distillation. The residue from this distillation comprises high-boiling alcohols and ethers and, in general, other oxygenated compounds and hydrocarbons. The treatment of this residue from a so-called carbonylation process to yield valuable organic compounds has been the subject of intensive and widespread research.

P.J. Ashworth; U.S. Patent 3,227,737; January 4, 1966; assigned to Imperial Chemical Industries Limited, England describes a process for the production of carboxylic acids from the alcohol-containing residue of a carbonylation process which comprises the steps of heating the residue with a caustic alkali, thereafter contacting the products so obtained with water to give aqueous and nonaqueous layers, treating the aqueous layer with carbon dioxide and removing the free carboxylic acids liberated.

The treatment of the residue from the carbonylation process is preferably carried out using sodium hydroxide as the caustic alkali. Preferably an excess, for example 10% by weight, of caustic alkali over that theoretically required is employed and the reaction temperature is suitably 260° to 350°C. On adding the product to water, there is a ready separation between insoluble materials such as ethers and hydrocarbons on the one hand and water-soluble soaps on the other. The aqueous layer is separated, washed if this is considered desirable with a light petrol fraction to remove neutral oil, and treated with carbon dioxide.

This treatment may be effected at atmospheric temperature and pressure or at any suitable elevated temperature and pressure. By operating in this manner, free carboxylic acids containing more than 10 carbon atoms are produced. These frequently contain occluded soaps of acids having 10 carbon atoms or less in the molecule, which may be removed by thorough washing with water. It is a particularly advantageous feature of this process that the liquid remaining after the carbon dioxide treatment, together if desired with the aqueous washings of the carboxylic acids having more than 10 carbon atoms in the molecule, may be acidified with a mineral acid, for example sulfuric acid or hydrochloric acid. This treatment liberates carboxylic acids containing 10 carbon atoms or less. It will be understood, of course, that carboxylic acids containing 10 carbon atoms or less may be liberated from the aqueous washings by acidification with a mineral acid, without bulking these aqueous washings with the liquid remaining after the carbon dioxide treatment. By using the overall process described above, the acids liberated from the soaps produced by treating the residue from a carbonylation process are automatically divided into 2 fractions, namely, those containing at most 10 carbon atoms and those containing more than 10 carbon atoms.

For instance, C_7 olefins may be carbonylated to give the mixture of branched chain alcohols known as isooctanol. The residue may be treated by the process of this method to give, as separate products, mixtures of C_8 and C_{16} carboxylic acids. Similarly, the residue obtained in the production of the mixture of branched chain alcohols known as nonanol may be converted into separate products, one comprising C_9 carboxylic acids and the other C_{18} carboxylic acids. Again, the residue obtained in a process for the production of mixed branched chain primary alcohols containing 7 to 9 carbon atoms may be treated by the process. In this way, there are obtained as separate products mixtures of C_7 to C_9 carboxylic acids and mixtures of C_{14} to C_{18} carboxylic acids.

Example 1: The starting material employed in this Example was the residue obtained in a process for the production of the mixture of branched chain alcohols known as isooctanol. The residue, of which 721 g. were employed, had an OH value of 98 mg. KOH per g. This residue was heated with caustic soda (60 g.) to 260°C. for 4 hours in a 1-liter flask equipped with a temperature point, a stirrer and a reflux condenser system. During the course of this reaction 13.8 grams of a light distillate were removed. To the product, 1,700 ml. of water were added and, after vigorous stirring, the mixture was allowed to stand and the aqueous phase was then removed.

In this way, there were obtained 2,025 ml. of the aqueous phase and 344 grams of neutral oil. Washing of the aqueous phase with light hydrocarbon removed a further 21.5 g. of neutral oil. The aqueous solution was then transferred to a baffled walled flask equipped with a temperature point, a gas outlet point and a cruciform stirrer through which carbon dioxide was passed at a rate of 20 liters per hour. After this treatment with carbon dioxide had been continued for 30 minutes, the outlet gas rate indicated that reaction was complete.

The crude C_{16} acid liberated was separated and washed with water to remove occluded sodium salts of C_8 carboxylic acids. In this way, 175 g. of C_{16} acid were obtained, this having an acid value of 195 mg. KOH per gram. This mixture on distillation gave 166 grams of C_{16} acid having an acid value of 220 mg. KOH per gram. The water which had been used for washing the crude C_{16} acid was treated with mineral acid, whereby 56.3 grams of crude C_8 acid were obtained, this product having an acid value of 326 mg. KOH per gram. Also, the aqueous layer remaining after the carbon dioxide treatment was acidified with sulfuric acid and yielded 72.8 grams of C_8 acid, this product having an acid value of 374 mg. KOH per gram. These crude mixtures of C_8 acid were bulked and distilled to give 113 grams of C_8 acid having an acid value of 385 mg. KOH per gram.

Example 2: The starting material employed in this example was the residue obtained in a process for the production of the mixture of branched chain alcohols known as nonanol. The residue, of which 836 grams were employed, had an OH value of 85 mg. KOH per gram. This residue was heated with caustic soda (60 g.) as described in Example 1. During the course of the reaction, 91.6 grams of a light distillate were removed. To the product, 1,700 ml. of water were added and, after vigorous stirring, the mixture was allowed to stand and the aqueous phase was then removed. In this way, there were obtained 2,010 ml. of the aqueous phase and 425 grams of neutral oil. The aqueous phase was transferred to a baffled walled flask and treated with carbon dioxide as described in Example 1.

The crude C_{18} acid liberated was separated and washed with water to remove occluded sodium salts of C_9 carboxylic acid. The residual product, which weighed 140 grams, consisted of 14% by weight of neutral oil, the remainder being C_{18} acid. The acid value of this product was 166 mg. KOH per gram. The water washings used to remove occluded sodium salts of C_9 carboxylic acid were bulked with the liquid remaining after the carbon dioxide treatment. To this liquid, sulfuric acid was added. 108 grams of acidic product were liberated. This contained 4% by weight of neutral oil but otherwise consisted almost entirely of C_9 acid, the acid value of the product being 538 mg. KOH per gram.

Oxidation with Cobalt Oxonation Catalyst

A process by R. Bearden, Jr. and J.K. Mertzweiller; U.S. Patent 3,409,648; November 5, 1968; assigned to Esso Research and Engineering Company is directed to an improved process for forming chiefly C_6 to C_{30} linear organic acids by first oxonating a C_5 to C_{29} alpha or internal olefin, preferably a linear olefin, selectively to aldehydes in the presence of a soluble cobalt oxonation catalyst and then contacting the aldehydes previously formed with the oxygen in the presence of the residue of the cobalt oxonation catalyst while maintaining an oxygen feed rate of at least 0.9 mol of oxygen per mol of aldehyde per unit time. This oxonation reaction can be conducted at temperatures of about 180° to 220°F. in the presence of a suitable oxonation catalyst, such as a cobalt soap or dicobalt octacarbonyl; but any suitable oxonation catalyst capable of selectively converting the olefins to their corresponding C_{n+1} aldehydes can be employed. The oxonation reaction is conducted for a sufficient period of time to substantially oxonate most of the olefins present in the feed stream to aldehydes. This time can vary widely, depending upon the specific reaction temperature, reaction pressure, olefins present in the feed stream, etc. However, in the case of a cobalt octacarbonyl catalyst employed in conjunction with C_6 to C_{26} alpha olefins (>90 weight percent of the feed stream being the alpha olefins) and when the oxonation temperature is 180° to 220°F. and when synthesis gas pressure is 100 to 150 atmospheres, oxonation can be conducted satisfactorily in a 60 to 180 minute reactor holding period. The lower temperatures and pressures are preferred as this favors linear aldehyde formation.

Carbon monoxide and hydrogen (synthesis gas) are fed to the oxonation reaction zone to supply the requisite materials for the aldehyde synthesis reaction; normally a considerable excess of both CO and H_2 are used. Thus, carbon monoxide is usually supplied to allow 2 to 20 mols of carbon monoxide per mol of olefin present in the feed stream per unit time. Preferably, the carbon monoxide feed rate is 5 to 10 mols of carbon monoxide per mol of olefin per unit time. Hydrogen can be fed at a feed rate of 2 to 20 mols of hydrogen per mol of olefin per unit time. Usually, the hydrogen feed rate ranges from about 5 to 10 mols per mol per unit time.

Normally the consumption ratio of H_2/CO is very near the theoretical 1/1 volume ratio for aldehyde synthesis; hence the mixed gases are best fed in this composition. In either batch or continuous oxonation processes, a continuous flow of the gas mixture is a convenient method of maintaining the gas composition essentially constant. The pressure in the oxo reaction stage is normally in the range of 50 to 300 atmospheres, preferably 65 to 200 atmospheres.

Subsequent to the oxonation step described above, the oxo reaction product, including the soluble cobalt octacarbonyl or other suitable oxonation catalyst, is discharged at a controlled rate from the oxonation reactor or other storage vessel into the oxidation reactor vessel, which can be a glass reactor equipped with appropriate agitation devices, such as a stirrer, and appropriate facilities for the feeding of the oxygen-containing gas thereto. The rate at which the oxygen is fed to the oxidation reaction zone is controlled by any suitable gas feeding and regulator device to insure that the proper concentration of oxygen with respect to aldehyde is maintained during the oxidation stage.

According to the process, at least 0.9 mol of oxygen per mol of aldehyde present in the oxo reaction product per unit time must be supplied in order to obtain the selectivity of reaction which the process is capable of attaining. Usually, the oxygen feed rate in a continuous flow operation ranges from about 0.90 to 3.2 mols of oxygen per mol of aldehyde per unit time, and preferably from 0.9 to 1.2 mol/mol/unit time. Use of oxygen supply rates below 0.9 mol/mol/unit time usually results in far inferior selectivities and acid yields. Thus, when the oxygen supply rate (oxygen feed rate) was reduced from 1.2 to 0.60 mol/mol/hr. in an oxidation stage having the same cobalt catalyst and conducted in the presence of n-heptane using the same weight concentration of catalyst at the same oxidation temperatures, the 0.6 mol/mol/hr. run resulted in an acid yield of 65.5 mol percent on aldehyde present in the oxo reaction product feed stream to the oxidation step versus a 80.6 mol percent acid yield when the oxygen feed rate was 1.2 mol/mol/hr.

Characteristically, the oxidation stage can be conducted at temperatures of about 86° to 122°F. One to 50 atmospheres pressure can be used for oxidation, but usually the pressure maintained during the oxidation step ranges only slightly above atmospheric, e.g., 2 to 4 psi above atmospheric pressure. However, oxidations carried out at elevated pressure would increase the solubility of oxygen in the reaction solvent, hence providing even more favorable oxygen to aldehyde ratios with improvements in acid yield. The oxidation reaction takes place essentially instantaneously so that reactor holding time is not a vital consideration.

Usually the catalyst is employed in the oxonation (first stage) step in concentrations ranging from about 0.05 to 0.5 weight percent cobalt catalyst (as cobalt metal based on olefins) present in the predominantly olefinic feed stream to the oxonation step. Preferably, the catalyst concentration on this basis ranges from about 0.1 to 0.2 weight percent. Essentially none of this catalyst is lost during the transfer from the oxonation vessel to the oxidation vessel, hence essentially the same catalyst concentration is present during the oxidation step as was present during the oxonation step. As soon as the oxygen is fed to the reaction products from the oxonation step, aldehyde oxidation to the corresponding organic acid, or mixtures thereof, takes place almost immediately. Thus, e.g., the dicobalt octacarbonyl oxonation catalyst from the olefin oxonation step is used directly and converted in situ directly to the active cobalt oxidation catalyst.

<u>Example:</u> A mixture of 273.5 g. (3.25 mols) of hexene-1 and 11.4 mmol. of preformed cobalt octacarbonyl in heptane (35 g. of solution) was charged to a 1-liter stainless steel autoclave. Oxonation was then begun at a synthesis gas pressure of 1,800 psig and at 212°F. using a synthesis gas blend containing a mol ratio of H_2 to CO of approximately 1.3:1. After 5 hours the uptake of synthesis gas had ceased and the reactor product, 416 g., was discharged. Analysis by gas chromatography showed a 95% yield of aldehyde product with 81% selectivity to the linear aldehyde.

Next, a mixture of 28 g. of the oxo product and 300 ml. of n-heptane was charged to a glass reactor equipped with stirrer and air inlet tube (frit). Dry air was passed into the mixture at 104°F. until the characteristic green color of the active cobalt oxidation catalyst occurred (7 minutes) and until ΔV measurements on the exit air indicated that oxygen was no longer being consumed, i.e., the initial aldehyde charge had been used up. At this point the remainder of the aldehyde charge, 172 g., was fed to the reactor at a rate of 0.1 mol aldehyde per hour. The air rate was regulated to supply 0.32 mol O_2 per hour.

After 312 minutes the reaction was no longer exothermic, and the temperature began to drop from the 104°F. mark held previously by means of an ice bath. At 360 minutes there was no further uptake of oxygen and the reaction was terminated. Cobalt catalyst was then removed. The acid products were then extracted into a 10% sodium hydroxide in water solution. Traces of hexane and alkaline insoluble by-products were removed from the alkaline extract by flash distillation (steam) and the crude acids were liberated by adding dilute hydrochloric acid. There was obtained 153 g. (75 mol percent based on olefin) of carboxylic acids. Linear acid content was determined by gas chromatography to be 86%.

Example 2: After conducting the oxonation reaction employing a C_8 refinery alpha olefin feed containing chiefly octene-1 and reaction conditions indicated in Example 1, an oxidation stage was conducted at 104°F. using n-heptane as solvent and employing a catalyst concentration of 0.2 weight percent cobalt. These runs were conducted to study the effect of oxygen feed rate variation upon selectivity as demonstrated by yield of acids. The table below summarizes the data obtained from 4 runs including a batch reaction (Run 1) and 3 continuous flow runs (Runs 2 to 4) wherein the aldehyde feed rate from the oxonation reaction to the oxidation step was controlled at 0.1 mol of aldehyde per hour. The pertinent data are tabulated in the following table.

Variable Studies — C_9 Aldehyde Air Oxidation

[Oxidation Temperature: 104°F.; Catalyst: 0.2 Weight Percent Cobalt; Solvent: n-Heptane]

Run No.	Aldehyde Feed Rate, Moles/Hr.	Ald. Conv. Rate, Moles/Hr.	Oxygen Feed Rate, Moles/Hr.	Oxygen Use Rate, Moles/Hr.	Overall Acid Yield, Mole Percent	Oxidation Yield, Mole Percent
1	(1)	0.07	0.32	0.03	51.0	57.6
2	0.1	0.08	0.06	0.06	58.0	65.5
3	0.1	0.09	0.12	0.09	71.5	80.6
4	0.1	0.10	0.32	0.09	73.0	82.4

[1] Batch Reaction 0.1 Mole Ald.

Complex Palladium Salt

N. von Kutepow, K. Bittler and D. Neubauer; U.S. Patent 3,437,676; April 8, 1969; assigned to Badische Anilin- & Soda-Fabrik AG, Germany report a carbonylation process in which an olefinically unsaturated compound is reacted with carbon monoxide and water to produce a carboxylic acid or with carbon monoxide and an alcohol or a phenol to produce a carboxylic acid ester, these reactions being carried out under the influence of a complex palladium salt as a catalyst in an amount of 0.01 to 1% by weight with reference to the olefinically unsaturated compound. For example, the catalyst may be bistriphenylphosphine palladium dichloride.

The preferred olefinically unsaturated initial materials are hydrocarbons with from 2 to 20 carbon atoms and up to 4 olefinic double bonds. They may have 1 acetylenic bond in conjugation with an olefinic linkage and may also contain an aromatic structure. They may bear as substituents 1 or 2 chlorine atoms, carboxylic groups, carboalkoxy groups having 2 to 5 carbon atoms, or alkoxy groups having 1 to 4 carbon atoms.

Pure carbon monoxide may be used. It is however also possible to react a commercial gas which contains inert components, such as saturated hydrocarbons or nitrogen. The amount of carbon monoxide, with reference to the olefinically unsaturated initial material, may vary within wide limits. Generally at least 1 mol of carbon monoxide is used for each double bond in the initial material. It is advantageous to use from 10 to 25 mols. The optimum ratio of carbon monoxide to olefinically unsaturated initial material also depends on the olefinically unsaturated initial material itself.

When reacting ethylene or substituted ethylenes it has proved to be an advantage to use 35 to 95 mol percent, with reference to the sum of ethylene and carbon monoxide or carbon monoxide and a corresponding amount of ethylene. When the reaction is carried out in the presence of water, carboxylic acids are obtained, and when in the presence of alcohols or phenols, carboxylic esters are obtained.

The catalysts for the process are complex palladium salts in which the palladium is generally divalent. Salt bonds and coordinative bonds are therefore present side-by-side. The following are some examples of suitable catalysts: bistriphenylphosphine palladium dichloride, bis-tri-o-tolylphosphine palladium acetate, bistributylphosphine palladium nitrate, triphenylphosphine piperidine palladium dichloride, etc. Compounds such as allyl palladium monochloride, triphenylphosphine palladium dichloride and ethylene palladium dichloride, which may possibly be in the dimeric form are also suitable as catalysts.

The process is advantageously carried out at a temperature of from 20° to 250°C. Within this temperature range, the temperatures used for the production of carboxylic acids are in general somewhat higher than those required when preparing esters of the same carboxylic acids. A preferred temperature range for the production of carboxylic acids is from 70° to 170°C. The process may be carried out at atmospheric pressure. In the interests of a higher rate of reaction however, it is advantageous to use super-atmosphere pressure. In general, pressures of from 25 to 1,000, preferably 75 to 1,000, atmospheres are used.

Example: 1 part of bistriphenylphosphine palladium dichloride, 160 parts of cyclohexene and 80 parts of 18% aqueous hydrochloric acid are charged into an autoclave of corrosion-resistant steel. The autoclave is closed, flushed out with nitrogen and 300 atmospheres of carbon monoxide is forced in. The temperature is brought to 120°C. and carbon monoxide is forced in up to a pressure of 700 atmospheres. The pressure and temperature are maintained for 14 hours after which the autoclave is cooled and released from pressure. The product amounts to 274 parts and the total absorption of carbon monoxide is 170 atmospheres.

Ether is added to the product, the aqueous phase is separated, the etheral layer is dried with calcium chloride and the ether then removed in vacuo, 217 parts of residue remains and is distilled over a short column in a high vacuum, 3.6 parts of first runnings boiling below 80°C. is obtained and 194 parts of cyclohexane carboxylic acid (boiling point 80° to 85°C. at 0.1 mm. Hg) having a melting point of 34°C.

Use of Halogenated Olefin

R.D. Closson and K.G. Ihrman; U.S. Patent 3,457,299; July 22, 1969; assigned to Ethyl Corporation describe a method for preparing unsaturated carboxylic acids and related compounds by reacting a halogenated olefin and carbon monoxide, using as a catalyst rhodium, iridium, platinum, palladium, osmium and ruthenium metal or mixtures thereof. It is preferred that the catalyst be in a fine state of subdivision. Metal turnings and finely divided metal powders can be employed. Colloidal dispersions of the catalyst in an inert liquid reaction medium are also applicable. Similarly, the metals and their salts can be dispersed and supported on an inert solid matrix such as charcoal, alumina, diatomaceous earth, bentonite, firebrick, kaolin, ground glass, silicon carbide, silica gel, and the like.

The reaction is carried out in the presence of a catalytic amount of one or more of the above catalysts; that is, from about 0.00015 to 0.15 mol of the catalyst per mol of olefinic halide, preferably in the range of from 0.0015 to 0.15 mol of the catalyst per mol of the olefinic halide.

Preparation by Oxo Synthesis

A wide variety of halogenated olefins can react with carbon monoxide according to this process. Thus, any halogenated olefin which (1) is stable under the reaction conditions employed, (2) contains a vinyl olefin radical C=C—X (wherein X is halogen), and (3) does not contain substituent groups which hinder or retard the process by undergoing competitive side reactions, are applicable. Preferred halogenated olefins which meet the above criteria have the formula:

$$R_1-\underset{R_2}{C}=\underset{H}{C}-X$$

wherein X is a halogen and R_1 and R_2 are selected from the group consisting of hydrogen and univalent organic radicals having 1 to about 28 carbon atoms, the organic radicals being selected from the group consisting of alkyl, cycloalkyl, and aryl radicals, such that at least one of R_1 and R_2 is hydrogen and the halogenated olefin has up to about 30 carbon atoms. Thus, olefinic chlorides, bromides, and iodides may be employed in the process, the olefinic chlorides being more highly preferred.

Some of the nonlimiting examples of the halogenated olefins applicable in the process are propenyl halides, eicosyl-1 halides, pentene-1 halides, tricosyl-1 halides and β-halo styrenes. An unsaturated carboxylic acid or related compound is prepared by the process. For example, if the reaction is carried out in the presence of water or alcohol, the corresponding carboxylic acid or an ester thereof is prepared. When the reaction is carried out in the presence of water, an ethylenically unsaturated carboxylic acid is obtained. It should be understood that the process can also be carried out in a liquid medium containing a mixture of two or more solvents, yielding a free acid, related compounds or mixtures, depending on the composition of the liquid reaction medium.

A temperature which affords a reasonable reaction time and which does not cause an excessive decomposition of the products or reactants is preferred. A preferred temperature range is from about 250° C. to the decomposition temperature of the halogenated olefin, and the most preferred range is from about 260° to 290°C. The process generally is carried out under super-atmospheric pressures. A readily obtainable pressure which affords a reasonable yield of product in a comparatively short reaction time is preferred. In many instances, best results are obtained when the reaction is carried out at pressures within the range of from about 2,000 to 5,000 psi.

The reaction time is not a truly independent variable and is dependent to some extent on the nature of the halogenated olefin reactant and the other process variables under which the reaction is conducted. For example, when high temperatures and high pressures are employed, the reaction time is usually reduced. Similarly, low temperatures and low pressures usually require a longer reaction time. In most instances, the reaction is complete within from about 2 minutes to 15 hours, and often with 30 minutes or less. In the following example, all parts are by weight unless otherwise indicated.

Example: An autoclave was charged with 360 parts of ethanol and 3 parts of palladium. After purging the autoclave with carbon monoxide, 140 parts of vinyl chloride was added, and the autoclave was pressured to 1,000 psi with carbon monoxide. Thereafter, the autoclave was heated to 270°C. After 2 hours, the pressure drop was 350 psi. The autoclave was cooled, vented, discharged, and the contents filtered. The filtrate was diluted with 500 parts of cold water and sodium chloride was added until the water was saturated. This mixture was then extracted with 2 portions of ether, 290 parts each. The combined extracts were dried over magnesium sulfate and filtered. Some of the ether was removed by the use of an aspirator. The remaining liquid was washed twice with 300-part portions of saturated sodium chloride solution and then dried over magnesium sulfate.

Distillation of the resultant solution gave the following fractions: (1) 570 parts of a mixture of an ether and and ester, BP 32° to 38°C.; (2) 110 parts, BP 70° to 79°C.; (3) 21.9 parts of a mixture of acid and ester, BP 80°C. at 33 to 60 mm.; (4) 3.6 parts, BP, 70° to 90°C. at 2 mm., which was discarded. Fraction 1 was distilled through a helices packed column to remove ether. Fraction 2 was diluted with 150 parts of cyclohexane and the resultant mixture distilled through a helices packed column. Two fractions were collected. One contained ethanol-cyclohexane azeotrope which was discarded, and the other contained excess cyclohexane and the product, which was retained. The residue from the distillation of Fraction 2 was combined with the residue of the first fraction and distilled through a helices packed column to give 30.6 parts of product, ethyl acrylate, BP, 96° to 99°C. It was identified by infrared analysis and by refractive index.

The cyclohexane fraction obtained in the distillation of Fraction 2 was diluted with ethanol and the ethanol-cyclohexane azeotrope was distilled and discarded. The residue was distilled to give an additional 8.1 parts of ethyl acrylate for a total of 38.7 parts of the product. Fraction 3 was diluted with 35 parts of ether and washed with 75 parts of 20% sodium carbonate. The basic wash was acidified with concentrated hydrochloric acid and extracted with ether to yield crude acrylic acid. This was distilled to give 4.9 parts of pure acid, BP 139° to 140°C. The unexpected presence of the acrylic acid in the product may be explained, without any intention of being limited to any theory, by hydrolysis of the acid chloride either in the autoclave or during the separation step.

High Partial Pressure of Carbon Monoxide

In a process by K.L. Olivier; U.S. Patent 3,505,394; April 7, 1970; assigned to Union Oil Company hydrocarbon olefins are oxidatively carbonylated by contacting the olefin, carbon monoxide and oxygen with a substantially anhydrous reaction medium containing a Group VIII noble metal and a redox agent for the Group VIII noble metal. This reaction can be performed without the necessity for a dehydrating agent by employing a high partial pressure of carbon monoxide in the reaction gas phase, e.g., from about 40 to 70% of the total reaction pressure.

Examples of olefins useful as reactants are the aliphatic hydrocarbon olefins having from 2 to 12 carbons such as ethylene, propylene, butene-1, butene-2, and pentene-2. Of these the aliphatic hydrocarbon olefins having from 2 to about 8 carbons are preferred. Also preferred are the alpha olefins since these olefins having an unsaturated terminal carbon are more reactive than the other olefins. The reaction is performed under liquid phase conditions in the presence of a liquid organic solvent which has a solvency for the catalyst and which, preferably, is inert to the reaction conditions. Various organic liquids can be employed for this purpose such as sulfones, amides, ketones, ethers and esters. Carboxylic acids such as the lower molecular weight aliphatic acids are preferred solvents and even when another solvent is used, it is preferred to maintain at least 10% of the solvent as an aliphatic carboxylic acid.

Illustrative of the preferred solvents are acetic, propionic, butyric, pentanoic, hexanoic, heptanoic, octanoic, pivalic, acrylic, beta-acetoxypropionic, etc. Of these, the aliphatic carboxylic acids having from about 2 to 6 carbons are preferred. The carboxylic acids are not entirely inert under the oxidation conditions in that the carboxylic acids add to the olefin double bond to form beta-acyloxy compounds. These materials, however, can be readily pyrolyzed to recover both the carboxylic acid for reuse as the reaction medium and the desired unsaturated acid.

Another class of organic solvents that have sufficient solvency for the catalyst salts, that are inert to the oxidative carbonylation, and that can be used in lieu of up to 90% of the aforementioned carboxylic acids are various amides such as formamide, dimethyl formamide, ethylisopropyl formamide, etc. Various alkyl and aryl ketones can also be employed in the reaction solvent, e.g., acetone, methylethyl ketone, diethyl ketone, diisopropyl ketone, etc. Various esters can also be employed in the solvent.

As previously mentioned, the reaction medium should contain catalytic amounts of a platinum group metal. The platinum group metal can be of the palladium subgroup or the platinum subgroup, i.e., palladium, rhodium or ruthenium or platinum, osmium or iridium. While all of these metals are active for the reaction, palladium is preferred because of its demonstrated greater activity. The platinum group metal can be employed in amounts between about 0.001 and 5 weight percent of the liquid reaction medium; preferably between about 0.04 and 2.0 weight percent. The platinum group metal can be added to the reaction medium as a finely divided metal, as a soluble salt or as a chelate. Preferably, the metal in its most oxidized form, i.e., as a soluble salt or chelate, is introduced into the reaction zone to avoid the formation of undesired quantities of water. Examples of suitable salts are the halides and carboxylates of the metals such as palladium chloride, rhodium acetate, ruthenium bromide, osmium propionate, iridium benzoate, palladium isobutyrate, etc.

To facilitate the rate of oxidation by rendering it more facile to oxidize the reduced form of the platinum metal, it is preferred to employ a reaction medium that contains a soluble halide, i.e., a bromide or chloride (preferably a chloride). The halide can be added as elemental chlorine or bromine; however, it is preferred to employ the less volatile compounds such as hydrogen, alkali metal or ammonium halides. Also, any of the aforementioned platinum group metals can be added to supply a portion of the bromide or chloride and, when the hereafter mentioned multivalent metal redox salts are employed, these too can be added as the chloride or bromide. Acyl halides which also serve as organic dehydrating agents can be added.

Thus, the use of acetyl chloride, serves to remove any undesired water and also provides a continuous source of hydrogen chloride, thereby replacing any chloride lost during the reaction by vaporization or side reactions. Examples of useful acyl halides include the chlorides and bromides having from 1 to about 10 carbons, preferably from 2 to 5 carbons. In general, sufficient of any of the aforementioned halides can be added to provide between about 0.05 and 5.0 weight percent halide in the reaction zone; preferably concentrations between 0.1 and 3.0 weight percent are employed. This amount of halide is preferably also in excess of the stoichiometric quantity necessary to form the halide of the most oxidized state of platinum group metal, e.g., in excess of 2 atomic weights of halogen per atomic weight of palladium present. In this manner, a rapid oxidation can be achieved.

As previously mentioned, various redox compounds can optionally be used in the reaction medium to accelerate the rate of reaction. In general, any multivalent metal salt having an oxidation potential higher, i.e., more positive than the platinum metal in the solution, can be used. Typical of such are the soluble salts of the multivalent metal ions such as the carboxylates, nitrates, halides of copper, iron, manganese, cobalt, mercury, nickel, cerium, chromium, molybdenum or vanadium. Of these, cupric and ferric salts are preferred and cupric salts are most preferred.

Preparation by Oxo Synthesis

In general the multivalent metal ion salt is added to the reaction medium to provide a concentration of the metal therein between about 0.1 and 10 weight percent; preferably between about 0.5 and 3.0 weight percent. Various other oxidizing agents can also be employed to accelerate the rate of reaction. Included in such agents are the nitrogen oxides that function as redox agents similar to those previously described. These nitrogen oxides can be employed as the only redox agent in the reaction medium or they can be employed jointly with one or more of the aforedescribed redox metal salts such as a combination of a nitrogen oxide and a cupric redox agent or ferric redox agent.

In general, between about 0.01 and 3 weight percent of the reaction medium; preferably between about 0.1 and 1 weight percent; calculated as nitrogen dioxide can comprise a nitrogen oxide that is added as a nitrate or nitrite salt or nitrogen oxide vapors. The nitrogen oxides can be added to the reaction medium in various forms, e.g., nitrogen oxide vapors such as nitric oxide, nitrogen dioxide, nitrogen tetroxide, etc., can be introduced into contact with the reaction medium during the oxidation to fix the aforementioned nitrogen oxide content therein or soluble nitrate or nitrite salts such as sodium nitrate, lithium nitrate, lithium nitrite, potassium nitrate, cesium nitrate, etc. can be added to the reaction medium.

The reaction can be conducted in the presence of carboxylate anions which can favor the reaction. Examples of useful anions are those of the low molecular weight acids such as acetic, propionic, butyric, isobutyric, valeric, isovaleric, pivalic, etc. Acetate ions are preferred. The concentration of the anions can be from about 0.01 to about 0.7 normality; preferably from about 0.04 to 0.3 normality. These values correspond to from about 0.05 to 7 weight percent; preferably from about 0.24 to 3 weight percent.

The soluble anion can be added to the reaction medium as a soluble salt such as an alkali metal or ammonium salt, e.g., sodium acetate, lithium acetate, potassium propionate, ammonium butyrate, diethyl ammonium acetate, tributyl ammonium valerate, pyridinium acetate, etc. The organic ammonia salts can include the salts of alkyl, aryl and heterocyclic amines having from 1 to 16 carbons. The identity of the organic portion of the ammonium salt is not significant in the reaction provided that the ammonium salt is soluble in the medium.

The process is operated continuously wherein the platinum group metal and redox agent participate in a catalytic manner. In this method, oxygen is introduced together with the olefin and carbon monoxide into contact with the liquid reaction medium. The carbonylation of the olefin and oxidation to the carboxylic acid results in the stoichiometric reduction of the platinum group metal. The introduction of oxygen serves to reoxidize the reduced metal to its more oxidized and active form. This oxidation is known to form a stoichiometric quantity of water. Surprisingly, water did not accumulate in the reaction medium nor did the course of the reaction become altered because of the presence of water to flavor the less desired products such as the unsaturated esters or carbonyl compounds. Instead, the water apparently participated in the oxidative carbonylation reaction to produce the desired alpha,beta-ethylenically unsaturated carboxylic acids and the beta-acyloxy carboxylic acids directly.

In the commercial application of this process, the oxygen introduction is controlled at a rate in response to the oxygen content of the exit gases from the reaction zone. Continuous or intermittent introduction can be employed; however, continuous introduction is preferred. Preferably, the rate of oxygen introduction is controlled relative to the olefin and carbon monoxide rates so as to maintain the oxygen content of the exit gases below the explosive concentration, i.e., less than about 10 and preferably less than about 3 volume percent. Under these conditions, the excess gas which comprises the olefin (when a gaseous olefin reactant is used) and carbon monoxide can be recycled to the liquid reaction medium.

When the olefin is a liquid under the reaction conditions, an inert gas such as nitrogen, air or mixtures of nitrogen and air can be employed to dilute the gas phase and exit gas stream from the reactor and thereby avoid explosive gas compositions. The reaction can be performed under relatively mild conditions, e.g., temperatures from about 30° to 300°C.; preferably from about 90° to 200°C. The reaction pressure employed is sufficient to maintain a liquid phase and preferably when gaseous olefins are employed, superatmospheric pressures are used to increase the solubility of the olefin in the reaction medium and thereby accelerate the reaction rate.

Superatmospheric pressures are even preferred with the olefins that are normally liquid at the reaction conditions so that the solubility and hence, reactivity, of carbon monoxide in the reaction system is promoted. Accordingly, pressures from atmospheric to about 200 atmospheres or more, preferably from 10 to 100 atmospheres, are used. An advantage of the process is that the use of high partial pressures of carbon monoxide in this oxidative carbonylation will insure the formation of the desired ethylenically unsaturated carboxylic acids and precursors thereof without the necessity to add an extraneous dehydrating agent to the reactants.

While the presence of water in the reaction medium will not completely preclude the desired oxidative carbonylation, it is nevertheless preferred to conduct the reaction under substantially anhydrous conditions, i.e., in reaction media containing less than about 5 weight percent water. Preferably, reaction media containing less than about 2 weight percent water are used and most preferably the reaction is initiated under essentially anhydrous conditions. The carbonylation is conducted at partial pressures of carbon monoxide from about 30 to 95% of the total pressure in the reaction zone. Preferably the partial pressure of the carbon monoxide is from about 40 to 70% of the total reaction pressure. During the oxidation a portion of the liquid reaction media can be continuously withdrawn and distilled to recover the desired products from the reaction medium which contains the catalyst salts and which is recycled for further contact to the reaction zone.

Preferably care is exercised to remove most quantities of water from this recycle reaction to thereby provide a substantially anhydrous recycle medium. The removal of water from this stream can be facilitated by azeotropic distillation, e.g., by the addition of a suitable azeotrope-forming agent such as a hydrocarbon, benzene, ester, e.g., ethyl acetate, etc. to remove all water in the distillation and/or by the addition of any of the known dehydrating agents such as acetic anhydride, phthalic anhydride, acetyl chloride, etc. to the reaction stream.

To permit recovery of the product by distillation, it is preferred to employ a high-boiling carboxylic acid or other high-boiling organic solvents in the reaction medium. It is preferred that a portion of the reaction medium comprise acetic acid in an amount from about 3 to 75%. Since the acetic acid is more volatile than the carbonylated products, the distillation recovery of the products necessitates the removal of the acetic acid. This acetic acid is recovered as a distillate and returned for further reaction. The carbonylated product can then be recovered by distillation of the remainder of the reaction medium that comprises the high-boiling acid which contains the catalyst. After distillation of the product, e.g., acrylic acid and a beta-acyloxy propionic acid, the distillation residue can be combined with the acetic acid and returned to the reaction zone.

Example: To determine the effect of carbon monoxide partial pressure on the course of the oxidation reaction, a series of experiments were performed wherein this variable was altered. In the experiments, a 1-gallon Teflon-lined autoclave was charged with 1 g. palladium chloride, 5 g. lithium chloride, 5 g. cupric chloride, 5 g. lithium acetate and 500 g. acetic acid. Carbon monoxide was introduced at varied amounts during the series of experiments and ethylene was then added to bring the total pressure to 900 psig. The autoclave was closed, heated to 280°F. and alternate addition of oxygen and nitrogen of about 20 psi increments were made during a 20-minute reaction period. After completion of the reaction, the autoclave was cooled, the gases were vented into a gas receiver, the liquid product was removed and distilled to separate the amounts of products indicated in the table shown on the following page.

	Reactants, p.s.i.		Products, grams				
Experiment	Ethylene	Carbon monoxide	Low boiling	Acrylic acid	Propionic acid	Beta-acetoxy propionic acid	CO_2
1	300	300	7	3.3	6	7	51
2	600	300	54	10	16	43	21
3	450	450	6	9	3	60	38
4	300	600	0	4	1.5	8	60
5	150	750	1	5	2.5	6	64
6	750	150	96	6	22	28	13

The low-boiling products comprised a mixture of acetaldehyde, vinyl acetate and slight amounts of saturated esters, i.e., methyl and ethyl acetates. The data indicate that the partial pressure of carbon monoxide in the reaction zone significantly influenced the yields of products. To illustrate, Experiments 4 and 5 which were performed at high carbon monoxide partial pressures produced acrylic and beta-acetoxy propionic acids as the major liquid products whereas performing the oxidation under high partial pressures of ethylene (Experiments 2 and 6) produced high yields of the low-boiling products. In the series of experiments, no dehydrating agent was added to the reaction zone and therefore, it can be seen that the course of the reaction was altered to favor the production of the carbonylated products simply by increasing the partial pressure of the carbon monoxide.

Pt or Pd, Aromatic Phosphine and Surface Active Agent

It is known that olefins can be hydrocarboxylated in liquid phase reactions using a catalyst comprising a palladium salt in complex association with a phosphine, e.g., triphenylphosphine, as shown in Netherlands Patent 6,409,121. This reaction, however, generally has a relatively low reactivity and produces acids having a high content of the iso or branched chain acids. Since the straight chain acid is generally the most useful product, being employed in the preparation of plasticizers, ester solvents, detergents, etc., it is desirable to provide a process that produces a higher yield of the normal or straight chain acid than of the isomer or branched chain acid.

A process by D.M. Fenton; U.S. Patent 3,530,155; September 22, 1970; assigned to Union Oil Company comprises hydrocarboxylation of olefins by contacting the olefin under liquid phase conditions with a catalyst comprising a platinum or palladium complex with an aromatic phosphine, water and carbon monoxide. High reactivity and high yields of the normal acid are obtained by incorporating in the reaction medium an anionic or nonionic surface active agent. The contacting is effected at relatively mild conditions including temperatures from 30° to 300°C. and pressures from 1 to 1,000 atmospheres, sufficient to maintain liquid phase conditions. The reaction is performed batchwise or in a continuous fashion and the products are recovered by any suitable method, e.g., distillation, extraction, etc.

The catalyst for the reaction is preferably formed in the reaction medium by charging thereto the phosphine and the platinum or palladium metal component. The platinum or palladium can be charged to the reaction medium as the metal, oxide or as a salt soluble in the particular reaction medium, e.g., as a halide, nitrate or carboxylate. Examples of suitable catalyst components are palladium, platinum, palladium oxide, platinum chloride, palladium bromide, platinum fluoride, palladium bromide, platinum iodide, palladium nitrate, or the platinum or palladium salts of carboxylic acids having from 1 to 20 carbons. The amount of the noble metal used in the reaction system can vary over wide limits from about 0.05 to 5 weight percent of the reaction medium; preferably from 0.5 to 1.5 weight percent.

The other component of the catalyst comprises an aromatic phosphine. Examples of suitable materials are triphenylphosphine, diphenylethylphosphine, phenyldimethylphosphine, etc. The reaction is performed under liquid phase conditions in the presence of a liquid organic solvent which has a solvency for the catalyst and which, preferably, is inert to the reaction conditions. Various organic liquids can be employed for this purpose such as hydrocarbons, sulfoxides, sulfones, amides, ketones, ethers and esters. As discussed above, however, the preferred reaction solvent is a carboxylic acid and most preferred is a fatty acid having from 2 to 20 carbon atoms.

The reaction is performed on an olefinic compound. Preferably hydrocarbon olefins are employed and these can be alpha olefins or internal olefins as well as nonconjugated diolefins. The olefinic compounds can have from about 2 to 25 carbons and in addition to the aforedescribed hydrocarbons, olefinic compounds containing inert functional groups in nonconjugated positions can also be employed. The lower molecular weight olefins having from about 2 to 12 carbons are a preferred class and the alpha olefins are also a preferred class of reactants.

The preferred class of surface active agents comprises the high molecular weight saturated fatty acids such as those having from about 12 to 25 carbons, e.g., lauric, myristic, palmitic, stearic, arachidic, behenic, etc. Other anionic surface active agents can be employed such as the anionic compounds obtained by sulfonation of fatty derivatives such as sulfonated tallow, sulfonated vegetable oils, sulfonated marine animal oils. Commercially available surfactants of this group are: Tallosan RC, Gamafon K, and Finish WFS.

Various sulfonated fatty acid esters of mono and polyvalent alcohols are also suitable such as: Nopco 2272R, Mekal N3, and Nopco 1471. Sulfated and sulfonated fatty alcohols are also useful as the surfactant employed. Typical of this class of anionic agents are: Duponal ME, Duponal L142, Duponal LS, Tergitol 4, Tergitol 7, etc.

Nonionic surface active agents can also be employed. Among the various nonionic surface active agents which are useful are various ethylene oxide condensation products with fatty acids, alcohols and glycerides, phenolic compounds, fatty amides, amines, fatty partial esters of hexitans and polypropylene glycols. Examples of ethylene oxide condensation products with fatty acids are the following: Nonisol 100, Nonisol 200, Nonisol 300, etc. Examples of ethylene oxide condensation products with fatty and rosin alcohols are: Brij 30, Synthetics D-37, etc. Examples of ethylene condensation products with alkyl and alkenyl phenols are: Igepal W, Igepal C, Antarox A-200, Triton TX45, etc. Examples of ethylene condensation products with fatty amines and amides are the Ethoamides prepared by condensation of ethylene oxide with fatty acid amides having from 8 to 18 carbons.

Ethylene oxide condensation products of fatty acid partial esters of hexitans are also suitable surface active agents. These agents are commercially available as the various Span and Tween products which are polyoxethylene derivatives of sorbitan monolaurate, sorbitan monopalmitate, sorbitan monostearate, sorbitan monooleate, sorbitan trioleate, etc. The surface active agent is employed in the reaction system at concentrations from about 0.5 to 50 weight percent of the reaction solvent. Preferably the concentration employed is from about 1 to 10 weight percent; however, a preferred higher concentration range can be employed when the surface active agent is one of the high molecular weight saturated fatty acids, e.g., from 5 to 25 weight percent.

The reaction is performed at relatively mild conditions including temperatures from about 30° to 300°C.; preferably from about 75° to 175°C. and most preferably from about 125° to 160°C. The reaction is performed at pressures from about atmospheric to 1,000 atmospheres. Pressures from about 5 to 100 atmospheres are preferred and these pressures are used to maintain liquid phase conditions at the reaction temperatures and in addition to improve the rate of reaction by increasing the solubility of the carbon monoxide reactant in the liquid phase.

The carbon monoxide concentration is not critical to the reaction. Thus, the partial pressure of the carbon monoxide in the reaction system can vary from 10 to 100% of the total pressure on the system. When the lower molecular weight olefins are used which have a substantial volatility at the reaction temperature, e.g., those olefins having from 2 to 6 carbons, it is preferred to employ the carbon monoxide partial pressures from about 10 to 90% of the total pressure on the reaction system. The partial pressure of the carbon monoxide can be adjusted if desired by the addition of an inert gas to the reaction zone such as nitrogen, carbon dioxide, etc., which serves as a diluent and thereby moderates the reaction. The reaction can be performed batchwise or in a continuous fashion.

When operating batchwise, the catalyst and the reaction medium is charged to the reaction zone and contacted therein with the olefin and the carbon monoxide. The olefin can be initially charged to the reaction zone which is then pressured with the carbon monoxide and heated to the desired reaction temperature. When performing the reaction in a continuous fashion, the reaction medium can be charged to the reaction zone to form a liquid phase therein and the olefin and carbon monoxide can be continuously introduced into the reaction zone to contact the reaction medium containing the catalyst.

The gaseous reactants can be withdrawn as a separate effluent, cooled, depressured and the noncondensibles, chiefly carbon monoxide, can be recycled to further contacting. The liquid product can be withdrawn separately from the reaction zone by withdrawing a stream of the liquid reaction medium contained therein and recovering the desired carboxylic acid therefrom by suitable processing such as extraction or distillation. Preferably distillation is employed, particularly with the lower molecular weight acid products, i.e., those having up to about 16 carbons and this distillation can be performed at atmospheric or subatmospheric pressures as apparent to those skilled in the art.

The reaction can also be performed in a continuous fashion by simultaneously introducing the liquid phase reaction medium, olefin and carbon monoxide into a tubular reaction zone and withdrawing the reaction medium and reacted gases therefrom, separating the gases from the reaction medium and subsequently distilling the latter to recover the desired product.

<u>Examples 1 through 3:</u> In these examples 1 g. palladous chloride, 10 g. triphenylphosphine, 400 g. acetic acid, 15 g. of water, 70 g. of a mixed C_6 to C_7 alpha olefin and 10 g. of the indicated surface active agent were added to a stirred, 1/2 gallon autoclave. The autoclave was pressured with 800 psi carbon monoxide initially, heated to 125°C. and maintained at that temperature for 2 hours. The results are shown in the following table:

TABLE 1

Example	Surface Active Agent	Product
1	Nonylphenol condensed with 10 mols ethylene oxide	α-Methylhexanoic acid, 15.5 g.; heptanoic and α-methylheptanoic acids, 43.4 g.; octanoic acid, 12.4 g.
2	Pluronics F-68 (1,500 to 1,800 MW polypropylene glycol condensed with 200 mols ethylene oxide)	α-Methylhexanoic acid, 12.2 g.; heptanoic and α-methylheptanoic acids, 34.6 g.; octanoic acid, 12.2 g.
3	Stearic acid	α-Methylhexanoic acid, 21.6 g.; heptanoic and α-methylheptanoic acids, 45 g.; octanoic acid, 10.6 g.

Examples 4 through 9: These examples show the effect of using stearic acid as the surface active agent when different aromatic phosphines are used as catalyst components. In each example 1/2 g. palladous chloride, 3 g. triarylphosphine, 400 ml. glacial acetic acid, 15 g. of water, 80 g. of 1-octene and the stearic acid, when used, were added to a stirred, 1/2 gallon autoclave which was initially purged with nitrogen. The autoclave was pressured with 800 psi carbon monoxide, heated to 125°C. and maintained at that temperature for 2 hours. The aromatic phosphine employed and results are shown in Table 2. It will be noted that use of the surface active agent resulted in each instance in either an increase in yield of acid or an increase in the ratio of normal to iso acid, or both.

TABLE 2

Example	Surface Active Agent	Triarylphosphine	Total Wt. Acid Produced, g.	Ratio of Normal to Iso Acid*
4	None	Triphenylphosphine	80	2.0
5	10 g. stearic acid	Triphenylphosphine	98	1.0
6	None	Tri-p-tolylphosphine	86	1.2
7	10 g. stearic acid	Tri-p-tolylphosphine	87	1.4
8	None	Tri-m-tolylphosphine	78	1.4
9	10 g. stearic acid	Tri-m-tolylphosphine	58	2.8

*Iso Acid is all the acid produced other than normal.

Removal of Cobalt Catalyst

A process by R. Bearden, Jr.; U.S. Patent 3,574,731; April 13, 1971; assigned to Esso Research and Engineering Company relates to the recovery of C_6 through C_{30} alkyl carboxylic acids from a mixture of oxidation products which are formed by the reaction of an olefin with carbon monoxide and hydrogen in the presence of an oxonation catalyst, i.e., cobalt, and thereafter oxidizing the oxonation product mixture with molecular oxygen to form the oxidation product mixture. The oxidation product mixture, containing carboxylic acids, oxides of the oxonation catalysts and oxidation by-products is reacted in a first stage with sulfur dioxide in the presence of water to convert the oxides of the oxonation catalyst to water-soluble catalyst sulfates dissolved in an aqueous phase.

Thereafter, the aqueous phase formed in the first stage is separated from the nonaqueous phase containing the carboxylic acids and the oxidation by-products and the latter reacted with a dilute aqueous alkali. The carboxylic acids are recovered as an aqueous solution of alkali carboxylates and the oxidation by-products separate as an alkali-insoluble phase.

Example 1: (a) Oxo Stage — A mixture of 168 grams (2 mols) of hexene-1 and 7 mmol. of preformed cobalt octacarbonyl in heptane (21 g. of solution) was charged to a 1-liter stainless-steel autoclave. Oxonation was then begun at a synthesis gas pressure of 1,800 psig and at 212°F. using a synthesis gas blend containing a mol ratio of H_2 to CO of approximately 1.3:1. After 5 hours the uptake of synthesis gas had ceased and the reactor product, 241 g., was discharged. Analysis by gas chromatography showed a 95% yield of aldehyde product with 81% selectivity to the linear aldehyde.

(b) Oxidation Stage — A mixture of 28 grams of the oxo product, stage (a), and 300 ml. of n-heptane was charged to a glass reactor equipped with stirrer and air inlet tube (frit). Dry air was passed into the mixture at 104°F. until the characteristic green color of the active cobalt oxidation catalyst occurred (7 minutes) and until ΔV measurements on the exit air indicated that oxygen was no longer consumed, i.e., the initial aldehyde charge had been consumed. At this point an additional amount of the oxo product, 172 g. was fed to the reactor at a rate of 0.1 mol aldehyde per hour. The air rate was regulated to supply 0.32 mol of O_2 per hour. After 5 hours the reaction was no longer exothermic, and the temperature began to drop from the 104°F. mark held previously by means of an ice bath. At 6 hours there was no further uptake of oxygen and the reaction was terminated. There was recovered 452 g. of oxidation mixture.

(c) Product Recovery Stage (Alkaline Extraction) — 100 g. of the oxidation mixture from stage (b) was extracted with 200 g. of an aqueous solution containing 20 g. (0.5 mol) of sodium hydroxide in order to separate the product acids from the alkali-insoluble oxidation by-products and heptane diluent. However, the extraction was complicated by the accompanying formation of a voluminous brown-black gel of cobalt hydroxide and/or cobalt oxides (most probably hydrated cobaltic oxide), which subsequently became suspended in the aqueous alkaline extract containing the product acid salts and which also collected at the interface between the aqueous and organic phases. The precipitate thus prevented clean separation of the phases.

Furthermore, when it was attempted to regenerate the product acids from a portion of the precipitate-laden alkaline extract by addition of an excess of dilute sulfuric acid, it was found that the cobalt precipitate dissolved very slowly and again created an ill-defined interface between the organic acid and aqueous phases. When the cobalt precipitate was dissolved by prolonged stirring with an excess of dilute acid, it was found that the organic acid phase took on color, indicating recontamination by cobalt. It was therefore necessary to remove the cobalt precipitate prior to separation of the organic and alkaline phases. The method chosen was filtration, a feat accomplished only with exceeding difficulty owing to the gelatinous nature of the precipitate. The procedure used was to make a crude separation of the organic and aqueous phase, allow several hours for the gel to settle in each phase and then decant as much of the clear liquids as possible. The resultant gel rich phases were then filtered separately. The alkaline aqueous phase present in both of the filtrates was separated, combined with the aqueous phase, decanted initially and then steam stripped to remove traces of organic by-products.

Upon addition of dilute hydrochloric acid to the alkaline solution of acid salts there was obtained 34 g. (71 mol percent based on starting olefin) of C_7 carboxylic acids. Neutralization Equivalent (mg. KOH/g.), Calculated: 432; Found: 433. The problems encountered in the purification of product acids by alkaline extraction, however, were eliminated by removing the cobalt catalyst prior to extraction according to the process of Example 2.

Example 2: With vigorous stirring, 80 g. of a 1.5 weight percent solution of sulfurous acid in water was added to 100 g. of the oxidation mixture obtained in Example 1, stage (b). After 5 minutes contact at 78°F., the phases were allowed to separate. The bottom aqueous phase, now pink in coloration due to the presence of cobalt salts (primarily $CoSO_4$) was drawn off and discarded. The remaining near water white organic layer was extracted with 200 g. of a 10 weight percent aqueous solution of sodium hydroxide. No precipitate was encountered.

The alkaline extract was separated, steam stripped to remove traces of heptane and alkali-insoluble organic materials, and then acidified with dilute sulfuric acid. There was recovered 36 g. (75 mol percent based on starting olefin) of C_7 carboxylic acids. Neutralization Equivalent (mg. KOH/g.), Calculated: 432; Found: 434. That the action of sulfurous acid on the cobalt catalyst to generate water-soluble cobalt salts is related to the reducing capabilities of the acid rather than its properties as a strong mineral acid is illustrated in Example 3.

Example 3: With vigorous stirring, 80 g. of a 1.5 weight percent solution of sulfuric acid in water was added to 100 g. of the oxidation mixture obtained in Example 1, stage (b). After 15 minutes contact at 78°F. there was no significant change in the organic layer, i.e., the deep green-black coloration resulting from the oxidation active cobalt catalyst was still present. The phases were allowed to separate and the organic phase was then extracted with 200 g. of 10 weight percent aqueous solution of sodium hydroxide. Precipitation of a cobalt gel occurred immediately, thus necessitating recovery of the product acids according to the procedure described in Example 1, stage (c). There was recovered 34.5 g. (72.3 mol percent based on olefin) of C_7 carboxylic acids.

Iridium Compound with an Iodide Promoter

J.H. Craddock, A. Hershman, F.E. Paulik and J.F. Roth; U.S. Patent 3,579,551; May 18, 1971; assigned to Monsanto Company describe a process for the preparation of carboxylic acids in the presence of catalyst compositions essentially comprising iridium compounds and complexes, together with an iodide promoter.

In accordance with the process, ethylenically unsaturated compounds are converted selectively to carboxylic acids by reaction in the liquid phase or vapor phase with carbon monoxide and water at temperatures from about 50° to 300°C., preferably 125° to 225°C., and at partial pressures of carbon monoxide from 1 psia to 15,000 psia, preferably 5 psia to 3,000 psia and more preferably 25 psia to 1,000 psia, although higher pressure may be employed, in the presence of a catalyst system comprised of an iridium containing component, and a promoter portion, i.e., an iodide. The iodide may be derived from iodine or iodine compounds. The process is particularly advantageous at lower pressures, although higher pressures may be used.

The catalyst as charged to the reactor is a solution containing an iridium component, an iodide (or iodine) promoter, and other moieties if desired. The catalyst essentially includes an iridium component, as the active component, such as $IrCl_3$, $IrBr_3$, $Ir_2(CO)_4Br_2$, IrI_3, $Ir[(C_6H_5)_3P]_2(CO)Cl$, $Ir[(C_6H_5)_3P]_2(CO)Cl(CH_3I)$, etc.; however, the catalyst may be composed of two distinct components, namely, the active catalyst portion, e.g., the aforesaid iridium compound, as the first component, and a promoting portion as the second component. The promoter portion of the catalyst system may or may not be catalytically active in itself, but promotes the reaction in various ways, such as by facilitating formation of the carbon-metal sigma bond, or by rendering the iridium species less volatile than the unmodified iridium carbonyl.

The active catalytic portion or first component of the catalyst is prepared from iridium species such as iridium metal, simple iridium salts, organo-iridium compounds, and coordination compounds of iridium. A preferred primary component of the catalyst system is a coordination compound of iridium, carbon monoxide, and a halide such as chloride, bromide and iodide, as well as suitable amine, organo-phosphine, organo-arsine, and/or organo-stibine ligands and, if desired, other ligands, e.g., halide such as chloride, iodide and bromide and trihalostannate such as the corresponding chloride, bromide or iodide, necessary to satisfy the coordination number of organo-stibine ligands and, if desired, other ligands, and thus form a coordination compound or complex of iridium such as $[(C_6H_5)_3P]_3IrI_3$, $Ir_2(CO)_4I_2$, etc.

The promoting portion or second component of the catalyst system as discussed herein consists of iodide and may be supplied as the free halogen or halogen compound such as hydrogen halide, alkyl- or aryl-halide (preferably having the same number of carbon atoms as the feedstock), metal halide, ammonium, phosphonium, arsonium, stibonium halide, etc., and may be the same or different from any halogen component already present in the precursor iridium component of the catalyst system. Iodine or iodide compounds are suitable for the promoter portion of the catalyst, but those containing iodide are preferred, with hydrogen iodide constituting a more preferred member.

The promoter portion or second component of the catalyst may alternatively be charged to the reaction separately from the active catalyst or first component, or it may be incorporated into the active component, e.g., $Ir(CO)I[(C_6H_5)_3P]_2$ or IrI_3. The preparation of the active catalyst complex which includes both iridium and iodide promoter components may be accomplished by a variety of methods. However, it is thought that a substantial part of the precursor medium component is converted to the monovalent state during the preparative treatment.

In general, in the process, it is preferable to preform the active carbonylation catalyst system which contains both iridium and iodide promoter components. For example, to prepare the catalyst system, the first component of the catalyst system, e.g., finely divided iridium metal (powder), a simple iridium salt or iridium compound as a precursor is dissolved in a suitable medium, and carbon monoxide is bubbled through the above iridium solution, preferably while maintaining gentle heating and stirring of the iridium solution. Then an acidic solution of the desired promoter source is added to form an active catalyst solution containing the necessary iridium and iodide promoter components.

Generally, the active catalyst containing the iridium and promoter components of the catalyst system may be preformed prior to charging the reactor, or it may be formed in situ in the reactor as discussed above. For example, to prepare the catalyst system, the first component of the catalyst system, e.g., an iridium salt such as $IrCl_3 \cdot 3H_2O$ is dissolved in a suitable solvent such as 2-methoxyethanol. Subsequently, carbon monoxide is bubbled through the solution where an intermediate, such as the dimer $[Ir(CO)_2Cl]_2$, is produced wherein the iridium is in the monovalent state. The second or promoter component is, for example, added to the above solution; e.g., as aqueous HI, elemental iodine, alkyl iodide (with alkyl radicals of 1 to 30 carbon atoms) or other iodine containing compound.

Alternatively, the iridium precursor, e.g., Na_2IrCl_6, Na_2IrBr_6 or $[Ir(CO)_2Cl]_2$, may be dissolved in 2-methoxyethanol containing a dilute aqueous acid, e.g., HCl, acetic acid, etc., as solvent. Then the solution of the iridium compound is heated, for example, to 60° to 80°C., or in general at a temperature below the boiling point of the solvent, with stirring. A reducing agent such as carbon monoxide is bubbled through the solution to obtain the iridium component at least in part in the monovalent state. Subsequently, the iodine promoter is added as described herein, although the iodine containing promoter may also be added first.

Example: A Hastelloy C batch reactor is charged with the following ingredients: 0.39 g. of an iridium compound having as a catalyst precursor the formula $Ir(CO)Cl(P\phi_3)_2$; 12.2 ml. of a promotor component consisting of 47 weight percent aqueous hydriodic acid (thereby providing a stoichiometric excess of water); 38 ml. of glacial acetic acid as solvent; and 14 grams of propylene having the structural formula $CH_2=CHCH_3$ as feedstock. The reactor is pressurized with carbon monoxide to a total pressure of 720 psia, corresponding to a carbon monoxide partial pressure of about 300 psia at the reaction temperature of 175°C. The reaction is carried out at constant pressure.

The reaction mixture is subsequently analyzed by gas chromotographic techniques to yield a solution containing (solvent and catalyst-free basis): 24 weight percent 2-iodopropane, 63 weight percent isobutyric acid, 13 weight percent n-butyric acid. The selectivity to the desired carboxylic acid product (defined as mols of carboxylic acid/total mols of olefin and/or olefin derivative consumed x 100) is greater than 99 mol percent at substantially 80% conversion level. No other organic oxygenated compounds such as alcohols, aldehydes, ketones, etc., are produced as determined by gas chromatographic analysis. No substantial amounts of other undesirable by-products such as methane, carbon dioxide, or higher carboxylic acids are formed.

The above experiment is repeated in separate tests except that the iridium component is supplied from several different compounds (on a molar equivalent basis):

$$[Ir(CO)_2Cl]_2$$
$$Ir(P\phi_3)_3H_3$$
$$Ir(CO)H(P\phi_3)_3$$
$$IrCl_3 \cdot 3H_2O$$
$$[\phi_4As]^+[Ir(CO)_2Cl_2]^-$$
$$[\phi_4As]^+[Ir(CO)_2I_2]^-$$

where ϕ is the phenyl group). Similar reaction rates and product distributions are obtained in all instances indicating that the various sources of iridium component give equivalent results. When this experiment is conducted with the equivalent molar quantity of cobalt chloride instead of iridium precursor as the catalyst, the selectivity and yield of the desired acid product are decreased significantly. It has been found that cobalt catalysts differ radically from iridium catalysts in that the cobalt catalysts also cause hydrogenation reactions such as hydrogenation of the desired carboxylic acid product to aldehydes and alcohols of the same number of carbon atoms. Consequently, the use of cobalt catalysts results in the substantial production of various undesirable by-products including higher carbon number alcohols, carboxylic acids, and derivatives. Still another distinction of the iridium catalysts compared to the cobalt and nickel catalysts is the fact that significantly lower carbon monoxide partial pressures can be used without encountering catalyst decomposition.

In related work, the same authors, J.H. Craddock, A. Hershman, F.E. Paulik and J.F. Roth; U.S. Patent 3,579,552; May 18, 1971; assigned to Monsanto Company describe a process for the preparation of carboxylic acids in the presence of catalyst compositions essentially comprising rhodium compounds and complexes, together with an iodide promoter. In this process, the catalyst as charged to the reactor is a solution containing a rhodium component, an iodide (or iodine) promoter, and other moieties if desired. The catalyst essentially includes a rhodium component which may contain the promoter, as the active component, such as:

$$[(n-Bu)_4P][Rh(CO)I_2]$$
$$RhI_3, RhBr_3, [(C_6H_5)_3P]_2Rh(CO)I, [Rh(CO)_2Br_2],$$
$$[(C_6H_5)_3P]_2Rh(CO)(Cl)(CH_3I),$$
$$[(C_6H_5)_3As]_2Rh(CO)Br,$$
$$[(n-Bu)_4N][Rh(CO)I_4],$$
$$[(C_6H_5)_3AsCH_3][Rh(CO)_2(I)_2], \text{ etc.}$$

The promoter portion of the catalyst system may or may not be catalytically active in itself, but promotes the reaction in various ways, such as by facilitating formation of the carbon-metal sigma bond, or by rendering the rhodium species less volatile than the unmodified rhodium carbonyl.

The active catalytic portion or first component of the catalyst is prepared from rhodium species such as rhodium metal, simple rhodium salts, organo-rhodium compounds, and coordination compounds of rhodium, by suitable chemical and/or physical treatment of the rhodium precursor in order to render the rhodium moiety in the proper valence state and ligand environment. For example, rhodium complexes containing stable chelating ligands such as trisacetylacetonato rhodium (III), may be treated chemically to remove or destroy the bidentate chelate ligands in order that transformation to the proper valence state and monodentate ligand configuration can be accomplished. The promoting portion or second component of the catalyst system consists of the same iodide defined in the previous patent, and the

Rhodium Compounds

D.M. Fenton; U.S. Patent 3,637,833; January 25, 1972; assigned to Union Oil Company outlines a process for preparation of carboxylic acids comprising reacting an olefin, carbon monoxide and water in the presence of hydrogen and a catalyst comprising rhodium. The olefin may be either an aliphatic olefin or a cycloolefin having from about 2 to 24 carbons, preferably from 2 to about 18 carbons. It may be any of the following: (1) ethylene and substituted ethylenes such as: $R_2R_1C=CR_4R_3$ wherein R_1, R_2, R_3 and R_4 are hydrogen, alkyl, cycloalkyl, aryl, alkaryl, aralkyl, alkenyl aryl, hydroxy, hydroxy alkyl, hydroxy aryl, etc.; (2) cycloalkenes and substituted cycloalkenes such as:

$$R_1C=CR_2 \atop () \atop R_5$$

wherein R_1 and R_2 are as previously mentioned and R_5 is an alkylene or isoalkylene group having from 2 to about 6 carbons.

The rhodium catalyst can be added to the reaction medium as a soluble salt, as a carbonyl compound or as a chelate. Examples of suitable salts are rhodium chloride, rhodium acetate, rhodium nitrate, rhodium bromide, etc. Examples of suitable chelates are rhodium acetyl acetonate and complexes of rhodium ion with such conventional chelating agents as ethylene diamine tetraacetic acid and its alkali metal salts, citric acid, etc.

When the rhodium is employed in the form of a salt it is believed that a carbonyl complex is formed in situ by reaction with the carbon monoxide reactant. The carbonyl complex may, however, also be formed externally and introduced into the reaction mixture as such. A catalytic quantity of the rhodium-containing catalyst is used. This is generally an amount sufficient to provide a concentration of rhodium which is between about 0.002 and 2.0 weight percent of the liquid reaction medium and preferably between about 0.05 and 0.5 weight percent.

The reaction is performed under liquid phase conditions and the reaction solvent may be water alone or a mixture of water and an organic solvent. Any conventional organic solvent that is inert to the reactants, the catalyst and the products, and which is miscible with water, may be used in combination with the water. Suitable solvents include ethers, esters, etc. Particularly effective solvents are fatty carboxylic acids of about 1 to 20 carbon atoms, including the acid that is to be prepared by the process of this method. It has also been found that a further increase in acidity of the reaction mixture, e.g., down to a pH of about 1, may result in increased yield of certain acids. This increased acidity may be readily achieved by addition of a mineral acid, such as hydrochloric acid. The reaction is performed under relatively mild conditions including temperatures from about 50° to 250°C.; preferably from about 70° to 175°C. Sufficient pressure is used to maintain the reaction medium in liquid phase. Although atmospheric pressure can be used, the rate of reaction is increased by superatmospheric pressures and, therefore, pressures from about 5 to 300 atmospheres and preferably from about 10 to 100 atmospheres are used.

Proportions of the reactants are not critical, although certain proportions may be optimum for a given olefin, catalyst and solvent. These are best determined empirically. In general, the amount of CO, based on the mols of olefin, will range from about 0.1 to 10 mol percent, the amount of hydrogen will range from about 0.1 to 100 mol percent and the amount of water will range from about 0.1 to 10 mol percent. Water should be present in an amount ranging from about 5 to 100% of the liquid phase.

The reaction conditions are maintained by conventional means. The pressure can be maintained by the pressure of the gases supplied to the reaction zone. If desired, however, a suitable inert gas, such as nitrogen, can also be charged to the reaction zone. The product acids may be readily separated from the reaction mixture by conventional means such as fractional distillation, chromatography, extraction, etc. The process is more specifically illustrated by the following examples.

Example 1: To 25 ml. concentrated hydrochloric acid, 75 ml. acetic acid, and 1/3 g. rhodium trichloride in a tantalum lined steel bomb of 300 ml. capacity were added ethylene to 300 psi and carbon monoxide to 800 psi. The mixture was rocked and heated to 100°C. for 2 hours and 175°C. for 2 hours. There was isolated some 2 g. of propionic acid.

Example 2: To 1/3 g. rhodium trichloride, 25 ml. concentrated hydrochloric acid and 75 ml. acetic acid in the above described bomb were added ethylene to 400 psi, carbon monoxide to 800 psi and hydrogen to 1,400 psi. The mixture was rocked and heated to 120°C. for 4 hours. There was isolated 17 g. of propionic acid.

OTHER CATALYSTS

Hydrogen Fluoride

A process by B.S. Friedman and S.M. Cotton; U.S. Patent 3,005,846;

October 24, 1961; assigned to Sinclair Refining Company relates to the synthesis of esters and carboxylic acids by the reaction of carbon monoxide and a monoolefin, straight or branched chain, in the presence of a hydrogen fluoride-alcohol mixture or a branched olefin in the presence of a hydrogen fluoride-water mixture. The products of this reaction are contacted with alcohol or water, the reagent being selected consistent with the catalyst mixture to produce the ester or the acid, respectively. The acid or ester is recovered while the hydrogen fluoride, usually containing certain proportions of water or low-boiling alcohol is recycled to the CO reaction.

In organic acid manufacture, a water-HF mixture containing about 5 to 30% water is used. This percentage figure represents either weight percent or mol percent, since water and HF have about the same molecular weight. A mixture of water and HF containing about this range of water is the mixture generally separated by fractional distillation from the organic acid product after the contact with additional water and this mixture may be recycled without further treatment to the carbonylation reaction with CO. The higher the proportion of HF in the mixture the greater the conversion of the branched or cyclic olefin to acid in each pass so that it may be preferred to add more HF or remove some water from the mixture but this is not necessary.

After the carbonylation reaction more water is added to the reaction product to bring the total amount of water used to the stoichiometric amount needed for conversion to organic acids. An excess of water is recovered with the HF when the organic acid product is fractionally distilled; in fact, water, as well as alcohols boiling in the neighborhood of about 100°C. or below are preferred to be present in the final reaction product in excess, e.g., in excess of the stoichiometric amount as determined by the mols of CO reacted. In this situation they actually aid in the recovery of the hydrogen fluoride when the reaction product is fractionally distilled.

The olefin, HF and water or alcohol are added to the reactor with agitation in the proportion of about 2 to 20 mols HF to 1 mol olefin, preferably about 2 to 5 mols HF per mol of olefin. The vessel is then pressurized with CO to a pressure of about 1 atmosphere to 100 or even 1,000 psig or more partial pressure of CO. If a countercurrent contact system is used for the CO, the partial pressure of this gas may measure less than 1 atmosphere in the exit gas line because this gas is being scrubbed out. It is advisable to operate at elevated carbon monoxide pressures in order to minimize olefin side reactions such as polymerization and cleavage. The CO may be mixed with an inert gas, such as hydrogen, carbon dioxide or CH_4, if desired.

The reaction with carbon monoxide can be conducted at a temperature of about 10° to 200°F. or more. The reactants, other than the CO are generally kept in the liquid phase. The most advantageous temperature to use is dependent on the concentration of HF in the mixture. For example, where the HF-water mixture contains about 5% water, a temperature of about 20 to 150°F. is preferred; about 10% water indicates a preferred temperature of about 50° to 150°F. while with about 25% water the reaction is best conducted at about 100° to 200°F. Where an HF-alcohol mixture is used, similar temperature ranges are advised.

The reaction is usually complete in 1 minute to 1 hour. This completion is signalled by a halt in the fall of the CO pressure. Agitation is discontinued and the contents of the vessel are transferred to another vessel where water, preferably at the contacting temperature of about 150° to 300°F., or alcohol, preferably at the contacting temperature of about 75° to 175°F., is added to supply the balance of the stoichiometric amount needed to give the acid or the ester. Alternatively, the water or alcohol may be added directly to the first vessel when the CO reaction ceases.

The acid or ester along with the HF and some excess water or alcohol is then conducted to a settler-still, wherein the mixture is allowed to settle, preferably at a depressed temperature. After removal of the lower layer heat is applied to vaporize the remaining HF, along with some water or alcohol if of low boiling point. The vapor may be recycled to the reactor.

Example 1: 183 g. of iosbutylene (3.27 mols) was charged with stirring for 44 minutes to the reactor along with a mixture containing 204 g. (10.2 mols) HF and 32 g. (1 mol) methanol. The reactor was pressurized with CO to 575 psig, and a water bath was placed around the reactor to maintain the contents at 80°F. The reaction mixture was stirred an additional 26 minutes, after which the CO was vented and the reaction mass conducted to a vessel which contained about 65 g. methanol at a temperature of 100°F. Subsequent separation gave a yield of 240 g. methyl trimethyl acetate.

Example 2: Where the same reaction was conducted using an HF-alcohol mixture containing 22 mol percent alcohol, the reaction with CO was slow below 130°F but quite rapid at 160°F. The product consisted largely of methyl esters of acids derived from polymers of isobutene, indicating that higher proportions of alcohol in the HF mixture may lead to some olefin polymerization.

Example 3: Butene-1 (193 g.) was contacted CO at 525 to 370 psig and 116°F. in the presence of 206 g. of anhydrous HF containing 32.5 g. of dry methanol. The amount of CO absorbed was 64 g. Methanol (64 g.) was then added during 15 minutes at 115° to 120°F. and the stirring continued for 10 minutes additional. Distillation yielded 103 g. methyl ester of 2-methylbutyric acid BP 116° to 120°C., 136 g. methyl ester of C_9 acids,

BP 185° to 188°C., and 28 g. methyl ester of C_{13} acids BP 257° to 269°C.

Example 4: A mixture of 213 g. HF and about 20 g. water, recovered from a previous reaction by distillation, is put in a stirred autoclave. The autoclave is charged with CO and maintained at 400 to 280 psig. 180 g. isobutylene is added at 75°F. during 70 minutes and the stirring continued for 30 minutes. The uptake of CO is about 63 g. The liquid product is added to about 40 g. water at -80°C., the mixture stirred, allowed to come to room temperature and heated to 200°F. with stirring for 1 hour. The product is predominantly pivalic acid plus some C_9 and C_{13} acids.

Oxidation of Oxo Synthesis Product Without Catalyst

K. Büchner and H. Tummes; U.S. Patent 3,047,599; July 31, 1962; assigned to Ruhrchemie AG, Germany found that mixtures of isomeric aliphatic or cycloaliphatic carboxylic acids having 5 to 10 carbon atoms may be obtained by oxidizing, in the absence of any catalyst and in the liquid phase, an aldehyde oxo-synthesis product having from 5 to 10 carbon atoms obtained by catalytically adding carbon monoxide and hydrogen to aliphatic or cycloaliphatic olefins having molecular sizes of from C_4 to C_9. The process is characterized in that raw aldehydes of C_5 to C_{10} molecular size are first freed from their metal content or, if desired, an aldehyde-rich fraction obtained by distillation of such a mixture is continuously passed as a thin film through empty reaction tubes or reaction tubes which have been packed with filling bodies having large surfaces.

The oxidation is effected in the absence of any oxidation catalyst and with the oxidizing gas either being passed through the fixed bed of inert filling bodies or, if the empty reaction tubes are used, through a foam formed from the oxidation product and the oxidizing gas. The temperature in the interior of the reaction tubes is maintained at 65° to 110°C. and preferably at from 80° to 100°C. by appropriate cooling. Demetallizing and purification of the raw aldehydes is effected by the hydrating treatment of the oxo product with water at an elevated temperature and an elevated pressure and may be effected in the manner described in German Patent 879,837. In this step, acetals which are present in the oxo product are simultaneously eliminated by the cleavage thereof.

An aldehyde fraction which is suitable for oxidation by the process may be obtained from the purified raw aldehyde fraction by distillation. First runnings, intermediate fractions and the distillation residue are recycled to the step for producing the aldehydes or aldehyde mixtures or used for the production of C_5 to C_{10} alcohols. This method ensures a particularly economical production of the aldehyde required. The aldehydes or aldehyde mixtures obtained from the oxo synthesis of aliphatic or cycloaliphatic olefins of from

C_4 to C_9 molecular size, after purification, are oxidized in the absence of any catalyst with oxygen-containing gases while the aldehyde or aldehyde mixture is in the liquid phase in form of a thin film. The thin liquid film either flows downwardly at the wall of a single oxidation tube or a plurality of oxidation tubes, combined to form a tube bundle, or is distributed in the form of a thin film within these tubes on a large-surface packing material. The volumes of aldehyde passed through these tubes are from 10 to 60% preferably from 20 to 40% by volume per hour of the reaction space.

The oxidation is only dependent upon the surface area. Therefore, the nature of the large-surface material is not critical. Materials which are suitable for the distribution of the aldehydes and aldehyde mixtures to be oxidized in accordance with the process include large-surface or porous inorganic and/or organic materials, such as pumice, asbestos, glass wool, ceramics, porous ceramics (as for example those known as Sterchamol or Stuttgart mass), coke, coal, cellulose, paper, cotton, cotton wool, porous synthetic resins and similar materials.

The oxidation may be effected with the oxidizing gas being passed in cocurrent or countercurrent flow relation with the liquid aldehyde. Air, admitted in countercurrent, causes the C_5 to C_{10} aldehydes, which are already partially oxidized by contact with the air, to foam. The oxidation may, therefore, also be effected in an oxidation tube filled with a column of foam. When the liquid aldehyde is supplied by dropping the same onto the column of foam, an upper limit of the height for the column of foam can be established. In this manner, the aldehyde, as the liquid phase of the foam bubbles, moves in the reaction tube countercurrentwise with respect to the admitted oxidizing gas stream. In this manner, a particularly ideal distribution of the aldehyde as a thin liquid film is achieved.

The temperature at which the oxidation is effected is of decisive importance to the yield of isomeric C_5 to C_{10} carboxylic acid which is obtained. The oxidation is effected at temperatures of between 80° and 110°C. At temperatures of below 80°C., the proportion of isomeric carboxylic acid recovered remains low and large amounts of nonoxidized aldehyde are present in the reaction product. The content of isomeric acid is likewise reduced when the oxidation is effected at temperatures above the optimum temperature range, due to the formation of hydrocarbons, as may be seen from Table 1 which shows the oxidation to be directly dependent upon the oxidation temperature of the iosmeric C_9 aldehyde.

Up to 77.6% of nonanoic acid is obtained in the optimum temperature range. In addition to the acid formed, small amounts of C_8 hydrocarbons are formed by cleavage of carbon monoxide. The nonoxidized aldehyde is preferably returned into the oxidation step after the separation thereof from the acid by distillation. Taking into account the quantities of aldehyde recycled to the reaction, acid yields of up to about 85% can be obtained. Similar results are obtained in the analogous production of other isomeric C5 to C10 acid mixtures.

TABLE 1

[Starting material charged: 220 g. per hour of C_9 aldehyde per 880 cc reaction space]

Oxidation Temperature, °C.	Hydrocarbons, weight-percent	Nonanoic Acid, weight-percent	Untreated Aldehyde, weight-percent
65	5.0	67.1	22.2
80	6.4	74.6	15.4
95	8.8	77.6	10.4
110	15.7	68.8	11.9

To maintain the oxidation temperature at the desired range, an auxiliary liquid boiling between 50° and 110°C., and preferably between 75° and 100°C., may be added to the aldehyde being processed. There are preferred as such auxiliary liquids the hydrocarbons. Suitable for the production of acid mixtures C6 to C9 are aldehyde-hydrocarbon mixtures which are most conveniently obtained by maintaining suitable fractionation temperatures in the separation of the C6 to C9 aldehydes from the reaction product of the oxosynthesis operation effected with C5 to C8 olefins, the aldehydes distilling simultaneously with the hydrocarbons. When using C5 to C10 aldehydes, the same may also be diluted in diluents such as benzene, toluene, cyclohexane, aliphatic hydrocarbons of C6 to C8 molecular size used alone or in mixture with each other.

Example: Catalytic addition of water gas to diisobutylene and subsequent treatment of the reaction mixture with water under pressure resulted in a practically metal-free and acetal-free raw aldehyde having the following characteristics:

Carboxyl number (CON)	250
Hydroxyl number (OHN)	61
Iodine number (IN)	14
Neutralization number (NN)	4.9
Saponification number (SN)	14.5

1,142 kg. of this raw aldehyde product were charged into a still of 2 m.^{3} capacity, provided with a column having a length of 4 m., and the aldehyde product was distilled therein. The results of the distillation are set out in Table 2, shown on the following page.

TABLE 2

Fraction	Head Temp., °C.	Pressure, mm. Hg	Distillate, weight-percent	IN	NN	SN	CON	OHN
1	41–62	300	16.3	41	0.5	0.5	0	4
2	63–83	50	5.2	48	0.9	15.5	216	16
3	83–85	50–40	42.5	0.7	4.1	8.8	385	9
4	80–85	40	3.8				316	
Residue	85	40	30.7	6.4	3.4	41.1	36	143

For the production of the branched nonanoic acid, use was made of fraction 3, while fractions 1, 2, 4 and the residue was recycled to the process cycle for the production of isononanol. The oxidation of the aldehyde fraction 3 was effected in a glass tube having a length of 2 m. and an inside diameter of 25 mm. which was constricted towards the center by indentation provided at distances of 15 cm. These indentations served the purpose of largely preventing the downflowing aldehyde material, which was being oxidized, from running down along only the wall.

The tube was packed with granular pumice of 2 to 5 mm. particle size. The tube was surrounded by a cooling jacket which was filled with water maintained at 80°C. and which was regulated by a thermostat. The aldehyde was charged to the top of the tube at a rate of 220 g. per hour by means of a metering pump constructed of glass. At the same time, air at a rate of 98 l. per hour was introduced into the bottom of the reaction tube. At this air rate, 70 to 80% of the oxygen present in the air was consumed in the reaction. The oxidation product was withdrawn from the base of the oxidation tube and distilled from time to time in a glass column having a length of 1 m., which was filled with packing rings.

The acid fraction recovered amounted to 74.6% by weight of the oxidation product charged and had the following characteristics: neutralization number, 347 (theoretically 354); saponification number 347; boiling range, 115° to 124°C. at 10 mm. Hg. All of the other fractions recovered from the distillation including the residue were returned into the process for preparation of isononanol. In runs repeated substantially as described, the oxidation was effected continuously at temperatures of 95°, 110° and 65°C. The yields of nonanoic acid, hydrocarbons and unconverted C_9 aldehyde obtained in these runs are set out in Table 1.

Phosphoric Acid

According to H. Koch and K.E. Möller; U.S. Patent 3,061,621; Oct. 30, 1962; assigned to Studiengesellschaft Kohle mbH, Germany it is possible to use phosphoric acid alone as the catalyst for specific olefins provided that definite conditions are complied with. It is decisive for the successful performance of the carboxylic acid synthesis using phosphoric acid alone as the catalyst that the addition of carbon monoxide to the olefin is effected in the absence of free water, i.e., with a phosphoric acid which contains less water than is contained in the compound $P_2O_5 \cdot 5H_2O$. Accordingly use must be made of at least 90% and preferably 95 to 100% orthophosphoric acid or derivatives thereof which are still poorer in water such as pyrophosphoric acid or higher polyphosphoric acids or mixtures thereof.

The temperatures required when operating with phosphoric acid are generally higher than those employed when using previously preferred catalysts. Temperatures of about 50° to 150°C. are used. However, if possible, the higher range is avoided in view of the corrosion which becomes serious at this level. The optimum with respect to the synthesis conditions, on the one hand, and the avoidance of corrosion, on the other hand, is reached at temperatures of 75° to 95°C. As regards the pressure of carbon monoxide pressures of 1 to 250 atmospheres may be used, the preferred pressure being 10 to 100 atmospheres.

The relative proportions of the olefin and phosphoric acid to be used in the process must be such that at least 1 mol of phosphoric acid is used per mol of olefin. In general, more than 2 mols and preferably 4 to 8 mols of phosphoric acid per mol of olefin will be used. However, even higher amounts of phosphoric acid may be advantageous in certain cases. Under these conditions, specific olefins can be converted into carboxylic acids with satisfactory to very favorable results, these olefins being those with 5 to 12 carbon atoms, it being rather unimportant whether they are straight-chained or branched-chained or cyclic.

Good to very good results are obtained with normal olefins having from 5 to 10 carbon atoms, branched olefins within this range of carbon numbers such as 2-methyl-pentene-1 and trimeric propene, and with cyclic olefins such as octalin or cyclododecatriene. The process offers the particular advantage that, upon completion of the addition of carbon monoxide, the reaction product readily separates into two layers, the upper of which contains the carboxylic acids desired. The lower phase is the catalyst which is returned into the process.

A further particular advantage of the process resides in the fact that single-stage operation is possible because of this readily occurring separation of layers, which is important in view of a completely continuous operation of the process. In this case, the synthesis is effected with a catalyst which contains a higher content of phosphorous pentoxide corresponding to the quantity of olefin to be converted. During the reaction, the quantity of water required for the stoichiometric formation of the carboxylic acid is introduced together with the olefin or separately. The separation of layers may also be promoted by using light hydrocarbons, e.g., commercial hexane, as diluents.

Example 1: 336 g. (4 mols) of hexene-1 diluted with 750 ml. of commercial grade n-hexane were injected within 1.5 hours and at a temperature of 85° to 90°C. into a 5 l. stainless steel autoclave equipped with a magnetic stirrer and containing 985 ml. = 19 mols of 100% H_3PO_4 and being under a carbon monoxide pressure of 100 atmospheres. Upon a total of 8 hours, the reaction product was removed from the autoclave and mixed with water in amount stoichiometrically required for the formation of the carboxylic acid (3 mols with a 75% yield) thereby completely separating the catalyst. The carboxylic acids were separated from the organic phase by way of the alkali salts. Their amount was 371 g. which, as evidenced by fractional distillation, consisted of 87% C_7 acids and 13% C_{13} acids. This corresponded to a total yield of 74% based on olefin charged. The recovered catalyst was used with the same success for 3 additional experiments.

Example 2: (a) Under the conditions described in Example 1, 392 g. (4 mols) of heptene-1 were converted on 985 ml. of a 100% H_3PO_4 used as the catalyst. The reaction product was diluted with 500 ml. of commercial grade hexane to aid the separation of phases. Upon separation of the catalyst, the reaction product was processed resulting in 437 g. of carboxylic acids by way of the alkali salts. As shown by the acid number, the carboxylic acids consisted of more than 90% of C_8 acids (theoretical acid number, 389) corresponding to a total yield of 77% based on olefin charged. The separated catalyst to which the water withdrawn for the formation of carboxylic acids was added again was used under the same conditions for 4 additional batches without a decrease in its activity taking place.

(b) When converting 1 mol of heptene-1 with 1,104 g. of a catalyst of the composition 4 mols H_3PO_4 + 4 mols $H_4P_2O_7$ (corresponding to a P_2O_5 content of 77.2%) under the same conditions as those used in Example 2 (a) with a 100% H_3PO_4, a 52% yield of carboxylic acids based on olefin charged was obtained.

Organic Sulfonic Acid

J. Devine and J.F. Davies; U.S. Patent 3,282,973; November 1, 1966; assigned to Lever Brothers Company describe a process for the synthesis of a carboxylic acid which includes reacting together an olefinic compound and carbon monoxide in the presence of an organic sulfonic acid catalyst and treating the reaction product with water. The organic sulfonic acid can be an aliphatic sulfonic acid, an aromatic sulfonic acid or mixtures thereof. The aliphatic sulfonic acid preferably has 1 to 20 carbon atoms in the molecule. Examples of such acids are D-camphor-10-sulfonic acid, and the alkyl sulfonic acids such as methane sulfonic acid and those sulfonic acids which are derived from sulfonation of paraffins. The aromatic sulfonic acid can be a benzene sulfonic acid with one or more sulfonic acid groups, for example, benzene sulfonic acid and benzene meta-disulfonic acid or a naphthalene sulfonic acid with one or more sulfonic acid groups, for example naphthalene-2-sulfonic acid. The aromatic sulfonic acid can be substituted in the aromatic nucleus by nitro or halogen groups; preferably only one such substituent is present. The aromatic sulfonic acid can alternatively or additionally be substituted in the aromatic nucleus by hydroxy or alkyl groups; more than one hydroxy or alkyl group can be present. Such alkyl aryl sulfonic preferably have 20 carbon atoms or less in the alkyl group and can be alkyl benzene or alkyl naphthalene sulfonic acids. Examples of substituted aromatic sulfonic acids which can be used in the process are meta-nitrobenzene sulfonic acid, phenol sulfonic acid, etc.

A particularly useful aliphatic sulfonic acid is methane sulfonic acid. A preferred aromatic sulfonic acid is dodecylbenzene sulfonic acid in which the dodecyl group is derived from oligomers (i.e., low multiple adducts) of the lower olefins. Such dodecyl benzene sulfonic acids are generally mixtures of isomers of indeterminate and varied structure and are differentiated by the degree of branching in the side-chain; acids with both straight and branched side-chains can be used in the process.

The organic sulfonic acid may be used alone or in combination with a suitable acid such as sulfuric acid or a phosphoric acid. When a mineral acid was used in combination with the organic sulfonic acid it was found convenient to have the molar ratio of mineral to sulfonic acid between 4:1 and 1:5 and more especially between 3:1 and 1:2. An advantage of using methane sulfonic acid and other organic sulfonic acid catalysts which melt at or near room temperature is that a major proportion of catalyst can be removed from the reaction mixture by freezing out. Olefinic compounds suitable for use in the process can have up to 30, particularly from 2 to 20, carbon atoms in the molecule. Such compounds, which can have more than one carbon-carbon double bond, may have other functional groups in the molecule.

Olefins with no other functional groups in the molecule which can be used in the process are 1-decene, cyclohexene, 1,5-cyclo-octadiene, etc. Examples of olefinic compounds with other functional groups in the molecule are 1,2-dichloroethylene and cinnamyl alcohol. The olefinic compound can be produced in situ. When it is required to subject normally solid olefinic compounds to the process, it may be found convenient to supply them to the reactor or reaction zone as solutions in inert solvents such as commercial normal hexane. In the operation of the process, the most suitable amount of catalyst will be dependent upon the nature and amount of olefin and the optimum amount of catalyst in any particular instance may be found by simple trial. Convenient mol ratios of catalyst to olefin are from 1:3 to 30:1; but it is preferred to work between 3:2 and 20:1. The carbon monoxide may be obtained from water gas or producer gas; even water gas or producer gas themselves may be used as such.

The process can be operated at room temperature, although a considerable variation in this factor is possible. Yields may be improved by raising the temperature, but in general temperatures above 200°C. should be avoided, lest other reactions occur, with consequent lowering of the quality and yield of the desired product. The temperature range 0° to 180°C. is that within which the best results have been obtained. Particularly good results have been obtained in the range 80° to 100°C., but when there was concentrated sulfuric acid in the reaction mixture, temperatures below about 70°C. gave the most satisfactory results as regards freedom from by-products such as polymers, coloring matter and odoriferous constituents.

The carbon monoxide should be under pressure and a convenient range is particularly in the range 50 to 125 atmospheres. The reaction between olefin and carbon monoxide should preferably be conducted under substantially anhydrous conditions. The presence of a substantial amount of water at this stage may have a deleterious effect. Carboxylic acids synthesized by the process can be obtained having greater mobility, lighter color and less offensive odor than comparable products made using concentrated sulfuric acid alone as catalyst.

It is desirable in carrying out this process to ensure that there is good contact between the carbon monoxide and the olefin. It may be advantageous in some instances to operate the process in solution in order to reduce the viscosity of the mixture of olefinic compound and catalyst, thus facilitating agitation. Processes can be operated as continuous processes or as batch processes. In the following example, the yields are calculated on the amount of olefin.

Example: A stainless steel autoclave fitted with an injection pump was charged with 150.4 g. (1.6 mols) of methane sulfonic acid. The autoclave was sealed, flushed out with carbon monoxide and pressurized with carbon monoxide to 100 atmospheres. The contents of the autoclave were heated to 100°C. and maintained at this temperature. Propylene tetramer was introduced into the autoclave by means of the injection pump at 0.56 to 1.12 ml./min. until a total of 33.6 g. (0.20 mol) of tetramer had been added. During the introduction of the tetramer the contents of the autoclave were continually agitated, and the carbon monoxide pressure varied between 92 and 100 atmospheres. When the addition of the tetramer had been completed, agitation was continued for a further 30 minutes after which 20 ml. of water were added by means of the injection pump, the autoclave being still under carbon monoxide pressure. After the autoclave had been allowed to cool the pressure was released. The reaction mixture was washed out of the autoclave with isopropanol and analyzed for carboxylic acid. The analysis indicated that 27.1 g. of carboxylic acid had been formed, a yield of 64%. The carboxylic acid product obtained was quite mobile and had a light color and an inoffensive odor.

Oxonium Tetraborate

A process by S. Pawlenko; U.S. Patent 3,349,107; October 24, 1967; assigned to Schering AG, Germany relates to the synthesis of carboxylic acids and their methylesters from olefins, carbon monoxide and —OH— containing compounds ROH, wherein R stands for H or CH_3. According to the process such syntheses can be carried out as a one-step process and with catalytic amounts of oxonium tetrafluoroborate $[ROH_2][BF_4]$.

Specifically, this is a process for the synthesis of aliphatic carboxylic acids having from 5 to 13 carbon atoms in the molecule and aliphatic carboxylic acid methyl esters having from 6 to 14 carbon atoms in the molecule, comprising reacting in a reaction space an olefin selected from the group consisting of monoolefins branched at the double bond and having from 4 to 12 carbon atoms in the molecule with CO and a reaction component selected from the group consisting of water and methanol, in the presence of a catalyst selected from the group consisting of aqueous solutions of 74 to 85% by weight of hydroxonium tetrafluoroborate $[H_3O][BF_4]$ and methanol solutions of 65 to 75% by weight of methoxonium tetrafluoroborate $[CH_3OH_2][BF_4]$. The reaction is carried out in the range of 50 to 200 atmospheres pressure and a temperature in the range of 20° to 50°C.

Example: In a pressure reactor of 2 liters, 435 g. catalyst consisting of 80.3% by weight of $[H_3O][BF_4]$, 19.4% by weight of water and 0.3% by weight of HF were placed. Into the pressure reactor within 130 hours 50,400 kg. (300 mols) of propylenetetramer and 5,310 kg. of H_2O were continuously introduced, keeping the reaction temperature constantly at 45°C. and the CO pressure at 150 atmospheres. The reaction product discharged during this period of time yielded 61,630 kg. of C_{13} carboxylic acid having a boiling point at 20 mm. Hg 167° to 182°C., an acid number of 263, n_D^{20} = 1.4478 and also 0.740 kg. of higher carboxylic acids. This corresponds to a yield of 96% by weight, based on the theoretical yield.

In carrying out the synthesis in the manner described in the average 9.6 g. $[H_3O][BF_4]$ and 3 g. of HF were carried over by the synthesis product. The crude synthesis product was always subjected to preliminary washing with feed water so that the carried over products were continuously reintroduced into the reactor. During the 130 hours of the synthesis reaction only 10 g. of fresh HF of 63% by weight and no additional catalyst at all were introduced into the reactor. At the end of the 130 hours period of the reactor contained 403 g. of catalyst consisting of 80.7% by weight of [H_3O][BF_4], 18.9% by weight of H_2O and 0.4% by weight of HF. The losses of catalyst amounted to 0.4 g. of [H_3O][BF_4] and 0.15 g. of HF per 1 kg. of pure C_{13}-carboxylic acid.

In purifying the synthesis product 3 parts by weight of the crude acid were diluted with 1 part by weight of n-heptane and treated with 85 g. of feed water per 1 kg. of crude acid. Subsequently, the crude acid was washed with NaCl-containing water, up to a pH of 4 to 5. As no olefin polymerizates or other by-products were present, any processing over the alkali salt was unnecessary. The washed crude acid was subjected to distillation and yielded n-heptane at 50 torr and the C_{13}-carboxylic acid at 20 torr.

PREPARATION FROM OLEFINS BY OTHER METHODS

OXIDATION OF OLEFINS WITH GASEOUS OXYGEN

Bromine and Heavy Metal Catalyst

E.F. Jason and E.K. Fields; U.S. Patent 3,054,814; September 18, 1962; assigned to Standard Oil Company prepare aliphatic acids from the various hydrocarbon fractions of dewaxed, water-extracted, hydrocarbon synthesis liquids by liquid phase oxidation with molecular oxygen in the presence of a catalyst system comprising a source of bromine and a heavy metal oxidation catalyst. By such an oxidation, especially of the fractions containing an average of more than 5 carbon atoms per molecule, aliphatic acids containing both keto groups and carboxylic acid groups are obtained.

The aliphatic acids are, in general, monoolefinic diketo monocarboxylic acids containing more carbon atoms than in the feedstock oxidized. The oxidation process is carried out at temperatures of from 200° to 500°F. at pressures to maintain a liquid phase. The precise pressure is not critical but is a matter of choice as long as a liquid phase is maintained. Pressures of from 100 to 1,000 psig or higher can be employed. It is also desirable to employ an acidic reaction medium or solvent.

For this purpose an aliphatic monocarboxylic acid of from 2 to 8 carbon atoms, preferably acetic acid because of its resistance to oxidation and its availability, is preferred. The oxidation process can be carried out in the absence of a solvent or reaction medium, but the aliphatic acids produced are sufficiently high in molecular weight and viscosity that the reaction products are more readily handled when a reaction medium is present.

Air is the most readily available source of molecular oxygen. However, substantially pure oxygen, i.e., commercial oxygen, oxygen plus ozone, mixtures of oxygen and inert gases, and mixtures of air and inert gases, can be employed as the source of molecular oxygen for the process. Molecular oxygen-containing gases having from 5 to 100% oxygen by volume can be employed.

The catalyst system comprises bromine and a heavy metal oxidation catalyst. The bromine may be employed as elemental, combined, or ionic bromine. More specifically, as a source of bromine for the catalyst system there may be employed molecular bromine, ammonium bromide, hydrogen bromide, and other bromine-containing compounds soluble in the reaction mixture. Satisfactory results can be obtained, for example, by the use of potassium bromate, tetra-bromoethane, benzyl bromide, and the like, as a source of bromine. The heavy metal oxidation catalyst portion of the catalyst system employed includes the heavy metals and derivatives thereof which are soluble in the reaction medium to the extent necessary to provide a catalytically effective amount of the heavy metal oxidation catalyst component.

The heavy metal oxidation catalyst component of the catalyst system may be provided by the addition of the metal in elemental form, as its oxide or hydroxide, or in the form of a salt of the metal. For example, the metal manganese may be employed as the manganese salt of an organic carboxyloic acid, such as manganese naphthenate, manganese toluate, manganese acetate, etc., or in the form of an organic complex, such as the acetylacetonate, the 8-hydroxy-quinolate and the ethylenediamine tetra-acetate, as well as inorganic manganese salts such as the borates, halides and nitrates. The catalyst system may also be provided by the use of a heavy metal bromide or mixtures of heavy metal bromides.

The amount of metal catalyst employed is not critical and may be in the range of about 0.01 to 10% by weight or more based on the feedstock reactant. Where the heavy metal is introduced as a bromide salt, for example as manganese bromide, the proportions of manganese and bromine will be in their stoichiometric proportions. The ratio of metal to bromine may be varied from such proportions within the range of about 1 to 10 atoms of heavy metal oxidation catalyst per atom of bromine to about 1 to 10 atoms of bromine per atom of heavy metal.

The amount of solvent or reaction medium employed will vary over wide limits as will be readily appreciated by those skilled in the art. The amount of solvent or reaction medium employed is not critical but typically will be in the range of from about 0.01 to 10, desirably 0.05 to 1.0 times the weight of oxidizable feedstock.

Example: A reaction system containing a reaction vessel having a means for measuring the temperature of the reactants contained therein, means for heating its contents, a bottom discharge port, a bottom air-charging line, a vapor conduit connecting its free-board space to a condenser, a condensate collector for separating condensate from uncondensed gases through a pressure control valve and a condensate return line connected to the reactor, is employed. The oxidizable feedstock is a C_{10} fraction of a dewaxed, water-extracted and aqueous alkali washed hydrocarbon synthesis liquid containing by weight:

20% Normal 1-olefins	8% Branched paraffins
12% Other normal olefins	9% Aromatics
11% Tertiary olefins	6% Carbonyl compounds
13% Other branched olefins	6% Hydroxyl compounds
6% Normal paraffins	9% Other oxygen compounds

The hydrocarbons contain 10 carbon atoms per molecule as do the "other oxygen compounds," the carbonyl compounds contain 8 carbon atoms per molecule, and the hydroxyl compounds are a mixture of C_7 and C_8 molecules. No molecule contains more than 10 carbon atoms. Such a mixture boils in the range of 159° to 184°C. at 757 mm. Hg.

To the reaction vessel there are charged 210 g. of the above C_{10} fraction of the hydrocarbon synthesis liquid, 11 g. of glacial acetic acid, 0.84 g. of tetrabromoethane and 10 ml. of an aqueous solution that is 0.25 molar in cobalt acetate and manganese acetate. The reactor is closed, and the pressure control valve is set about 400 psig. The reaction mixture is heated to about 300°F. and air is passed into the reaction mixture at 2.74 liters per minute. Air flow is continued for about 5 hours during which time the temperature is maintained between 303° to 318°F. by the removal of heat by the reflux condenser system.

The reactor contents are cooled to about 30°C., filtered to remove a small amount of insoluble material, and then distilled. A forerun consisting of water and 43 ml. volatile organics is removed at atmospheric pressure. The remainder is stripped in vacuo and 28 g. of liquid are collected over a range of 38° to 91°C., at 1.5 mm. Hg. The residue is taken up with an excess of 5% aqueous potassium hydroxide. The insoluble material, 3 grams, is extracted with ether. The organic acid is liberated from the aqueous solution with dilute hydrochloric acid and is separated from the aqueous mother liquor.

The sprung acid is taken up with ether, the ether solution washed with water, dried and stripped in vacuo at 130° to 140°C. and 1.0 mm. Hg. The residue, 108 grams, is a viscous, heavy, light-colored liquid. The analysis of this liquid product shows 68.17% carbon and 9.01% hydrogen, a molecular weight of 308 ±10 and a neutral equivalent of 266. From this carbon and hydrogen analysis and oxygen by difference, the product is a monoolefin diketo monocarboxylic acid having the empirical formula $C_{16}H_{26}O_4$ whose calculated carbon is 68.05% and hydrogen is 9.22% with a molecular weight of 282 and a neutral equivalent of 282.

Similarly other fractions of dewaxed, water and alkali washed hydrocarbon synthesis liquid, especially fractions whose aliphatic hydrocarbons (olefins and paraffins) contain 7 to 15 carbon atoms per molecule, may be converted to olefinic keto monocarboxylic acids of higher carbon content than the feedstock oxidized.

A related process by E.F. Jason and E.K. Fields; U.S. Patent 3,076,842; February 5, 1963; assigned to Standard Oil Company specifically pertains to the oxidation of certain alkene-1 hydrocarbons to aliphatic monocarboxylic acid and a keto derivative thereof of one less carbon atom than in the alkene-1 hydrocarbon.

This process is conducted in the liquid phase at a temperature below 200°C., preferably at a temperature in the range of about 50° to 200°C. The temperature at which the process is carried out will determine to an appreciable extent the minimum pressure to be employed to maintain the liquid phase of the reaction mixture. The pressure at any specific temperature will be governed by the vapor pressures of the materials in the reaction mixture. When the reaction mixture contains the alkene-1 hydrocarbon, the pressure to be maintained will be that required to keep at least a portion of the alkene-1 in the liquid phase.

It is advantageous during the course of the reaction to subject the vapors in contact with the reaction mixture to partial condensation to condense out of the vapors at least the alkene-1 hydrocarbon contained therein. However, there are also advantages in carrying out the process in the presence of a reaction solvent or diluent. For this purpose any inert solvent may be employed. It is preferred that the solvent or reaction medium dissolve at least a portion of the alkene-1 being oxidized and also dissolve the heavy metal oxidation catalyst. Monocarboxylic acids containing 2 to 8 carbon atoms can be used as reaction solvents or reaction media.

Such monocarboxylic acids include benzoic acid and the lower aliphatic monocarboxylic acids such as acetic acid, propionic acid, butyric acid, valeric acid, enanthic acid and caprylic acid. It will be appreciated that many of these acids are produced in the process. Whether or not the acids used as the reaction solvents or reaction media are produced in the process, the separation of the desired products from the reaction mixture can be readily accomplished. Because of its resistance to oxidation under the conditions of the process, acetic acid is the preferred lower aliphatic monocarboxylic acid for use as the reaction solvent or reaction medium.

The use of such a reaction solvent or reaction medium either permits a convenient means for removing heat of reaction since the vaporized reaction solvent can be condensed and returned to the liquid phase or, in the case of the use of the higher boiling monocarboxylic acids, a lower pressure reaction can be conducted and still maintain the liquid phase.

Example: As an oxidation reactor there is employed a vertical tubular reactor into the bottom of which air or other source of molecular oxygen-containing gas can be charged. The bottom of the reactor is also suitably adapted to the removal of the mixture resulting from the oxidation process. The top of the reactor is provided with a means for closing the reactor through which is connected a vapor line for transfer of vapors to a condenser from which condensate may be recycled to the reaction zone.

A condenser is provided with means for removing the uncondensed materials through a pressure regulating valve with which the reaction pressure is maintained to obtain a liquid phase throughout the reaction. The reactor is constructed of corrosion-resistant material such as highly corrosive resistant alloys, or is glass lined. To such a reactor there is charged a mixture containing 112.2 g. (1 mol) of 1-octene, 120.1 g. (2 mols) glacial acetic acid and 10 ml. of an aqueous solution containing cobalt acetate and manganese acetate, each in a 0.25 molar concentration. There is also added 1.0 ml. of 5 molar ammonium bromide dissolved in water.

The resulting mixture is heated to 170°C. in the presence of sufficient nitrogen so that the resulting pressure is 400 psig. Air at a pressure of about 400 psig is introduced into the reactor at a flow rate of about 3 l. per minute. After 5 hours of air addition, the reactor contents are cooled and distilled.

As a first fraction there are collected all materials boiling up to 50°C. at 140 mm. Hg. This mixture contains primarily formic acid, acetic acid and water. The total amount of acetic acid collected in this mixture is 128 g. As a second fraction there is collected material boiling in the range of 63°C. at 2.2 mm. Hg to 94°C. at 1.8 mm. Hg. This fraction when redistilled has a boiling point of 200° to 203°C. and has a refractive index of n_D^{20} of 1.4218. This second fraction is n-heptanoic acid for which the literature reports a boiling point of 202°C. and a refractive index of $n_D^{19.8}$ of 1.4216.

As a third fraction there is collected material boiling at 121° to 143°C. at 1.7 mm. Hg. This material has a refractive index of n_D^{20} of 1.4464. Analysis of this material (third fraction) shows 60.0% carbon and 9.4% hydrogen. The neutral equivalent of this fraction is 146. Acetyl pentanoic acid has a calculated neutral equivalent of 145 and a calculated carbon and hydrogen content of 58.0 and 9.0%, respectively. The third fraction is substantially all 5-acetyl pentanoic acid. Only a small amount of residue remains, about 7.3 g., which was not further characterized.

When the process is carried out at a temperature of 150°C., the yield of n-heptanoic acid is increased, and the yield of the keto acid is decreased. By carrying out the process of the foregoing example at a temperature of about 180° to 185°C., the yield of the keto acid is increased while the yield of n-heptanoic acid is decreased.

The use of manganese bromide in place of ammonium bromide in the process in an amount to provide an equivalent amount of metal will produce substantially equivalent results. Also in place of employing both manganese acetate and cobalt acetate there may be employed either manganese acetate or cobalt acetate. Other members of the heavy metal oxidation catalyst can be employed to produce substantially the same results. As additional feedstocks of the process there may be specifically employed 1-hexene, 3,3-dimethyl hexene-1, 1-decene, 1-hexadecene, 1-heptadecene, and the like.

Cerium Salt-Nitric Acid Mixture as Catalyst

In a process by E.F. Lutz; U.S. Patent 3,407,221; October 22, 1968; assigned to Shell Oil Company alpha- and beta-olefins are oxidized to carboxylic acids by intimately contacting the olefin in liquid phase with an oxygen-containing gas in the presence of an oxidation catalyst consisting of a cerium salt and nitric acid.

The alkenes oxidized according to the process are preferably olefins in which the unsaturation occurs in the alpha- or beta-position. However, the charge to the oxidation zone may be mixtures of olefins which are terminally or internally unsaturated, and in which the unsaturation occurs in positions other than the alpha- or beta-position. The olefins may be straight chain or branched chain alkenes, and contain from about 4 to 20 or more carbon atoms in the chain.

The oxidation of the olefin mixture, i.e., the mixture of α-, β-, γ-, etc. alkenes, is carried out in liquid phase in the presence of a cerium-nitric acid catalyst. Cerium may be charged as either Ce(III) or Ce(IV), as long as the cerium-containing compound is soluble in the reaction medium. Cerium salts of either inorganic or organic acids can be used, e.g., cerous nitrate and cerous acetate. Cerous nitrate is particularly useful because of its high solubility in the solvent employed, and because of its compatibility with nitric acid, its co-catalyst.

In general, it is preferred to use substantially less than a stoichiometric amount of catalyst for the oxidation. While the mol ratio of cerium to olefin may satisfactorily be varied between about 1:15 and 1:0.5, it is generally preferred to use a ratio of between 1:1.5 and 1:1.0. Within the co-catalyst system itself, mol ratios of cerium/nitric acid of between 1:6 and 1:0.2, preferably between 1:2 and 1:1 are satisfactory.

The particular solvent employed is chosen based on the solubility of the catalysts, and the stability and inactivity of the solvent under the reaction conditions. Paraffins, such as hexane and heptane, are not satisfactory, because of the low solubility of the cerium salts. In general, primary and secondary alcohols, likewise, are unsatisfactory because of their reactivity and tendency to be oxidized. Nitriles, such as acetonitrile and butyronitrile, tend to favor nitration rather than oxidation, and low yields of product acid are obtained.

It has been found that the most satisfactory solvents for the reaction are the low molecular weight, especially normal, paraffinic acids, such as acetic, propionic, n-butyric and n-valeric acids. Some ester formation occurs during the reaction, by reaction of the olefin reactants with the paraffin acids, the acids adding to the olefin at the point of unsaturation, thus producing an ester. The ester by-product may undergo nitration, to form a nitro-substituted ester. Thus, the nitration and esterification by-products are the two major contaminants in the acid product. Because of its availability and low cost, it is preferred to use acetic acid as the solvent. The acid may be used in an essentially concentrated form, or diluted with water; however, it is preferred that the water content of the solvent not exceed about 10% by weight.

The upper temperature at which the oxidation is effected is limited only by the boiling point of the solvent. For example, when acetic acid is used as solvent, it is preferred to operate at temperatures between about 110° and 115°C.; with propionic acid, temperatures up to about 140°C. are permissible; with butyric acid, the upper limit of the temperature range would be about 160°C.; and so forth. It is preferred, in general, to operate at temperatures above about 100°C., preferably above 110°C., in order to minimize the reaction time. Temperatures below about 85°C. are conducive to low oxidation yields. The reaction time is limited not only by the temperature employed, but also by the rate of olefin addition to the catalyst/solvent mixture. The reaction is permitted to continue until

Fatty Acids

at least 75%, preferably 85%, of the reactants are converted and is run between atmospheric pressure and 30 psig. The olefin is added slowly, maintaining low concentration, to minimize formation of by-products.

Example: Into a 3-neck round-bottom glass flask equipped with a magnetic stirrer was introduced a mixture of cerium (III) nitrate and concentrated nitric acid (70%) in acetic acid. Olefin was introduced dropwise through a dropping funnel through one neck of the flask; a second neck of the flask held a dip tube through which oxygen was introduced. The third neck of the flask contained a reflux condenser. The table below summarizes the pertinent reaction conditions and product yields obtained from several runs using this apparatus. All runs were made at atmospheric pressure.

Olefin, mols	Solvent, cc	Catalyst, mols	Rate of O_2 Addition, cc/min.	Temp., °C.	Time, hr.	Conversion, Percent (Basis Olefin)
1-Hexadecene, 0.1	Acetic acid, 200	$Ce(NO_3)_3 \cdot 6H_2O$, 0.0375 + Conc. HNO_3, 0.125	~25	111-114	(*2 / 4)	84
1-Hexadecene, 0.1	Acetic acid, 200	$Ce(NO_3)_3 \cdot 6H_2O$, 0.0625 + Conc. HNO_3, 0.125	~37	114	(*1.5 / 2.0)	92
1-Hexadecene, 0.1	Acetic acid, 195	$Ce(NO_3)_3 \cdot 6H_2O$, 0.0625 + Conc. HNO_3, 0.125	~55	113	(*3.5 / 4.0)	--
1-Hexadecene, 0.15	Acetic acid, 250	$Ce(NO_3)_3 \cdot 6H_2O$, 0.125 + Conc. HNO_3, 0.125	55-90	110-114	(*3.0 / 3.5)	94
1-Hexadecene, 0.2	Acetic acid, 450	$Ce(NO_3)_3 \cdot 6H_2O$, 0.075 + Conc. HNO_3, 0.25	40	113	(*3.0 / 4.0)	67
1-Octene, 0.3	Propionic acid, 185	$Ce(NO_3)_3 \cdot 6H_2O$, 0.025 + Conc. HNO_3, 0.125	25	108-120	4.5	27
1-Octene, 0.3	Propionic acid, 205	$Ce(NO_3)_3 \cdot 6H_2O$, 0.0375 + Conc. HNO_3, 0.125	75	104-118	(*3.75 / 12)	24.4
1-Octene, 0.3	Acetic acid, 205	$Ce(NO_3)_3 \cdot 6H_2O$, 0.0375 + Conc. HNO_3, 0.125	25	104-111	(*3.75 / 4.5)	25
1-Octene, 0.07	Propionic acid, 144	$Ce(NO_3)_3 \cdot 6H_2O$, 0.0375 + Conc. HNO_3, 0.125	25	116-120	(*0.83 / 1.25)	**
2-Octene, 0.2	Acetic acid, 205	$Ce(NO_3)_3 \cdot 6H_2O$, 0.0375 + Conc. HNO_3, 0.125	~25	111	(*3.0 / 4.0)	**
2-Butene, 0.32	Butyric acid, 219	$Ce(NO_3)_3 \cdot 6H_2O$, 0.125 + Conc. HNO_3, 0.125	~25	110-115	(*2.33 / 3.33)	54.9

*Olefin addition discontinued after this time period; second number indicates total reaction time.
**Only acid portion of product analyzed.

Use of Dinitrogen Tetroxide

D.R. Lachowicz, T.S. Simmons and K.L. Kreuz; U.S. Patent 3,415,856; Dec. 10, 1968; and U.S. Patent 3,458,582; July 29, 1969; both assigned to Texaco, Inc. describe a process for preparing nitroperoxy, nitroketone, alkanoic and alkanedioic compounds from alkenes and alkenoic acids comprising contacting an alkene with a mixture of dinitrogen tetroxide and oxygen to form the nitroperoxy intermediate, contacting the nitroperoxy intermediate with a denitrating agent to form the nitroketone intermediate and acidifying the nitroketone intermediate under aqueous conditions to form the alkenoic and alkanedioic acid.

In the first stage of the reaction, the reaction temperature employed is advantageously between about −40° and 20°C. Higher reaction temperatures tend to facilitate the decomposition of the peroxy nitrate product and at temperatures below the prescribed range the dinitrogen tetroxide would not function due to its inability to dissociate into monomeric nitrogen dioxide. The reactant mol ratio of olefin to dinitrogen tetroxide to oxygen is normally between about 1:0.5:1 and 1:1.5:30. However, the important aspect of the reactant ratio is that the mols of oxygen be at least equivalent and preferably in excess to the mols of dinitrogen tetroxide.

If the ratio of N_2O_4 is above that of oxygen another NO_2 group forms rather than the desired peroxy group. Excess oxygen even in excess of the stated range does not deleteriously affect the reaction. The reaction time is normally between about 1/2 and 10 hours, although longer and shorter periods may be employed. The formed nitroalkylperoxy nitrate or peroxynitrato alkanoic acid depending on the initial olefin reactant is recovered, if desired, by standard means, for example, via stripping volatiles.

It is to be noted that the nitrating agent, dinitrogen tetroxide, is actually an equilibrium mixture of dinitrogen tetroxide and nitrogen dioxide with the equilibrium being driven to essentially 100% dinitrogen tetroxide at 0°C. and essentially 100% nitrogen dioxide at 140°C. Under advantageous conditions, the nitrating agent is normally introduced into the reaction system at a rate of between about 0.002 and 0.02 g./min./g. olefin, however, the actual rate depends in large measure upon the rate of heat removal from the reaction system.

To promote contact of the reactants in the first stage, the reaction is desirably carried out under conditions of agitation in the presence of an inert liquid diluent, for example, inert liquids having a boiling point between about 30° and 100°C., such as n-hexane, n-heptane, carbon tetrachloride and diethylether. The olefinic reactant employed should be of at least 6 carbons and preferably less than about 55 carbon atoms, although higher molecular weight olefins may be utilized. The contemplated olefinic materials can be derived from many sources such as wax cracking and olefin polymerization.

In the second stage, the nitroalkylperoxy nitrate or nitratoperoxy alkenoic acid of at least 6 carbons recovered from the first stage is contacted with a denitrating agent. The reactant contacting is conducted, preferably with agitation, at a temperature between about −60° and 70°C. in a mol ratio of denitrating agent to peroxy compound of at least about 1:1, and preferably less than about 20:1. The reaction of the second stage is more or less instantaneous after addition of reactants. The particular mode of bringing the reactants together depends on many things such as molecular weight of reactants and reactivity of the peroxy material. Normally, with the more reactive peroxy materials, the contacting of reactants is accomplished by slow addition of the peroxy intermediate to the denitrating agent.

The nitroketone intermediate product can be recovered by standard recovery processes, for example, via filtration of the solid intermediate after the addition of the reaction mixture to water or via distillation. Normally, inert diluent is not employed in the second stage of the overall process if one of the reactants is in liquid form. However, if both reactants are in the solid state, then to facilitate interaction inert liquid diluent is employed, for example, inert liquid diluent having a boiling point between about 30° and 100°C., such as pentane, hexane, carbon tetrachloride and diethylether. Agitation of the reaction mixture is also a preferred condition.

Specific examples of the denitrating agents contemplated here are dimethylformamide, diethylformamide, dimethylacetamide, dimethylsulfoxide, diethylsulfoxide, tetramethylurea and tetraethylurea.

In the third stage of the process the nitroketone recovered from the second stage is contacted with water in the presence of an acid member selected from the group consisting of mineral acid, hydrocarbon sulfonic acid and halo acetic acid having a dissociation constant in excess of 10^{-2} at a temperature of between about 0° and 150°C. in a mol ratio of nitroketone to acid member of between about 1:1 and 1:10, and in a mol ratio of nitroketone to water of at least about 1:2 to form a carboxylic acid.

This third stage of the reaction is normally conducted for a period in the range of 15 minutes to several hours. However, the actual reaction time will be dependent in large measure on the kind and strength of the acid member employed. Under preferred conditions, the reaction mixture is agitated in order to facilitate contact between the reactants. Further, if both the acid and ketone are of the solid nature, in order to afford better reactant contact, inert liquid diluent is advantageously employed, for example, inert liquid diluent having a boiling point between about 50° and 150°C., such as acetic acid.

The water contact in the third stage is normally accomplished by first forming the final nitroketone-acid reaction mixture and then contacting with an excess of water, e.g., pouring the reaction mixture into a stoichiometric excess of cold water. The carboxylic acid product is recovered by standard means such as by filtration or extracting the formed carboxylic acid, e.g., with ether, followed by stripping off the extractant from the extract solution to leave the carboxylic acid as residue.

Specific examples of the acid catalyst contemplated in the third stage are sulfuric acid, phosphoric acid, nitric acid, trichloroacetic acid, methane sulfonic acid, and ethane sulfonic acid. The acids employed are advantageously of an acid strength in respect to aqueous dilution of at least about 70 weight percent of the concentrated state.

Example 1: This example illustrates the first stage of the overall process, namely the preparation of the intermediate peroxy compounds from olefins. Through a mixture of 5 ml. of 1-dodecene and 60 ml. of n-hexane maintained at 0°C. there was bubbled oxygen at a rate of 56.5 ml./min. together with the simultaneous introduction of about 2.2 g. of dinitrogen tetroxide over about a 4 hour period. The volatiles in the final reaction mixture were removed under reduced pressure and the residual product was identified by infrared and nuclear magnetic resonance spectroscopy as 1-nitro-2-dodecylperoxy nitrate.

Example 2: This example illustrates the second stage of the overall process, namely the conversion of the peroxy compound of Example 1 into the corresponding nitroketone. In an amount of 7.22 g. (0.023 mol) 1-nitro-2-dodecylperoxy nitrate of Example 1 was added to 25 ml. of dimethylformamide with agitation at 20° to 27°C. and the mixture was immediately added to water. The resultant aqueous mixture was filtered and a solid product weighing 4.68 g. was recovered. The solid product was identified as 1-nitro-2-dodecanone representing a yield of 90 mol percent based on the initial dodecene reactant.

Example 3: This example illustrates the third stage of the overall process, namely the conversion of the nitroketone of Example 2 to the corresponding carboxylic acid. To 4.68 g. of 1-nitro-2-dodecanone prepared in Example 2 there was added 50 ml. of concentrated sulfuric acid and the mixture was heated with stirring for 15 min. and then added to a stoichiometric excess of water. A solid product weighing 2.65 g. was recovered by extraction of the resultant aqueous mixture with ether followed by ether evaporation leaving the product as residue. The residual product was identified as undecanoic acid in a yield of 70 mol percent based on the initial dodecene reactant.

Example 4: This example further illustrates the overall process and subprocesses. To a magnetically stirred flask there was added 5.4 g. of oleic acid and 60 ml. of n-hexane. The mixture was cooled and maintained at 0°C. and simultaneously bubbled through were oxygen at a rate of 56.5 ml./min. and 1.4 ml. of dinitrogen tetroxide. When all the N_2O_4 had been added, the solvent and excess NO_2 were removed by vacuum and the residual product was identified as a mixture of 9-nitro-10-peroxynitrato octadecanoic acid and 10-nitro-9-peroxynitrato octadecanoic acid.

The above residual product was cooled to about -20°C. and 25 ml. of dimethylformamide were added and the resultant mixture was stirred for about 0.5 hour in a temperature range between -20° and 16°C. The stirred mixture was then poured into 150 ml. of H_2O and filtered. The filtered solids were water washed and weighed 6.5 g. They were identified essentially as a mixture of 9-nitro-10-keto octadecanoic and 10-nitro-9-octadecanoic acid representing a yield of 98.5%. This nitroketone product was further purified by successive extractions with water, carbon tetrachloride and ether.

To 30 ml. of glacial acetic acid there was added 1 g. of the above purified nitroketone mixture and 10 ml. of 35% HNO_3. The resultant mixture was stirred and heated 3 hours at 110°C. and then poured into cold water (large stoichiometric excess). The resultant aqueous mixture was extracted with ether and the ether extract solution was subjected to distillation to remove the ether leaving a yellowish oil. The yellowish oil was subjected to fractional distillation under reduced pressure and 0.3 g. of pelargonic acid and 0.5 g. of azelaic acid were recovered. This represented a yield of 60 mol percent for pelargonic and 90 mol percent for azelaic based on the nitroketone reactant.

Selective Oxidation

G.C. Robinson; U.S. Patent 3,557,169; January 19, 1971; assigned to Ethyl Corporation describes a process for producing straight chain unsubstituted monobasic carboxylic acids having from about 7 to 19 carbon atoms per molecule with improved selectivity by oxidation of selected olefins. Alpha olefins are dimerized to produce ethylenes containing at least 1,1-disubstitution with a methylene group in the alpha position of at least one of the substituting radicals. The ethylenes are oxidized selectively to produce cleavage of the molecule at the linkage of the methylene group of the radical to the balance of the substituted ethylene molecule. The oxidizing of the olefins to produce acids is carried out at a temperature from 75° to 110°C.

As oxidation catalysts, one may use various conventional systems such as tertiary butyl hydroperoxide, manganous stearate, of about 0.1 to 1.0%, mixtures of 0.1 weight percent of cobalt or cobalt-containing material and an equal molar amount (cobalt to bromine) of bromine or bromine-containing material such as cobalt acetate and ammonium bromide, cobalt bromide, cobalt naphthenates, etc. In addition, copper and vanadium salts, organic as well as inorganic, may be used.

One will note that the oxidation is performed at low temperatures, such as from about 75° to 110°C. at which temperatures nondirected attacks on random carbon atoms are virtually avoided. A typical preferred temperature is about 105°C. In certain instances the oxidation is advantageously performed in inert diluent media, typical reasonably inert diluents being acetic acid and propionic acid.

Example 1: 30 parts of 2-n-butyl-1-hexene of 99% purity was oxidized with oxygen at 106°C. for approximately 4 hours. Tertiary butyl hydroperoxide (1%) was added at the start. Approximately 20% of the olefin reacted. To this mixture was added 1% manganous stearate and oxidation continued for approximately 5 hours at approximately 106°C. when the total olefin oxidized was approximately 75% of the starting amount. The product had an acid number of 56.

The acids were extracted with a 7% sodium carbonate solution. The sodium carbonate extract was extracted twice with ether and acidified with HCl. The acids were extracted with ether and the extract distilled to remove the ether. The resulting crude acids which were of a light straw color were analyzed by vapor phase chromatography yielding major amounts of n-propionic acid (52 weight percent), normal butyric acid (12.6%), normal pentanoic acid (9.3%) and normal hexanoic acid (11.4%) with no other major peaks. The crude acids were 10% by weight of the starting material and corresponded to an average molecular weight of 100. In this experiment, identification of major products was of main concern and the overall yield was not of great significance.

Example 2: To a stirred reaction flask was added 31.0 g. of tetradecene dimer (80% vinylidene plus tri-substituted), 25 g. of glacial acetic acid and 0.3 g. manganous stearate. This mixture was oxidized for 14 1/2 hours at about 106°C. Oxygen uptake was slow for the first half hour, rapid during the next two hours, and tapering off to virtually zero during the balance of the period. 36.3 g. of reaction product (exclusive of acetic acid) was recovered. This product was 33.7% fatty acid (weight), with 75% of those acids falling in the C_{11}-C_{15} range.

Example 3: To a stirred reaction flask was added 48.5 g. of tetradecene dimer of Example 2 and 0.5 g. of manganous stearate. This mixture was oxidized for 12 1/2 hours at 106°C. The crude oxidate weighed 52.0 g., and was 17% crude acids. Of the crude acids 43 weight percent was fatty acids (straight chain saturated monofunctional carboxylic acids) with 36% of the crude or 84% of the fatty acids falling in the range of 11 to 15 carbon atoms per molecule. Distribution by carbon atoms per molecule was as follows:

Acids (carbon atoms per molecule)	Weight Percent
6	0.44
7	0.83
8	1.25
9	2.14
10	3.16
11	5.45
12	9.8
13	7.4
14	7.9
15	4.9

Continuous Atomization

E.J. LeMaster; U.S. Patent 3,590,058; June 29, 1971 disclosed a method for the oxygenation of liquid hydrocarbon compounds to fatty acids by atomizing a preheated and pressurized mixture of the hydrocarbon, steam, and air to a vapor-foam, and passing such vapor-foam mixture through a catalytic bed at a temperature above atmospheric temperature but below the boiling point of the hydrocarbon.

Figure 2.1 shows partly diagrammatically a pilot plant for operation of the process. Hydrocarbons to be converted are supplied through conduit (56), and then pass through a hot water heat exchanger (81) and a steam heat exchanger (82). For oxidizing olefins, one heat exchanger, as for example (81), is sufficient. After passing through the heat exchangers, the hydrocarbons to be reacted are supplied through conduits (83) and (84) to the inner concentric tube (85a) of coaxial conduit (85) and then through atomizer (59) into the top of oxidation reaction vessel (51). The vessel (51) is provided with an upper dome (86) and a lower dome (87). It is

FIGURE 2.1: APPARATUS FOR CONTINUOUS ATOMIZATION

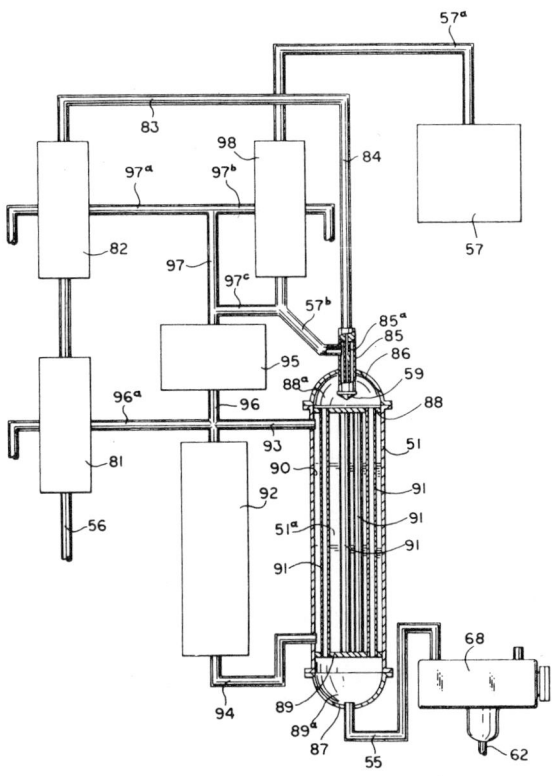

Source: E.J. LeMaster; U.S. Patent 3,590,058; June 29, 1971

supplied interiorly of the upper dome with a perforated head plate (88) and interiorly of the lower dome with a perforated head plate (89). Each of the perforations of head plate (88) corresponds with a similar perforation through head plate (89), and tubes (91) connect corresponding perforations in the two plates. The tubes (91) are all packed with granules of catalyst such as cobalt. The incoming hydrocarbon which is to be reacted, entering the reaction vessel from conduit (85), goes first through atomizer (59) and then to the space (88^a) between the upper dome and the upper plate. The space (51^a) in reaction vessel (51) surrounding the tubes (91) is a water jacket (or if desired a jacket for other heat controlling fluid) by which the temperature of the catalyst and of the reacting hydrocarbons in the tubes during reaction is maintained approximately constant at optimum temperature. The water jacket is sealed from the space (88^a), from the interior of tubes (91) and from the space (89a), because the ends of the tubes (91) are connected in sealing relationship with all the perforations in heads (88) and (89), and these heads are also sealed to the sides of the vessel (51). For the purpose of maintaining the appropriate temperature, thermostats or other temperature controls are provided. Hot water is constantly circulated from a boiler (92) through conduit (94) and conduit (93) to and from the water jacket portion (51a) of the reaction vessel. Hot water is also supplied from the boiler (92) to steam superheater (95) by means of a conduit (96) which is provided with a branch conduit (96a) supplying steam to heat exchanger (81).

Supply conduit (93) is shown extending from conduit (96). From steam superheater (95), a main steam conduit (97) supplies superheated steam and is subdivided into branch conduits (97a), (97b), and (97c). Branch conduit (97a) supplies steam to heat exchanger (82), and conduit (97b) supplies steam to heat exchanger (98) whose purpose will be later described. Conduit (97c) supplies superheated steam to the outer portion of coaxial conduit (85) and thus to space (88a). An air compressor (57) supplies the air under pressure through conduit (57a) to heat exchanger (98) where the air is heated by the superheated steam.

The heated air then passes through conduit (57b) to a Y connection with conduit (97c) and then to the outer portion of coaxial conduit (85). The heated hydrocarbons, air and steam are mixed in and as they are ejected from the atomizer (59) which could be, if desired, an external mix nozzle. The mixture, after being atomized by atomizer (59), passes into space (88a), then through the catalyst packed tubes (91), and into space (89a). The space (89a) is between the lower dome (87) and the lower plate (89). From space (89a), the reacted product passes through outlet conduit (55) to accumulator (68) where the product is drawn off and separated by any separation and purification process desired.

Example 1: Oxo aldehydes are formed as an intermediate product in the manufacture of oxo alcohols by oxonation and subsequent hydrogenation of olefins. Such intermediate products were preheated and pumped at a flow rate of 2 to 4 liters per hour at a pressure of 3 to 15 atmospheres through an atomizing nozzle with steam at a molar ratio of 2:1 to 10:1 and an air flow of 1.7 to 1.9 scfm into a reactor (reaction vessel) at a pressure of 1 to 10 atmospheres, the reaction vessel being composed of 19 3/4" tubes 42" long filled with 1.9 liters of 15% Co and 4% Mn catalysts on alumina or pumice. The reaction vessel was substantially identical with that shown in Figure 2.1. In such reaction vessel, the tubes are enclosed in an overall outer shell, the shell being filled with hot water or hot water and steam to allow reactor heat regulation between the optimum temperatures of 110° to 180°C. The reaction resulted in an average weight percent conversion of 30% across the reactor to iso-octyl and decyl alcohols and acids. A total conversion of over 70% to alcohols and acids was achieved by recycle of the unreacted product.

Example 2: This involves oxidizing olefins with various isomers of different configuration and branching and with a carbon atom content of 7 to 20 with the apparatus used in Example 1 to dihydroxy alcohols with simultaneous oxidation and chain cleavage to yield monocarboxylic acids with a carbon atom content of 2 to 19.

This process was also more advantageously used by the oxidation reaction taking place in two stages. Mixed nonenes, being used as an example, are preheated and pumped at a pressure of 3 to 15 atmospheres at a flow rate of 1 to 3 liters per hour through the atomizing nozzle with steam at a molar ratio of 2:1 to 4:1 and an air flow of 1.7 to 1.9 scfm into the reactor at a pressure of 1 to 10 atmospheres and a reaction temperature of 120° to 200°C., resulting in a first stage effluent averaging 15 to 20 weight percent conversion to dihydroxy alcohols by using in such first stage the higher pressure, steam ratio and liquid flow rate with the lower temperature.

The dihydroxy alcohols were separated from the first stage effluent and pumped to the second stage reactor where the lower pressure, steam ratio and liquid flow rate were used with higher reaction temperature, resulting in over 80% total conversion to C_2 through C_8 monocarboxylic acids, provided unreacted effluent from each oxidation stage be recycled.

OZONOLYSIS OF OLEFINS

Formic Acid Solvent

P.S. Bailey; U.S. Patent 3,238,250; March 1, 1966; assigned to Esso Research and Engineering Company prepares fatty acids by ozonolysis of an olefin in solution in a reactive ozonolysis solvent at a temperature within the range of about 30° to -100°C. to form a peroxidic ozonolysis intercondensation product of the olefin with ozone and the solvent, followed by oxidation of the peroxidic intercondensation product in a formic acid-containing solution with molecular oxygen in the presence of catalytic amounts of ozone, whereby the desired carboxylic acid is substantially selectively provided.

Ozonolysis of an olefin of the type containing at least one hydrogen atom on the carbon atoms linked by the olefin double bond in solution in a reactive solvent will result in the formation of a peroxidic intercondensation product involving the reaction of 1 mol equivalent of ozone and from 1 to 3 mol equivalents of solvent with each olefinic bond in the molecule. Conversion of the peroxidic intercondensation product to a carboxylic acid product presents a serious problem when it is desired to conduct the conversion by oxidation with molecular oxygen. Thus, the peroxidic intercondensation product will contain functional groups other than peroxide groups such as aldehyde groups or hydroxyl groups. As a consequence, there is a tendency for such additional functional groups to become involved in side reactions which lead to the formation of intractable oxidation products contaminated with by-products other than carboxylic acids. Moreover, such by-products are generally separated from the desired carboxylic acid product only with difficulty.

Molecular oxygen may be successfully used with a substantially selective conversion of the peroxidic intercondensation product to carboxylic acids by conducting the oxidation in a particular manner. Thus, in accordance with the process the peroxidic intercondensation product is dissolved in a solvent consisting of formic acid or a mixture of formic acid with acetic acid, such solvent containing at least 2 mol equivalents of formic acid per mol equivalent of peroxide group in the peroxidic intercondensation product. Thereafter, molecular oxygen which contains a catalytic amount of ozone is passed through the solution at a temperature from about 20°C. to about reflux temperatures preferably intermediate about 50°C. and reflux temperature until substantially all of the peroxide groups have disappeared.

Temperatures may range from about 20° to 70°C. with particular peroxidic intercondensation products. As a consequence, the peroxidic intercondensation product is substantially selectively converted to a desired carboxylic acid product. If formic acid is not utilized as a solvent or if catalytic amounts of ozone are not present during the oxidation, the desired selectivity is not obtained.

The starting olefinic material for the process may be defined as an olefin containing at least one hydrogen atom attached to the carbon atoms linked by the olefinic double bond. Representative olefins of this nature include straight chain and branched chain mono-olefins and polyolefins, monocyclic and polycyclic mono-olefins and polyolefins. In general, the feed materials should be an olefin which is at least partially soluble in the solvent under reaction conditions, such as an at least partially soluble olefin containing 4 to 20 carbon atoms in the molecule. Representative open chain olefins that may be utilized include materials such as butene-1, 1,5-hexadiene, pentene-1, straight and branched chain heptenes, etc.

The term "reactive solvent" may be defined in its accepted sense as a solvent containing a C_1 to C_4 alkyl alcohol, formic acid, acetic acid, a mixture thereof, or a mixture of one or more such reactive solvents with a cosolvent such as acetone, chloroform, carbon tetrachloride, etc., which is substantially completely unreactive with the zwitterion formed by reaction of the ozone with the olefin under the ozonolysis conditions employed.

However, such mixture should contain at least 2 mol equivalents of reactive solvent per mol equivalent of olefin. The ozonolysis reaction is preferably conducted at temperatures within the range of about 100° to 30°C. by passing a mixture of oxygen with ozone through a solution of the olefin in an excess, e.g., 2 to 20 mols, of the reactive solvent. For example, the mixture of oxygen with ozone may contain from about 2 to 6 weight percent of ozone and the oxygen-ozone mixture may be passed through the solution at a rate within the range of about 0.01 to 0.5 cubic foot of gaseous mixture per liter of solution per minute. The ozonolysis reaction should, of course, be conducted above the freezing point of the solvent employed.

Example 1: Dissolve about 4.1 g. (about 0.05 mol) of cyclohexene in about 50 ml. of anhydrous methanol and cool the resultant solution to a temperature of about -70°C. Pass dried oxygen through an ozonator under conditions to form a gaseous mixture of ozone and oxygen containing about 2 to 6% by weight of ozone and pass the resultant mixture through the methanol solution at the rate of about 20 liters of gas per hour. Continue the passage of the ozone-oxygen mixture until about 1 mol of ozone per mol of cyclohexene has been absorbed. This may readily be determined by testing the tail gas from the reaction zone. When the tail gas gives a strong test for the presence of ozone, the reaction is substantially complete.

After about 1 mol of ozone per mol of cyclohexene has been absorbed, evaporate the methanol from the reaction product at room temperature at a pressure of about 0.5 ml. A clear viscous syrup is obtained with substantially quantitative yield. The syrup consists essentially of a mixture of a monomeric ω-aldehydemethoxyhydroperoxide, the acetal of the substance and hemiperacetal and peracetal trimers and tetramers of these substances.

The structure of the products has been verified by infrared analysis, the infrared analysis showing the presence of carbonyl groups and hydroxy groups. The product releases oxygen when treated with lead tetra-acetate, thus definitely establishing the presence of hydroperoxides. Analysis of the product showed about 50.7% of carbon, about 9.15 weight percent of hydrogen, and about 26.30 weight percent methoxy. The predominant products, when the methanol is removed from the reaction product as soon as possible after ozonolysis, are the hemiperacetal polymers. This reaction product is mildly reactive with methanol as is shown by a change in product composition, favoring the formation of the peracetal polymers when the methanol solution of reaction product is permitted to stand.

Example 2: In order to prepare adipic acid, dissolve the reaction product of Example 1 in about 55 ml. of 80% formic acid (the remainder being water) at room temperature, pass a mixture of about 0.9 weight percent of ozone in oxygen through the formic acid solution at the rate of about 20 liters per hour, allowing the temperature to rise quickly to a temperature of about 35°C. and then cautiously raise the temperature to about 70°C. over a period of about 1.5 hours.

Spontaneous reaction of the aldehyde groups with oxygen occurs during this period. About 0.15 mol of ozone per mol of methoxy hydroperoxide is absorbed during this period. Next pass a charge stream consisting of oxygen and a trace amount of ozone through the solution while raising the temperature of the solution to reflux temperature over about a 15 minute period and maintain the refluxing solution at this temperature for about 30 minutes. Cool the resultant product to about 0°C. in an ice water bath to precipitate the adipic acid reaction product and recover the adipic acid by filtration. Additional adipic acid may be recovered by evaporating the filtrate and recrystallizing the residue from a minimal amount of water. The product is substantially pure adipic acid (MP 143° to 148°C.), the yield of adipic acid based on the cyclohexene starting material being about 73%.

Alkoxyalkanol Solvent

L.C. Mitchell; U.S. Patent 3,362,971; January 9, 1968; assigned to Ethyl Corporation describes a process for preparing carboxylic acids (and ketones) from olefins by (1) ozonizing the olefins in an alkoxyalkanol, and then (2) oxidizing the ozonized olefin with an oxygen-containing gas in the same alkoxyalkanol solvent. The addition of an aqueous acid organic or mineral in step (2) improves the yield of product obtained. Noncyclic olefins having from 6 to 30 carbon atoms are suitable reactants. A preferred alkoxyalkanol is 2-methoxy ethanol; sulfuric acid is a preferred mineral acid. The process can be carried out as both a batch and continuous process. In the following examples, all parts are parts by weight unless otherwise noted.

Example 1: Into a reaction vessel equipped with efficient cooling means is charged 13.46 parts of 1-dodecene and 65 parts of methoxyethanol. An ozone-oxygen stream, 0.935 millimol ozone per liter, is bubbled into the resultant mixture until a 25% excess of ozone is admitted. During the bubbling the temperature of the reaction vessel is maintained within the range of -20° to -30°C. After the ozone contacting has been completed, the resultant mixture is warmed to room temperature. The reaction product is admixed with 40 parts of water and 1.86 parts of concentrated sulfuric acid. The resultant mixture is then heated to reflux and oxygen bubbled through the heated mixture for 5 1/4 hours. The oxygen is bubbled through at a rate of 80 cc per minute. The resultant mixture is cooled to ambient temperature.

The reaction mixture is extracted three times with petroleum ether. The petroleum ether portions used are successively, 70, 52.5 and 35 parts. After extraction, the combined organic layers are washed with water. The water layer is separated and the resultant organic fraction dried over anhydrous sodium sulfate. After drying, the organic material is separated by filtration. The filtrate is distilled at ambient temperature and aspirator pressure to yield a residue of crude undecanoic acid. The crude product is further purified by fractional distillation.

When the above procedure is repeated except that the reaction mixture obtained from the ozonization step is not admixed with sulfuric acid and water prior to carying out the reaction with oxygen, the yield of product is slightly reduced. Similar results are obtained when the ozone stream contains 5.0 or 20.0 millimols of ozone per liter. High yields of undecanoic acid are obtained when the procedure of the above example is followed except that the ozone is admixed with carbon dioxide, nitrogen or air.

Example 2: The process of Example 1 is repeated except that ethoxyethanol (ethylene glycol monoethyl ether) is employed instead of methoxyethanol. Similar results are obtained. Similar results are also obtained when ethylene glycol monopropyl ether is employed.

Example 3: The procedure of Example 1 is followed except that 3.72 parts of concentrated sulfuric acid is added to the ozonization product prior to contacting the product with gaseous oxygen. Similarly, high yields of undecanoic acid are obtained when 0.5 or 5.0 parts of concentrated sulfuric acid is added to the ozonization product prior to the secondary oxidation reaction. Similar results are obtained when the reaction of oxygen with the ozonization product is carried out at a temperature of 150°C.

Example 4: The process of Example 1 is repeated except that the ozonization reaction is carried out at a temperature of -80°C. and 5.0 parts of orthophosphoric acid is employed in place of the sulfuric acid in the second oxidation step. Similar results are obtained with hydrochloric acid, metaphosphoric acid, pyrophosphoric acid, and triphosphoric acid are employed. Similar results are obtained when the above acids are employed in a concentration range of from 0.001 to 5.0 mols per mol of starting olefin.

Example 5: The procedure of Example 4 is followed except that the ozonization step is carried out at a temperature of 10°C. Similar results are obtained if a stoichiometric amount of ozone is employed in the reaction.

Example 6: The procedure of Example 2 is followed except that trichloroacetic acid is added prior to oxidizing the ozonization product. Similar results are obtained when n-butyric acid, isobutyric acid, n-valeric acid, and isovaleric acid are employed. Similarly, mixtures of acetic and sulfuric or orthophosphoric acid yield good results.

Example 7: The procedure of Example 6 is followed except that the second step, the reaction of the ozonization product with oxygen, is carried out at a temperature of 50°C. Similar results are obtained when the reaction is carried out at a temperature of 180°C.

Example 8: Decene-1 is reacted according to the procedure of Example 1 except that the second reaction mixture comprises, in addition to the methoxymethanol, a mixture of 10 parts of water, 70 parts of glacial acetic acid, and 1.68 parts of sulfuric acid. Pelargonic acid is obtained. The reaction is repeated except that the second reaction medium contains 5 parts of water, 80 parts of glacial acetic acid and 3 parts of sulfuric acid. Similar results are obtained when 90 parts of water, 10 parts of glacial acetic acid and 6 parts of sulfuric acid are present in the second reaction medium. Similar results are obtained when octadecene-1 is employed to yield heptadecanoic acid.

Example 9: A mixture of olefins, 26.92 parts, consisting of 65 weight percent dodecene-1, 25 weight percent tetradecene-1 and 10 weight percent hexadecene-1 is oxidized according to the procedure of Example 1. The product consists of approximately 65/25/10 weight percent mixture of undecanoic acid, tridecanoic acid and pentadecanoic acid. Similar results are obtained when 1,6-hexylene glycol monomethyl ether is employed in place of the methoxyethanol.

Example 10: A 26.92 part portion of an olefinic mixture consisting of 73.4 mol percent dodecene-2, 9.9 mol percent dodecene-3, 5.4 mol percent dodecene-4, 5.6 mol percent dodecene-1, and 5.7 mol percent dodecane is oxidized according to the procedure of Example 4. The product consists of a mixture of the corresponding carboxylic acids derived by a cleavage of the double bond within the olefinic starting materials. A similar product is obtained when the procedure is carried out using an olefinic mixture having the following composition: 6.9 mol percent dodecene-1, 75.2 mol percent dodecene-2, 4.8 mol percent dodecene-3, 6.0 mol percent of a mixture of dodecene-4 and dodecene-5, and 7.1 mol percent dodecane. Similar results are obtained when 1,4-butylene glycol monopropyl ether is employed.

Phosphoric Acid Promoting Agent

H. Mihara, I. Miwa, K. Ueno and S. Morita; U.S. Patent 3,060,211; October 23, 1962; assigned to Toyo Koatsu Industries, Incorporated, Japan provide for the production of saturated aliphatic acids such as azelaic acid, pelargonic acid and caproic acid from unsaturated fatty acid materials such as rice bran oil fatty acid, tall oil fatty acid and commercial grade oleic acid, by the process of treating the unsaturated fatty acid with ozone and decomposing and oxidizing the resulting ozonide. A radical increase in the yield is achieved by conducting the process and particularly the decomposition step in the presence of a reaction promoting agent.

The reaction promoting agents which may be advantageously employed are the phosphoric acids such as orthophosphoric acid, pyrophosphoric acid, metaphosphoric acid, phosphorus acid, polyphosphoric acid and phosphoric anhydride and derivatives thereof such as the organic esters trioctyl phosphate, ethylmetaphosphate, butyl pyrophosphate, tricresyl phosphate, etc. The reaction promoting agent may be individually employed or a mixture of two or more may be employed and may be added to the unsaturated fatty acid prior to ozonization thereof or to the ozonide prior to decomposition thereof. The amount of promoting agent should be between 0.01 and 10% by weight of the unsaturated fatty acids.

The following example is given as illustration of the process. The fatty acid materials being treated in the example have the following analysis:

(a) Rice bran oil fatty acid:	Percent	
Oleic acid	40.2	
Linoleic acid	29.8	
Palmitic acid	17.5	
Undecomposed oil	4.2	
Wax	7.2	
Moisture and others	1.1	
(b) Tall oil fatty acid:	Percent	
Oleic acid	52.9	(continued)

	Percent
Linoleic acid	44.1
Saturated fatty acid	1.0
Rosin acid	1.0
Unsaponifiable matters	1.0

Example 1: 50 grams of rice bran oil fatty acid, 250 grams of glacial acetic acid and 0.5 gram of orthophosphoric acid of 89% purity are placed in a chamber and maintained at a temperature of 20°C. A 2% ozone concentration oxygen is fed into the bottom of the chamber at the rate of 2 liters per minute until no more ozone is absorbed as evidenced by the ozone content of the outlet gas. The amount of ozone required was 1.3 times the quantity calculated from the iodine number of the treated material. The reacted materials are heated to 100°C. for one hour to completely decompose the resulting ozonides after which 0.01 gram of manganese acetate, an oxidation catalyst, is added and oxygen fed therethrough at the rate of 1 liter per minute for three hours while maintaining the temperature at 100°C. to completely oxidize the decomposition products, mainly aldehydes.

The resulting oxidized product is then distilled at normal pressure to remove the solvent, acetic acid, and is then subjected to vacuum distillation. There were produced 5.0 grams of caproic acid having a boiling point of 105° to 110°C. at 15 mm. Hg and a neutralization number of 487 and 8.9 grams of pelargonic acid having a boiling point of 142° to 147°C. at 15 mm. Hg and a neutralization number of 353, leaving a distillation residue of 40 grams having a neutralization number of 385. The distillation residue is extracted four times with five times its weight of hot water and the extract treated with activated carbon in the hot state and filtered. The filtrate is concentrated by evaporation and upon cooling produced 19.1 grams of crystal azelaic acid in the form of white flakes having a neutralization number of 595 and a MP of 104° to 105°C.

By contrast, when the above procedure and conditions were closely followed with the exception that the promoting agent, orthophosphoric acid, was omitted, there were produced from 50 grams of rice bran oil fatty acid, 4.3 grams of caproic acid having a boiling point of 105° to 110°C., at 15 mm. Hg and a neutralization number of 487, 7.7 grams of pelargonic acid having a boiling point of 142° to 147°C. at 15 mm. Hg and a neutralization number of 353 and 45 grams of distillation residue with a neutralization number of 355 from which no more than 16.1 grams of azelaic acid were obtained. It is obvious from the above that the use of the promoting agent in the process greatly increases the yield of the saturated aliphatic acids.

Pyridine Solvent

In a process by D.W. Peck and L.W. Newton; U.S. Patent 3,383,398; May 14, 1968; assigned to Union Carbide Corporation, the reaction of an olefinically unsaturated compound containing a vinylene group (—CH=CH—) with ozone, when conducted in the presence of pyridine or an alkyl derivative thereof as a solvent, results in the conversion of each carbon atom of the vinylene group to a carboxyl group. Thus, cyclododecene, when reacted with ozone in the presence of pyridine, is converted directly to 1,12-dodecanedioic acid.

The pyridines which are employed in the process are pyridines and its alkyl-substituted derivatives of up to about 10 carbon atoms. These monocyclic pyridines can be considered as consisting of one nitrogen atom, from 5 to 10 carbon atoms and sufficient hydrogen to provide a compound having no unsaturation except in the heterocyclic pyridine ring thereof.

Although the process is applicable to all reactions in which an olefin can be reacted with ozone to convert both of the carbon atoms of the vinylene group to carboxyl group, it is especially applicable to monoolefinically-unsaturated aliphatic and cycloaliphatic compounds having no unsaturation other than one vinylene group and containing up to about 20 carbon atoms. Suitable olefins in this group include aliphatic monoolefins such as ethylene, butene, hexene, and the like; alicyclic monoolefins such as cyclopentene, cyclohexene, cyclooctene, cyclododecene, and the like; and monoolefinically unsaturated aliphatic monocarboxylic acids and their lower alkyl esters such as oleic acid, methyl oleate, linoleic acid, methyl linoleate, and the like.

Example 1: A mixture of a crude oleic acid ozonide produced by the ozonolysis of oleic acid and pyridine was charged to a test tube and the test tube was immersed in a constant temperature bath maintained at 50°C. The resulting mixture was titrated for ozonide periodically and, after about 1 hour, the ozonide was essentially completely decomposed. Similar results were obtained when methyl ethyl pyridine was substituted for pyridine. When the ozonide alone was charged to the test tube no decomposition was observed even after 4 hours.

Example 2: A stream of oxygen containing about 4% ozone was passed through a charge containing 100 grams of oleic acid, 200 grams of pyridine and 30 grams of water, which was heated at 50°C. Several duplicate runs were conducted, but were terminated at different levels of ozone input to the reaction mixture. The product acids were recovered by stripping the reaction product under reduced pressure to remove pyridine and water followed by a vacuum distillation to recover pelargonic acid. The distillation residue was extracted with hot water and azelaic acid was recovered on evaporation of the water from the aqueous extract. The results of these runs are summarized in Table 1.

TABLE 1

Run No.	Ozone Charged, percent of Theoretical	Yields, percent	
		Azelaic Acid	Pelargonic Acid
1	73	49	42
2	109	64	55
3	139	71	59
4	141	68	68
5	151	67	73
6	176	67	64

As can be seen from the data presented above, optimum yields of azelaic and pelargonic acids are obtained when about 40 to 50% excess ozone is employed, based on the theoretical amount necessary to convert all of the oleic acid charged to its ozonide. Maximum yields of the product acids are obtained at this level, and yields are not significantly increased with additional ozone.

Example 3: A stream of 3.5% ozone in oxygen was passed through a mixture of 45 grams (0.2 mol) of 1-hexadecene, 100 grams of pyridine and 15 grams of water at 28° to 31°C. until 14 grams (0.29 mol) of ozone had been added. After flash evaporation of the reaction product to remove pyridine and water and then washing the residue with aqueous hydrochloric acid, there were recovered 46 grams (0.19 mol) of pentadecanoic acid, MP 45° to 47°C., for a yield of 95%. After recrystallization from pentane the melting point of the product acid was 50.5° to 51.5°C., as compared with the literature value of 51° to 53°C.

Example 4: A stream of 3.5% ozone in oxygen was passed through a mixture of 18 grams of cyclohexene, 100 grams of pyridine and 15 grams of water at 28° to 31°C. until 14 grams of ozone had been added. After flash evaporation and washing the residue with 100 ml. of benzene and then two 100 ml. portions of pentene, there were recovered 18 grams of adipic acid, MP 137° to 150°C. On recrystallization from aqueous nitric acid the melting point of the adipic acid was 151° to 152°C. compared with the literature value of 151° to 153°C.

Example 5: A stream of 3.5% ozone in oxygen was passed through a solution of 22 grams of cyclooctene, 120 grams of pyridine, and 15 grams of water at 42° to 56°C. until 14 grams of ozone had been added. After flash evaporation and slurrying the residue first in pentane, then in water, there were recovered 19 grams of suberic acid melting at 139.5° to 140.5°C. as compared with the literature value of 140°C.

Example 6: A stream of 1.3% ozone in air was passed through a solution of 100 grams of 86% cyclododecene (0.52 mol) in cyclododecane, 200 g.

of pyridine, and 30 grams of water at 27° to 37°C. until a total of 37 grams (0.77 mol) of ozone had been added. After flash evaporation at 20 mm. pressure to remove pyridine and water, recrystallization of the residue from benzene and a pentane wash, there were recovered 67 grams of crude 1,12-dodecanedioic acid. After water washing, there were obtained 59 grams of the diacid, MP 125° to 126°C. Recrystallization of a small sample increased the melting point to 127° to 128°C.

The mother liquor from the recrystallization from the benzene was evaporated to dryness and the solids, after washing with pentane, were found to be 48 grams of crude diacid. After water washing twice, there were obtained 43 grams of diacid, MP 123° to 125°C.

Example 7: A stream of 3.5% ozone in oxygen was passed through a solution of 33 grams of 85% cyclododecene in cyclododecane (0.17 mol cyclododecene), 67 grams of pyridine and 10 grams of water at 28° to 31°C. until 14 grams (0.29 mol) of ozone was added. The reaction product, which weighed 122 grams, was flash evaporated to remove 48 grams of pyridine and water. The residue was slurried in pentane and then water to provide 31 grams of 1,12-dodecanedioic acid melting at 124° to 126°C., representing a yield of 80%. Employing similar techniques, several additional runs were conducted employing different reaction conditions. The data for these runs are summarized in Table 2, with the data for the above-described run being included as Run No. 1.

TABLE 2

Run No.	Reaction Conditions					Product	
	Charge, gm.			Ozone Cyclododecene Mole Ratio	Temp., °C.	Yield, percent	Melting Point, °C.
	Cyclododecene	Pyridine	Water				
1	33	67	10	1.7	28-31	80	124-6
2	33	[1] 67	10	1.7	28-59	85 / [2] 70	119-22 / 126-7
3	33	54	23	1.7	27-35	91	126.5-7.5
4	51	100	100	1.7	28-36	87	121-3
5	33	77	0	1.7	26-37	74 / [2] 59	115-9 / 122-3.5
6	33	67	10	1.7	45-55	88	125.5-126
7	33	67	10	2.4	26-9	87	124.5-125
8	[3] 33	67	10	1.7	22-54	96	126-6.5
9	33	67	10	1.7	28-29	[4] 62	129-30

[1] 2-methyl-5-ethylpyridine substituted for pyridine.
[2] After recrystallization from benzene.
[3] 97% pure cyclododecene.
[4] The residue from the flash distillation was slurried first in 74 ml. of benzene and then in two 50-ml. portions of pentane.

A comparison of Runs 1 and 2 illustrates the superiority of pyridine over alkyl-substituted pyridines, such as 2-methyl-5-ethylpyridine, in providing good yields of high purity diacid, and Runs 1 and 3-5, when compared, show the necessity of maintaining water in the solvent system to obtain high yields of high purity acid. A comparison of Runs 1 and 6 discloses that a slight improvement in yield is obtained at slightly higher temperatures, and Run 7, when compared with Run 1, illustrates that a slight improvement in yield of acid is obtained when the molar ratio of ozone to cyclododecene is increased from about 1.7 to 2.4. Run 8, when compared with Run 1, shows that a purer feedstock results in improved yields of acid, and Run 9, when compared with Run 1, indicates that the use of benzene to purify the crude ozonolysis residue results in a considerable loss of acid.

Lower Alkanol Reaction Medium

M. Dubeck and L.C. Mitchell; U.S. Patent 3,414,594; Dec. 3, 1968; assigned to Ethyl Corporation describe a process for preparing carboxylic acids and ketones by (a) ozonizing olefins in a lower alkanol reaction medium; (b) then oxidizing the ozonized olefin in the presence of an aqueous mineral acid, using an oxygen-containing gas. Nonvinylidene olefins yield carboxylic acids; vinylidene olefins yield ketones. Air or oxygen are preferred as oxidizing agents in step (b). An example of a suitable mineral acid is sulfuric acid. The acids or ketones produced have at least one carbon atom less than the starting olefin. The process is described as a batch process and a continuous process.

The first step of this process comprises reacting one or more olefins with ozone. It is preferred that the ozone be in the gaseous state and more preferably admixed in a minor amount with an inert carrier gas. Carrier gases which may be employed are the inert gases such as argon and neon, and the like, and most preferably nitrogen, oxygen, air, carbon dioxide and mixtures thereof.

In a preferred embodiment, the carrier gas contains at least 20% by weight oxygen and more preferably is substantially pure oxygen. In other words, in this more preferred embodiment the ozone reactant is an ozone-oxygen gaseous stream. The concentration of the ozone in the carrier gas is not critical and may range from about 0.001 to 30% by weight. Most preferably the concentration is within the range of about 0.001 to 20% by weight. In a highly preferred embodiment the ozone concentration is from 0.01 to 10% by weight.

The first step of this process can be carried out by contacting a molar equivalent ratio of olefin and ozone; however, it is not necessary to do so. Thus, good results are obtained if a slight excess of olefin is employed; for example, from about 1.20 mols of olefin per each mol of ozone. However, in many instances, higher yields are obtained when an excess of ozone is used. In general, it is preferred that from 1 to 2 mols of ozone be employed per each mol of olefin. Greater excesses of ozone, such as 3 mols per mol of olefin, can be employed if desired. However, in many instances, significant advantages are not obtained with these higher mol ratios. The first step of this process can be conducted at atmospheric, superatmospheric, or subatmospheric pressures. The exact atmosphere employed is not critical, and in most cases the reaction is effectively carried out at substantially atmospheric pressure.

The reaction of ozone with an olefin in this process is carried out at a temperature within the range of from about -100° to 50°C. More preferably, the reaction temperature is within the range of -70° to 35°C. The most preferred reaction temperatures are within the range of about -10° to 35°C. In most instances, heat is evolved during the reaction of ozone with the olefin; hence, efficient cooling means are usually desired.

In this process, the reaction of ozone with an olefin is conducted in the presence of a lower alkanol as a reaction medium. Preferred alkanols have from 1 to 3 carbon atoms and no olefinic unsaturation. These preferred lower alkanols are methanol, ethanol, n-propanol, and isopropanol. Methanol and ethanol are preferred and methanol highly preferred. A small amount of water in the lower alkanol can be tolerated. In general, the amount of water should be less than about 3% by weight. Sufficient lower alkanol should be employed to produce a readily fluid reaction mixture. Generally, a weight of alkanol amounting to at least the weight of olefin reactant is required, and in most cases, at least twice this amount is desirable. Up to 20 or more times the weight of the olefin reactant can be employed if desired.

The time of reaction between ozone and an olefin is not a truly independent variable but depends at least to some extent on the other reaction conditions employed such as the concentration of ozone. For example, efficient agitation of the reaction mixture usually results in a lessening of reaction time. On the other hand, inefficient contacting of the reactants usually lengthens the reaction time. In most instances, the reaction is complete after a reaction time within the range of from about 15 minutes to 35 hours.

After the ozonization of the olefin is completed, a catalytic quantity of a mineral acid is added to the resultant reaction mixture. Typical mineral acid catalysts which can be employed include hydrochloric acid, sulfuric acid, metaphosphoric acid, triphosphoric acid, orthophosphoric acid, pyrophosphoric acid, and the like. In general, an amount of mineral acid between about 0.0001 and 15 mols per each mol of starting olefin is employed. A preferred acid concentration is from 0.001 to 1.0 mol and a most preferred range from 0.001 to 0.3 mol per mol of olefin.

Water can be added with the mineral acid. In general, from 0.01 to 10 mols of water per mol of starting olefin is added, most preferably from 0.1 to 5.0 mols. The second chemical reaction in this process comprises the oxidation of the products of the ozonization reaction (admixed with the mineral acid, and optionally, water as described above) with an oxygen-containing gas. The oxygen-containing gas may be pure oxygen or air or oxygen admixed with an inert carrier gas. Carrier gases which may be employed are the inert gases such as argon, neon, and the like; nitrogen, carbon dioxide, steam, and mixtures thereof. In a preferred embodiment, the carrier gas contains at least 20% by weight oxygen. Highly preferred oxygen-containing gases are pure oxygen and air.

It is preferred that the amount of oxygen employed be sufficient to oxidize all of the ozonization residue to the corresponding carboxylic acids. In general, at least a stoichiometric equivalent of oxygen is employed. A slight excess of oxygen frequently increases the yield. Most preferably, the amount of oxygen employed is within the range of from about 1.0 to 2.5 mols. In general, it is desired that a much larger excess of oxygen be bubbled through the reaction mixture, about 50 to 100 or more mols of oxygen per mol of starting olefin to insure the completeness of the oxidation. The oxidation step can be carried out in the presence of metal salts if desired.

The oxidation of the ozonization residues is carried out at a temperature which affords a reasonable rate of reaction and a minimum of by-product formation. In general, suitable reaction temperatures are within the range of about 30° to 180°C. More preferably, the reaction temperature is within the range of about 40° to 175°C., and most preferably between 50° to 150°C.

The oxidation step is conveniently carried out by bubbling oxygen through the liquid reaction mixture. In many instances, the bubbling action causes sufficient agitation to insure sufficient contact of the reactants. If desired, other agitation means such as stirring and rocking can be employed. The time of reaction is not a truly independent variable, but is dependent at least in part on the other reaction conditions employed. In most instances the reaction is substantially complete in about one-half to 60 hours. In the following examples, all parts are parts by weight unless otherwise noted.

Example 1: Into a reaction vessel equipped with efficient cooling means, gas inlet means, and a reflux condenser was charged 3.36 parts of 1-dodecene and 126 parts of methanol. Thereafter, an ozone-oxygen stream, 1.07 millimols per liter, was bubbled into the resultant mixture until a slight excess of ozone had been admitted. During the bubbling the reaction temperature was maintained between -20° and -30°C. After the ozone-contacting had been completed the resultant reaction mixture was warmed to room temperature and divided into two equal portions. One portion was added to a reaction vessel equipped with gas inlet means, cooling means, and a refluxing condenser. The mixture was refluxed and stirred and oxygen bubbled in at the rate of 80 cc per minute. The oxygen addition, at reflux, was allowed to continue overnight. A sample of the resultant reaction mixture was taken and analyzed for active oxygen. The analysis indicated that no substantial reduction to active oxygen had taken place and an appreciable amount of undecanoic acid had not been formed.

When the reaction is repeated except that 100 parts of water and between 0.0001 and 15 mols per each mol of starting olefin of sulfuric acid is added to the ozonization product, an appreciable yield of undecanoic acid is produced demonstrating the catalytic action of sulfuric acid in the second oxidation step.

Example 2: Into a reaction vessel equipped as in Example 1 was charged 13.46 g. of dodecene-1 and 64 parts of methanol. Thereafter, ozone was reacted with the resultant mixture as in Example 1. After the ozonization had been completed, 10 parts of water and 1.86 parts of sulfuric acid was added to the reaction mixture. The acidified mixture was then contacted with oxygen while maintaining the mixture at reflux. The reaction with ozone was carried out by bubbling in oxygen at the rate of 80 cc per minute for a period of 18 hours.

After the reaction with oxygen, 200 parts of water was added and the resultant reaction mixture was extracted three times with petroleum ether. The petroleum ether portions used were successively 70, 52.5 and 35 parts. After extraction, the combined organic layers were dried over anhydrous sodium sulfate. After drying, the organic material was separated by filtration. The filtrate was distilled at room temperature and 20 mm. pressure to yield a residue of crude undecanoic acid. Vapor phase chromatographic analysis of the crude product indicated that it contained 79% undecanoic acid and the yield was 67%. When the reaction is repeated, except that no sulfuric acid is added to the reaction mixture, the yield of product is substantially reduced.

Example 3: The process of Example 1 is repeated except that ethanol is employed instead of methanol. Similar results are obtained. Similar results are also obtained when n-propanol and isopropanol are employed.

Example 4: The procedure of Example 1 is followed except that 3.72 parts of sulfuric acid is added prior to the oxidation with gaseous oxygen. Similar results are obtained when 0.5 and 5.0 parts of sulfuric acid are employed in the procedure of Example 1.

Example 5: The process of Example 1 is repeated except that the ozonization reaction is carried out at a temperature of -80°C. and 5.0 parts of orthophosphoric acid is employed in place of the sulfuric acid in the second oxidation step. Similar results are obtained when hydrochloric acid, metaphosphoric acid, pyrophosphoric acid, and triphosphoric acid are employed. Similar results are obtained when the above acids are employed in a concentration range of 0.001 to 5.0 mols per mol of starting olefin.

Example 6: The procedure of Example 5 is followed except that the ozonization step is carried out at a temperature of 10°C. Similar results are obtained if a stoichiometric amount of ozone is employed in the reaction.

Example 7: The procedure of Example 4 is followed except that the second step, the reaction of the ozonization product with oxygen, is carried out at a temperature of 50°C. Similar results are obtained when the reaction is carried out at a temperature of 150°C.

USE OF OXIDIZING AGENTS

Metal Salt of Oxyhalide Acid

K.A. Keblys and M. Dubeck; U.S. Patent 3,409,649; Nov. 5, 1968; assigned to Ethyl Corporation provide a process for catalytic oxidation of an olefin which comprises cleaving the olefin at the carbon-to-carbon double bond using a catalyst system consisting essentially of (1) ruthenium or a ruthenium compound, (2) alkali or alkaline earth metal salt of an oxyhalide acid, and (3) an alkali, the process being carried out in a basic aqueous medium. Olefins having up to 100 carbon atoms are useful. Sodium or calcium hypochlorite are examples of suitable salts while sodium hydroxide and calcium hydroxide are examples of useful alkalis. The products obtained in this process are carboxylic acids, ketones and keto acids.

The ruthenium-containing material can be a ruthenium metal or organic and inorganic ruthenium compounds. Of the ruthenium-containing materials, ruthenium metal, ruthenium trichloride, and ruthenium dioxide are the most highly preferred.

An important and necessary part of the catalytic system of this process is an oxidizing agent which is a metal salt of an oxyhalide acid, the metal being selected from the group consisting of the alkali metals and the alkaline earth metals. Although any oxyhalide acid may be employed, hypohalous acids and halous acids are preferred. For economic reasons, the most preferred metals to be used in conjunction with oxyhalide acids are sodium and calcium. Thus, the most preferred metal salts of oxyhalide acids are sodium hypochlorite, sodium chlorite, calcium hypochlorite, and calcium chloride. Another necessary component of the catalytic system is an alkali. Although any alkali such as lithium hydroxide, sodium hydroxide, potassium hydroxide, rubidium hydroxide, or cesium hydroxide may be employed, for economic reasons sodium hydroxide and calcium hydroxide are preferred.

The reaction of this process is carried out in the presence of a catalytic amount of the ruthenium-containing material which is usually up to about 20 mol percent. Amounts as low as 0.01 mol percent can be employed, but usually the preferred range is between 1 and 5 mol percent. The oxidizing agent, that is, a metal salt of an oxyhalide acid, should be used in the amount of at least 1 mol per mol of olefin. Although much larger amounts may be employed, a large excess of the oxidizing agent is undesirable because it tends to promote side reactions. The preferred amount of metal salt of an oxyhalide acid is from about 1 to 5 mols per mol of the olefin. It is important that the aqueous reaction medium in which the reaction is carried out be alkaline, and most preferably, have a pH of at least 11. A pH considerably higher than 11 is undesirable since under such conditions, the production of lower carboxylic acid is favored.

In the following examples, all parts are by weight unless otherwise indicated.

Example 1: Oxidation of 1-Hexene with Ruthenium Trichloride-Sodium Hypochlorite — To 600 parts of 1.81 molar sodium hypochlorite solution containing 18.8 parts of sodium hydroxide was added 2.12 parts of ruthenium trichloride. A flask equipped with a high-speed stirrer, a condenser, a thermometer, and an addition funnel was charged with 33.7 parts of 1-hexene. The above sodium hypochlorite-ruthenium trichloride solution was added to the reaction flask from the addition funnel in 5 to 10 part increments. The reaction mixture was stirred at high speed while the temperature was maintained at 16° to 22°C. by cooling with a water bath.

After all of the sodium hypochlorite-ruthenium trichloride solution had been added, the reaction mixture was stirred for one hour at 17° to 20°C. After the addition of 17 parts of hexene-1, the layers were separated and filtered to remove the gray solid. The glassware and the solid were washed with heptane and the washings were combined with the organic layer. The analysis of the organic layer by vapor phase chromatography showed that 51% of unreacted 1-hexene was recovered. Thus, only 49% of hexene had reacted.

The aqueous layer was treated with 20 parts of concentrated sodium sulfite solution, producing a black precipitate which was filtered off. A sodium hydroxide solution was added to the filtrate until the pH of 11 was obtained. It was then saturated with sodium chloride and extracted with four 70-part portions of ether which were discarded. The aqueous portion was acidified to a pH of 1 with hydrochloric acid, saturated with sodium chloride, and likewise extracted with four 70-part portions of ether. This ether extract was dried over magnesium sulfate and concentrated to about one-tenth of its original volume. Vapor phase chromatography showed that the product was butyric acid, 9.9% yield, and valeric acid, 26% yield. The above yields are based on reacted olefin.

Example 2: Oxidation of 1-Hexene with Ruthenium Dioxide-Sodium Hypochlorite — A flask equipped as in Example 1 was charged with 33.7 parts of 1-hexene and 1.9 parts of ruthenium dioxide. To this mixture was added, in 1 to 10 part increments, 650 parts of 1.82 molar sodium hypochlorite solution containing 19.2 parts of sodium hydroxide. The reaction was carried out at 16° to 22°C. as described in the preceding example.

At the end of the reaction, the mixture was filtered to remove the black solid and the solid was washed with heptane and water. The heptane layer was analyzed by vapor phase chromatography and indicated that 30% of unreacted hexene was recovered. The reacted mixture was treated as in Example 1. The product, containing valeric acid in 46% yields, based on reacted 1-hexene, was obtained.

Example 3: Oxidation of 1-Hexene with Ruthenium Metal-Sodium Hypochlorite — To 775 parts of 1.55 molar sodium hypochlorite solution containing 18.4 parts of sodium hydroxide (pH 11.7) was added 0.5 part of ruthenium metal. The resulting solution was cooled to -2°C. and stirred. 18 parts of 1-hexene dissolved in 17 parts of n-heptane was then added over a period of 4 hours. The ice bath was removed and the reaction mixture allowed to warm to room temperature. After 4 hours at a temperature of 20° to 30°C., the reaction mixture was filtered and the solid washed with n-heptane. The filtrate was separated into two layers, and vapor phase chromatography of the organic layer disclosed that 13% of n-hexene was recovered.

The aqueous layer was extracted with two 35-part portions of n-heptane and then with four 70-part portions of ether. Both extracts were discarded. After acidification of the aqueous layer with concentrated hydrochloric acid, the solution was saturated with sodium chloride and extracted with four 70-part portions of ether. The examination of this ether extract by vapor phase chromatography showed that C_2-C_5 acids were present in the following yields: acetic acid, 2%; butyric acid, 7.3%; propionic acid,

2.3%; and valeric acid, 51%. The yields are based on the reacted olefin.

Example 4: Oxidation of 1-Dodecene — A flask equipped as in Example 2 was charged with 44.19 parts of 1-dodecene and 2.0 parts of ruthenium trichloride. 600 parts of 1.66 molar sodium hypochlorite solution containing 17.2 parts of sodium hydroxide was added over a 7-hour period to the reaction flask from the dropping funnel. The reaction temperature was maintained at 20° to 30°C. for the first 24 hours and then increased to 30° to 40°C. for the final four hours. The reaction product was then filtered giving a black solid. The solid and the aqueous filtrate was washed with three 35-part portions of n-heptane. The washings were combined and submitted to vapor phase chromatography analysis which showed that 22.4 parts of dodecene was recovered.

The black solid was dispersed in 300 parts of ether, acidified with concentrated hydrochloric acid and filtered. The filtrate was separated into layers and the ether layer washed once with about 100 parts of water before being dried over magnesium sulfate. This solution was distilled to about one-third of its volume and then submitted to vapor phase chromatography analysis which showed that it contained 2.6 parts of dodecene, 0.7 g. C_{10} acid, and 18.1 parts of C_{11} acid. Thus, the combined recovery of 1-dodecene was 25.0 parts or 57%, and the yield of decanoic and undecanoic acids, based on consumed olefin, was 4 and 90%, respectively.

Periodic Acid or Potassium Permanganate

In a process by C.M. Starks and P.H. Washecheck; U.S. Patent 3,547,962; December 15, 1970; assigned to Continental Oil Company, tertiary amines are disclosed as excellent phase transfer agents for oxidation of olefins with oxidizing agents in a mixed aqueous phase oxidation.

In carrying out the process, it is only necessary that the reactants, e.g., olefin and oxidizing agent aqueous solution, be in the liquid state. Preferably the olefin will be in a hydrocarbon solvent. The pressure can vary over a wide range as well as can the temperature. Normally, ambient temperature will be utilized and sufficient pressure to maintain the olefin in the liquid state. In most cases, atmospheric pressure is utilized except with such low boiling olefins such as ethylene, propylene, and the like. Thus the normal temperature range will be 30° to 100°C. and only sufficient pressure utilized to maintain the system in the liquid state.

The reaction can be carried out at subambient temperatures or even under vacuum; however, as with most reactions, temperature and pressure enhance the reaction so no advantage is gained by lowering temperature or pressure. The reaction proceeds normally at ambient conditions, and thus, economically, one would not normally choose to use high temperature and pressures. The reaction is exothermic, therefore the temperature will be in excess of room temperature after the reaction is initiated.

The olefins which can be oxidized by the method of this reaction include those compounds having one or more olefinic unsaturations and can be aliphatic, cycloaliphatic, or aryl olefins. The aromatic olefins and cyclo-olefins can have alkyl substituents, and the aliphatic olefins can be normal or branched. These olefinic compounds can vary in molecular size over a wide range so long as they are liquid at reaction conditions. It should be obvious that the molecular size would not affect the oxidation. For example, the aliphatic olefins can contain 2 to 50 carbon atoms or more. Most generally, the olefins of interest will contain 4 to 30 carbon atoms.

The cyclo-olefins generally contain preferably 4 to 8 carbon atoms. The aryl olefins can be mono- or polynuclear but most generally will contain one or two rings. Here, again, the carbon atom range can be up to 50 carbon atoms or more, the lower limit being obviously 8, e.g., styrene, and most generally they will be styrene or alkyl-substituted styrene of 8 to 18 carbon atoms.

Suitable oxidizing agents are periodic acid or potassium permanganate, although other aqueous oxidizing agents can be developed for use in this process. The catalysts which are useful are the tetraoxides of osmium and ruthenium; however, the osmium or ruthenium can be added as the pure metal in finely divided state, the lower oxides or as a salt such as the halides, preferably chlorides, sulfates, acetates, adipates, nitrates, citrates, hydroxides, and the like, or the paraperiodic acid will oxidize the metal to the active tetraoxide. Obviously, it is preferable to add the metal as the tetraoxide since any paraperiodic acid utilized for oxidizing the catalyst is not available for oxidizing the olefin. As is true with most catalysts, only small quantities are employed, usually 0.05 to 2%.

A wide variety of tertiary amines can be used in this process. The compound can contain three identical alkyl or aryl groups or three dissimilar groups. The substituents can be acyclic, alicyclic, bicyclic or aryl groups or the nitrogen can be contained in one or more rings. At least one of the alkyl groups would preferably be a rather large organic moiety (8 to 30 carbon atoms) to insure greater solubility in the organic phase.

Sufficient tertiary amine is utilized to solubilize the metallic catalyst and to stabilize the oxidizing agents and will depend somewhat on the particular tertiary amine and the amount of catalyst present. Generally it is preferred to use 0.1 to 5% tertiary amine based on the olefin containing solution (olefin and solvent).

Example: Two reactions (A and B), identical in all respects except for the presence of a tertiary amine, were carried out. An aqueous solution, 500 ml., or paraperiodic acid (100.30 g., 0.44 mol) was placed in each of two 3-necked flasks equipped with magnetic stirrers, thermometers and condensers. To each flask was added solid ruthenium dioxide (0.0535 g., 0.004 mol). The black solid immediately reacted to form a yellow solution of ruthenium tetraoxide.

To flask A was added a solution of 1-octene (11.22 g., 0.1 mol) dissolved in 100 ml. of hexane. The mixture was stirred at 27°C. The temperature of the reaction mixture slowly rose to 32°C. and then declined.

To flask B was added a solution of 1-octene (11.22 g., 0.1 mol) and tri-dodecylamine (0.5 g.) dissolved in 100 ml. of hexane. The reaction mixture was stirred at 27°C. The reaction mixture exothermed to 35°C. and then slowly declined.

Aliquots of each reaction mixture were withdrawn periodically and analyzed by gas chromatography. The thermal response factors of 1-octene and heptanol were determined from standard solutions assuming the thermal response factor of heptanoic acid was 1.0. The thermal response factors for all impurities were assumed to be 1.0. The data listed in the table indicate the weight percent of the three major components versus time.

Oxidation of Olefins

Time (hours):	Reaction A (no promoter)			Reaction B (tertiary amine)		
	1-octene	Heptanal	Heptanoic acid	1-octene	Heptanal	Heptanoic acid
½	91.5	4.9	1.7	97.9	1.0	0.0
1	87.2	8.5	3.5	90.9	2.9	4.3
2	84.3	6.7	7.9	75.7	5.0	15.9
4	81.0	8.6	9.3	46.5	7.6	39.4
6	78.2	15.6	5.7	20.7	6.6	63.2
8	78.1	6.1	14.3	0.0	2.2	87.4
24	72.6	12.8	13.6	0.0	0.0	93.2

The experimental conditions described above are only representative. Tridodecylamine is only typical of many tertiary amines which would be effective. The concentrations of paraperiodic acid and ruthenium dioxide are only representative. It would be advantageous to operate at a high periodic acid concentration to insure maximum rate of reaction. However, it would be advantageous to use as low a concentration of ruthenium dioxide as feasible and which would still maintain a reasonable reaction rate since ruthenium dioxide is expensive. The solvent, hexane, is not an essential part of the process although it has been shown that ruthenium tetraoxide attacks most common solvents except paraffins and chlorinated hydrocarbons such as carbon tetrachloride and chloroform. Only one temperature (25° to 30°C.) was examined. The process is operable in other ranges and would proceed more rapidly at higher temperatures. Although 1-octene was used in the example, the process would not be limited to only 1-olefins. Internal olefins could also be oxidized by this method. It is to be noted that in this experiment the tertiary amine acts as a promoter of the reaction and does not appear to be acting as a phase transfer agent in the true sense.

REACTION WITH FORMIC ACID

Sulfuric Acid Catalyst

B. Yeomans; U.S. Patent 3,515,737; June 2, 1970; assigned to The Distillers Company Limited, Scotland has found that the process for the preparation of neocarboxylic acids from olefins by reaction with formic acid and sulfuric acid, followed by addition of water, is improved by using a molar ratio of olefin:formic acid:sulfuric acid, in the range of between 1:1:2 and 1:4:12 and by the use of a small amount of water in the last step, that is, between 3 and 25% of the weight of the sulfuric acid present in the reaction mixture containing water. The acids are easily isolated from the organic phase. The sulfuric acid may be recycled after addition of sulfur trioxide and the process may be operated continuously.

By "neo acid" is meant a tertiary aliphatic carboxylic acid where the α-carbon atom is attached directly to 4 further carbon atoms, i.e., the α-carbon atom is a quaternary carbon atom. It is particularly preferred to use acyclic olefins. The olefin is preferably a monounsaturated compound having a branched carbon skeleton, such as types (1), (2) and (3):

(1) −C−C=C(H)(CH₃) with C,H substituents   (2) −C−C=C−C with C,H substituents   (3) (C)(C)C=C(C)(C)

Where the olefin contains the group:

(4) −C−C=C(H)(H) with H substituent   (5) −C−C=C−C with H,H substituents

the molecule should also contain a group having a carbon skeleton as shown on the following page.

(6)
```
    C
    |
  C-C-C
    |
    H
```
(7)
```
    C
    |
  C-C-C
    |
    C
```
or (8)
```
    C C
    | |
  C-C-C-C
```

In any event it is preferred that the olefin should contain one or more of these carbon skeletons (6), (7) and (8). The olefin preferably contains any number of carbon atoms from 5 upwards, but olefins having from 8 to 20 carbon atoms in the molecule are particularly preferred.

In place of the olefin there may be used other compounds containing from 5 to 20 carbon atoms, for example, tertiary halides, alcohols such as a primary, secondary or tertiary octanol, tertiary mercaptans such as 2,2-dimethylpentyl mercaptans and mixture of an isoparaffin such as isoheptane and an isoparaffin such as isobutene. These compounds will react with formic acid in the presence of concentrated sulfuric acid as though they are true olefins.

The olefin may be added to the reaction mixture in solution, for example, in cyclohexane or an aliphatic chloro-carbon solvent. It is preferred to use a solvent which does not contain hydrogen atoms, for example, carbon tetrachloride or tetrachloroethylene.

In the process, the formic acid is added to the sulfuric acid catalyst at about 0° to -20°C. A small amount of the olefin may be also added during this step in order to help stabilize the formic acid. The remainder of the olefin is then added at a temperature between 0° to +20°C., and after completion of the reaction, phase separation is obtained. It is necessary to add a small amount of water at this stage to assist phase separation. The amount of water should not exceed 25% w./w. based on the sulfuric acid present in the mixture of the water. It is preferred to add more than about 3% of water, the particularly preferred range being between 5 and 15% w./w. It is critical to add only the minimum amount of water necessary to achieve phase separation in order to avoid expensive reconcentration of sulfuric acid.

It has also been found that addition of more formic acid facilitates separation. It is preferred to add one mol of formic acid per mol of olefin used in the reaction stage. When operating with the preferred ratio of olefin to formic acid of 1:2, one mol of formic acid is used up in the reaction stage and one remins in solution in the sulfuric acid. Addition of one mol more of formic acid assists in the separation of the neo acid and restores the concentration of formic acid in the sulfuric acid to the optimum value. Use of appreciably more than one mol of formic acid per mol of olefin used in the reaction stage will result in too high a concentration in the sulfuric acid and reduced yields of neo acid. Consequently the amount added should not exceed 3 mols, and is preferably less than 2 mols and most preferably is 1 mol. The separated organic phase is decanted and the catalyst raffinate is extracted with a suitable solvent, for example, cyclohexane or an aliphatic chlorocarbon solvent such as carbon tetrachloride or tetrachloroethylene.

As the sulfuric acid is diluted to only a minor extent to achieve phase separation, the recovered sulfuric acid solution may readily be refortified with sulfur trioxide and recycled to the reaction stage. The sulfur trioxide used to refortify the recovered sulfuric acid may be added in solution, preferably in a solvent which does not contain hydrogen atoms. An aliphatic chlorocarbon solvent such as carbon tetrachloride or preferably tetrachloroethylene, or alternatively liquid sulfur dioxide may be used. The refortification is carried out at a temperature in the range of 0° to −30°C., preferably between −15° and −20°C.

The comparatively small surplus of acid made during refortification may be separated from the recycle stream for use in subsequent neo acid purification procedures, for example, regeneration of the neo acids from their aqueous solutions in sodium or potassium hydroxide. When the preferred molar ratio of reactants is used, approximately 20% of the refortified acid is so used, and little or no surplus sulfuric acid has to be disposed of. Any sulfonic acid produced in the process may be separated from the neo acid product by trituration with water. By recycling the sulfuric acid to the reaction stage there is the further advantage that the bulk of any neo acids which may be left in the sulfuric acid phase are not lost to the process.

Example 1: Formic acid (2 mols) was added to 99% w./w. sulfuric acid (3.88 mols) at −10°C. with stirring, over a period of 25 minutes. During this period about 10% of a mixture of propylene trimer (1 mol) and cyclohexane (0.93 mol) was also added and the remaining 90% was added over a further 135 minutes at +10°C. The mixture was stirred for a further 10 minutes and then aliquots (50 ml.) were withdrawn and mixed with water. The ease of phase separation obtained is illustrated in the table below.

Percent w./w. water added based on sulphuric acid present	58.0	11.6	8.3	6.0	2.9
Volume (ml.) of organic phase separated in 'x' minutes 'x'					
Do. 1	[1]26	26	26	6	3
Do. 5	26	26	26	18	11
Do. 13	26	26	26	26	12
Do. 34	26	26	26	26	21
Do. 64	26	26	26	26	21
Do. 124	26	26	26	26	24

[1] 26 ml. = theoretical volume of organics present in the 50 ml. sample of reaction product.

The results indicate that additions as small as 6% w./w. of water to the sulfuric acid present in the reaction product are sufficient to give adequate and speedy phase separation.

Example 2: Formic acid (2 mols) was added over a period of 25 minutes to 99% w./w. sulfuric acid (3.88 mols) at -10°C. with stirring. During the period about 7% of a mixture of propylene trimer (1 mol) and cyclohexane (0.93 mol) was added and the remaining 93% was added over 130 minutes at +5°C. The product was stirred for a further 10 minutes and then treated with water (1 mol) added over 20 minutes as a fine spray at about 0°C. The product was separated and extracted with cyclohexane (3 x 150 ml.). The organic extracts were bulked and neodecanoic acids were separated from neutral reaction products by extraction with aqueous 12% w./v. potassium hydroxide (3 x 20 ml.). The caustic extracts were acidified with mineral acid, extracted with cyclohexane (3 x 150 ml.), dried and concentrated free of solvent, yielding a distillation residue (110.3 g.) which contained 0.57 mol of neodecanoic acids.

A repeat experiment was carried out exactly as described above except that the water treatment step comprised adding the reaction product to ice (500 g.) and the neodecanoic acids were then isolated as above, as a distillation residue (104.1 g.) which contained 0.44 mol of neodecanoic acids. These experiments demonstrate that neo acids may be separated without loss of yield, by the addition of a small quantity of water to the reaction mixtures.

In a related process by B. Yeomans; U.S. Patent 3,703,549; Nov. 21, 1972; assigned to BP Chemicals Limited, England di-neo acids are produced by treating a mono-neo acid containing at least 10 carbon atoms and no tertiary hydrogen atoms with strong acid. The process for the production of a di-neo acid comprises treating a mono-neo acid containing 10 to 21 carbon atoms of the formula:

$$R_1-\underset{\underset{COOH}{|}}{\overset{\overset{R_2}{|}}{C}}-R_3$$

where R_1, R_2 and R_3 are all alkyl groups which may be the same or different and which do not contain tertiary hydrogen and which each contain from 1 to 7 carbon atoms, with strong acid. By "tertiary hydrogen atom" is meant a hydrogen attached to a carbon atom whose other valencies are satisfied by carbon atoms. It will be understood that for an alkyl group to contain no tertiary hydrogen it may be a straight chain alkyl group or any branching must be gem branching, i.e., two branches on the same carbon atom. The mono-neo acid used in the rearrangement reaction is preferably derived from an olefin by reaction with formic acid or carbon monoxide in the presence of strong acid. The olefin may be an acyclic one containing 9 to 20 carbon atoms with one alkyl substituent only in the chain.

Example 1: Production of Mono-Neo Acid — Formic acid (1.5 mol of 99% w./w.) and 2-methyloctene-4 (1 mol) dissolved in tetrachloroethylene (1 mol) were added under stirring to a round bottom flask (1 l.) which contained sulfuric acid (6 mol of 99% w./w.) so that a slight excess of formic acid to olefin was always present in the reactor. The additions were carried out over 2 hours at +2° to +15°C. The reaction product was then diluted with water. The neo acid (0.880 mol) produced was chemically separated from neutral reaction by-products by forming the sodium salts and selectively dissolving in water. The neo acid was shown to mainly consist of 2,2-dimethyloctanoic acid.

Production of Di-Neo Acid — 2.2-dimethyloctanoic acid (0.20 mol) was mixed with 99% w./w. sulfuric acid (0.40 mol) at 22°C. and was then allowed to stand for 11 days. The mixture was poured into two volumes of water and the precipitated 2,2,6,6-tetramethylpimelic acid (0.00144 mol) was separated by filtration. Neutral by-products (0.42 g.) were isolated by chemical separation and these largely consisted of 2-methyloctane (39.1% w./w.), 3-methyloctane (28.2% w./w.) and 4-methyloctane (16.5% w./w.).

Example 2: Production of Mono-Neo Acid — Formic acid (1.5 mol of 99% w./w.) and 2-methylnonene-4 (1 mol) dissolved in tetrachloroethylene (1 mol) were added under stirring to a round bottom flask (1 l.) which contained sulfuric acid (6 mol of 99% w./w.) so that a slight excess of formic acid to olefin was always present in the reactor. The additions were carried out over 2 hours at +1° to 13°C. The reaction product was then diluted with water. The neo acid product (0.896 mol) was chemically separated from neutral reaction by-products. The neo acid product mainly consisted of 2,2-dimethylnonanoic acid.

Production of Di-Neo Acid — 2,2-dimethylnonanoic acid (0.010 mol) was mixed with 99% w./w. sulfuric acid (0.200 ml.) at 23°C. and was then allowed to stand at ambient temperatures for 8 days. The mixture was poured into two volumes of water and the precipitated 2,2,7,7-tetramethylsuberic acid (0.00135 mol) was separated by filtration. Neutral by-products (0.425 g.) largely consisted of 2-methylnonane (38.9% w./w.), 3-methylnonane (24.8% w./w.), 4-methylnonane (17.2% w./w.) and 5-methylnonane (7.9% w./w.).

Free Radical Initiator

A process by W.A. Mueller and R. Swidler; U.S. Patent 3,637,478; January 25, 1972; assigned to Armour Industrial Chemical Company produces aliphatic acids by reaction of terminally unsaturated aliphatic compounds or monocyclic monounsaturated aliphatic compounds with formate ion in the presence of a free radical initiator. The aliphatic acids formed are useful in the production of lubricants, paper coating, rubber compounding or for the formation of derivatives such as soaps, amines and the like.

The process is advantageously conducted in a homogeneous medium, in which the source of formate ions, the olefin, and the initiator are dissolved. The reaction will proceed under conditions where a portion of reactant may not be in the homogeneous system. The solvent must be sufficiently polar to dissolve the source of formate ions, while having sufficient solvent power to accommodate the required concentration of olefin. Aqueous solutions of aliphatic alcohols having from 1 to 6 carbon atoms are especially satisfactory as solvents. Aqueous solutions of methanol and ethanol are especially preferred. The concentration of alcohol in water may vary from about 40 to 90%, from about 60 to 80% being especially preferred.

The reaction between the unsaturated compound and formate ion may be initiated by free radicals which may be obtained from any suitable source including chemical or photoinitiators, known in the art as free radical initiators. Chemical free radical initiators are selected to afford a continuous supply of radicals throughout the reaction period. Therefore, an initiator is selected so that under reaction conditions of time and temperature not more than 2 to 4 half lives of the initiator elapses. Specific chemical initiators which are especially useful in the process include dialkyl peroxides such as di-tert-butyl peroxide and dicumyl peroxide, and peresters such as tert-butyl perbenzoate. Suitable concentrations of the chemical initiators are from 0.1 to 2 mol percent based upon the formate ion concentration. Photoinitiation such as ultraviolet radiation may be used alone or in conjunction with photosensitizers such as dialkyl ketones and organic peroxides. Diethyl ketone is particularly useful as a photosensitizer when using Quartz Mercury resonance lamps.

The reaction may be conducted by dissolving the olefinic and formate reactants in aqueous alcohols. Concentration of formate ion and olefin may be adjusted to produce maximum yields of the desired product. In general, a high mol ratio of formate to olefin tends to produce 1:1 adducts, and a low mol ratio tends to produce telomeric acids. However, these ratios may vary according to the reactivity of the olefinic reactant. Certain olefins produce substantial amounts of 1:1 adducts each at low ratios of formate ion to olefin while others produce telomeric acids even at high formate to olefin ratios. Thus, the ratios of formate ion to olefin may be varied over wide limits to derive high yields of desired product. It is preferred that the formate ion be present in an excess of from about 5 to 20 mols of formate ion per mol of olefin. Lower amounts of formate ion relative to olefin present tend to promote undesirable side reactions, especially telomerization of the olefin. Molar amounts of formate ion relative to olefin of greater than 20 to 1 may be used to promote formation of the 1:1 adduct, but become economically undesirable. When the olefinic material is a solid or liquid it may be simply added to the aqueous alcohol medium to provide a suitable concentration relative to the formate ion. When the olefinic material is gaseous, the gas may be charged into the closed reaction vessel after flushing with nitrogen. The chemical initiator is added in a mol percent of from 0.1 to 2, based upon formate ion concentration.

The formate ion, olefin, and chemical initiator in aqueous alcohol solution is flushed with nitrogen to remove residual oxygen from the system, sealed in the vessel, stirred and heated to reaction temperature suitable to the nature of the initiator employed, as is well known in the art, at autogenous pressure until the reaction is substantially completed. Preferred temperatures are from about 120° to 160°C., when di-tert-butyl peroxide or tert-butyl perbenzoate is used as an initiator.

When the olefinic material is gaseous, such as ethylene, the formate ion producing substance and chemical initiator may be added to the aqueous alcohol in an autoclave, flushed with nitrogen, and then the gaseous olefin added to a pressure affording the desired concentration of olefin in the reaction mixture, usually from about 50 to 1,000 psig, followed by stirring and heating. The olefin and/or the source of free radicals may be added gradually or stepwise throughout the course of the reaction in order to maintain a favorable rate of formate ion to olefin mol ratio.

When the reaction is conducted in the presence of irradiation, the formate ion producing material and an olefinic material may be dissolved in aqueous alcohol, and alternatively, ultraviolet radiation either alone or in conjunction with sensitizer may be used at convenient temperatures of between 0° to 120°C. The reaction should be continued until the olefinic material is substantially consumed by the reaction. The following examples are presented to illustrate the process.

Example 1: Sodium formate, 1-octene, and di-tert-butyl peroxide in mol ratios of 100:10:1 were added to and mixed with 50% aqueous ethanol in a glass bomb. The solution of reactants and free radical initiator in aqueous ethanol were flushed with nitrogen, sealed and heated to and maintained at about 130°C. for 15 hours. The bomb and contents were then cooled to room temperature, the contents transferred to a steam distillation apparatus, and the material steam distilled to remove excess ethanol and higher aliphatic alcohols until the distillant became clear. The residue made up principally of an aqueous solution of sodium pelargonate, was then acidified with hydrochloric acid and steam distilled yielding pelargonic acid in 50% yield, based upon 1-octene reactant. The products were analyzed and identified by infrared and gas chromatographic data compared with synthesized pure sample materials.

Example 2: 27.2 grams sodium formate, 3.3 grams 1-hexene, 0.36 gram di-tert-butyl peroxide and 100 ml. 70% methanol were added to a 300 cc stainless steel stirred autoclave. The mixture was flushed with nitrogen and heated to and maintained at 130°C. for 15 hours. Using the same recovery technique as described in Example 1, heptanoic acid was obtained in 23% yield, determined by analysis described in Example 1.

Example 3: 27.2 grams sodium formate, 7.3 grams undecylenic acid, 1.6 grams sodium hydroxide, and 1 gram of di-tert-butyl peroxide were added to 100 ml. 50% aqueous methanol in a glass bomb. The mixture was flushed with nitrogen, sealed and heated to and maintained at about 140°C. for 15 hours. The bomb and contents were cooled to room temperature, acidulated with hydrochloric acid, and 1,12-dodecanedioic acid was recovered by filtration. 80% crude mass yield, based upon undecylenic acid reactant was obtained. The product melted at 117° to 126°C., and had a neutralization equivalent of 130 (119 theoretical).

Example 4: 386 grams sodium formate, 8.25 grams di-tert-butyl peroxide and 1,421 ml. 70% aqueous methanol were added to a 1-gallon stainless steel stirred autoclave. The mixture was flushed with nitrogen, sealed, and ethylene was added to a pressure of 750 psig. The reaction mixture was stirred and heated at about 130°C. for about 18 hours. The contents were cooled to room temperature and a pressure of 400 psig was observed. The autoclave was opened and the contents transferred to a steam distillation apparatus and steam distilled until the distillant was clear to remove excess methyl and higher aliphatic alcohols. The residue was acidulated with hydrochloric acid and the acid solvent extracted. The acids were then esterified with ethanol and separated from insoluble and nonesterifiable materials by filtration and washing with sodium carbonate solution. The yield of aliphatic acids was 88% based upon ethylene consumed. The distribution of ethyl esters obtained as determined by gas chromatographic analysis was as follows:

Ethyl propionate	31.3%
Ethyl valerate	29 %
Ethyl enanthate	16 %
Ethyl perlargonate	11 %
Ethyl hendecanoate	7 %
Ethyl tridecanoate	5 %

TRANSADDITION REACTION WITH SATURATED CARBOXYLIC ACIDS

Alkali Metal Catalyst

L. Schmerling and W.G. Toekelt; U.S. Patent 3,075,010; Jan. 22, 1963; assigned to Universal Oil Products Company describe a process for the preparation of a carboxylic acid which comprises reacting a polyolefinic hydrocarbon with a compound selected from the group consisting of alkali metal salts of saturated carboxylic acids and alkaline earth metal salts of saturated carboxylic acids, the acids being characterized by the presence of at least one hydrogen atom on an alpha carbon atom. The reaction takes place in the presence of a catalyst selected from the group consisting of alkali metals, alkali metal hydrides, alkali metal amides, alkali metal alkyls and alkali metal aryls at a temperature in the range of from about 50° to 300°C. The resultant product is hydrolyzed to form the salt of a carboxylic acid, thereafter acidifying the product, and recovering the desired carboxylic acid.

The olefins which may be used in this process include polyolefinic hydrocarbons comprising both straight and branched chain alkadienes containing from 4 to 12 carbon atoms. Butadienes and isoprenes are the preferred reactants due to their relatively greater availability and correspondingly lower cost. The alkali metal salts or alkaline earth metal salts of saturated carboxylic acids which may be reacted with the olefinic compound include the following: RR'CHCOOM, MOOCCHR(CR'R")$_n$COOM, (RR'CHCOO)$_2$M' and [OOCCHR(CR'R")$_n$COO]$_2$M' in which R, R' and R" are independently selected from the group consisting of hydrogen, alkyl, cycloalkyl and aryl radicals, M is an alkali metal, M' is an alkaline earth metal and n is an integer of from 0 to 10.

Generally speaking the reaction between the alkali metal salt of a saturated carboxylic acid or the alkaline earth metal salt of a saturated carboxylic acid and a diolefin, in the presence of a catalyst, is effected at a temperature in the range of about 50° to 300°C., and preferably at a temperature in the range of about 150° to 250°C., the particular temperature being dependent upon the reactants and the catalyst which are used. In addition the reaction will proceed at an elevated pressure, usually in the range of from about 25 to 200 atmospheres or more. This pressure will generally be supplied by the olefin, if in gaseous form. The pressure may also be supplied by the addition of an inert gas. In each case, however, the pressure will be sufficient to maintain a substantial portion of the reactants in liquid form.

The process may be effected in any suitable manner and may comprise either a batch or a continuous type operation. For example, when a batch type operation is used a quantity of the alkali metal salt of a saturated carboxylic acid or the alkaline earth metal salt of a saturated carboxylic acid along with the catalyst or the diolefin if in liquid form, and the diluent or solvent, if any is used, is sealed in a suitable apparatus such as, for example, a rotating autoclave. If the diolefin is in gaseous form, it is pressed in, until the desired pressure has been reached, after the autoclave is sealed. The reaction vessel is heated to the desired temperature and maintained there for a predetermined period of time after which the autoclave and contents are cooled to room temperature, the excess pressure is vented and the reaction product is recovered by conventional means such as, for example, by dissolving the reaction product in water to hydrolyze the product thereby forming the desired salt of a higher molecular weight organic acid.

The aqueous solution may then be extracted with a suitable organic solvent such as ether to separate the diluent and to remove traces of water-insoluble material after which the aqueous solution is concentrated and the desired salt is separated by fractional crystallization. If, as is usually the case, the higher weight molecular acid itself is desired, the aqueous solution is acidified by conventional means using acidifying agents such as inorganic acids including hydrochloric acid, sulfuric acid, nitric acid, etc., and recovered, one method consisting of extraction of the acid with a solvent such as ethyl ether, followed by fractionation of the extract.

Example 1: A mixture of 30 g. of potassium acetate and 10 g. of sodamide was placed in the glass liner of a rotating autoclave. The glass liner was sealed into the autoclave and 70 g. of 1,3-butadiene charged thereto, the initial pressure being 5 atmospheres. The autoclave was heated to a temperature of 250°C. during a period of 4.5 hours, the maximum pressure reaching 20 atmospheres. At the end of this time the autoclave and contents thereof were cooled to room temperature, the final pressure at room temperature being 5 atmospheres. The excess pressure was vented and the recovered product was dissolved in water yielding an aqueous solution and an upper layer, which were steam distilled.

The aqueous residue was then acidified with hydrochloric acid, extracted with ether and the ether solution was subjected to fractional distillation under reduced pressure. The cut boiling at 77° to 78°C. at 1.4 mm. pressure comprising a hexanoic acid (mixed with some hexenoic acid) was recovered and analyzed.

Found: C, 62.30; H, 10.26.
Calculated for $C_6H_{12}O_2$:   C, 62.04; H, 10.41;
Calculated for $C_6H_{10}O_2$:   C, 63.13; H, 8.99.

Example 2:   A mixture of 50 g. of sodium propionate and 10 g. of sodamide along with 200 g. of benzene was sealed into a turbomixer which was heated with stirring to 204°C. Butadiene (75 g.) was then added gradually during two hours. The initial pressure was about 17 atmospheres and reached about 27 atmospheres at the end of the addition, at which time the temperature was 238°C. Stirring was continued for an additional two hours after which the turbomixer and contents were cooled to room temperature, the excess pressure was vented and the turbomixer was opened. The recovered product was dissolved in water yielding an aqueous layer and an upper layer, which were steam distilled.

The aqueous residue was then acidified with hydrochloric acid, extracted with ether, and the ether solution was subjected to fractional distillation under reduced pressure. The cuts boiling at 87° to 150°C. at 4.6 mm. pressure were combined, pentane was added and the solution was washed with water, the solution was dried over sodium sulfate and redistilled through a Minical column. Most of the material boiled at 119° to 121°C. at 3.2 mm. (about 264° to 265°C. at atmospheric pressure). Titration with alkali indicated that it had a molecular weight of 178.3; that calculated for a bisbutenylpropionic acid is 182.3. The material was analyzed:

> Found: C, 72.30; H, 9.94.
> Calculated for $C_{11}H_{18}O_2$:   C, 72.37; H, 9.96.

Some lower boiling material from this fractionation was again redistilled through the Minical column. Product boiling at 108° to 110°C. at 26 mm. (204° to 206°C. at atmospheric pressure) was recovered and analyzed:

> Found: C, 64.30; H, 10.13.
> Calculated for $C_7H_{14}O_2$:   C, 64.58; H, 10.83;
> Calculated for $C_7H_{12}O_2$:   C, 65.60; H, 9.43.

The above analyses clearly indicated that the latter compound comprised 2-methylhexanoic acid mixed with methylhexenoic acid while the former compound comprised 2,2-bis-(2-butenyl)-propionic acid.

Example 3:   In this example a mixture of 50 g. of sodium propionate and 75 g. of isoprene along with 10 g. of sodamide and 200 g. of benzene is placed in a condensation apparatus provided with heating and stirring means. The mixture is gradually heated to a temperature of about 240°C. and maintained there for a period of about 5 hours while stirring constantly. At the end of this time the apparatus and contents are allowed to cool to room temperature. The recovered product is dissolved in water thereby yielding an aqueous solution and an upper layer which are steam distilled. The aqueous residue is then acidified with hydrochloric acid, extracted with ether and the ether solution is subjected to fractional distillation under reduced pressure. The cuts comprising the isomeric dimethylhexanoic acids and the isomeric 2,2-bis-(methylbutenyl)-propionic acids are separated and recovered.

Water-Soluble Initiator

C.C. Hobbs, Jr. and A.F. MacLean; U.S. Patent 3,470,219; Sept. 30, 1969; assigned to Celanese Corporation have found that in effecting a transaddition reaction between an olefin and a saturated aliphatic monocarboxylic acid, which reaction is carried out in an aqueous system containing a water-soluble initiator such as a persulfate, the efficiency of the reaction is enhanced by minimizing contact of reaction products with the initiator. A preferred embodiment comprises continuously extracting the reaction products from the reaction zone, substantially as rapidly as they are formed, with a liquid extractant which is a selective solvent for the reaction product and which is substantially immiscible with the reaction medium contained in the reaction zone. Another embodiment comprises adding the initiator gradually in stages to a mixture of the reactants whereby, even at unusually high reaction temperatures, efficiency of utilization of the initiator is kept at a high level while degradation of the products by the initiator is kept at a low level.

Examples 1 through 4: In carrying out the runs of Examples 1 through 4, 150 ml. of aqueous acetic acid of the strengths stated and containing 7 milliequivalents of sodium acetate was charged to a 250 ml. Magne Dash reactor together with 30 ml. of n-decane. The air in the reactor was purged by flushing with ethylene. The system was then heated to the desired temperature (80°C.) and pressured to the desired level with ethylene. When everything was operating at a steady level or state (i.e., the pressure was maintained at a steady level and the temperature was maintained at a steady 80°C., neither rising nor falling significantly), 3 millimols of $Na_2S_2O_8$ in 15 ml. of aqueous solution was pumped into the reactor. The reaction conditions were maintained for 2 1/2 to 3 hours.

The reaction mass separated into an aqueous phase and an organic phase upon discontinuation of stirring. Analyses were made by gas chromatography of both the aqueous and organic (mainly n-decane) phases. The distribution coefficient for butyric acid between 50 weight percent HOAc-50 weight percent H_2O and n-decane was about 0.15. The distribution coefficient is the ratio of concentrations of a component in two phases when equilibrium has been established with respect to that component. All the other components were transferred substantially completely to the n-decane layer.

The data and results of Examples 1 through 4 are summarized in Table 1.

TABLE 1

Example Nos.	1	2	3	4
Ml. aqueous HOAc (a)	150	150	150	150
Wt. Percent HOAc in aqueous HOAc	50	50	50	10
Organic extractant, specifically n-decane, ml	30	30	30	30
NaOAc,[b] milliequivalents	7	7	7	7
$Na_2S_2O_8$, millimoles	3	3	3	3
Temperature, °C	80	80	80	80
Ethylene pressure, p.s.i.g	30	100	400	100
Product, millimoles:				
Butyric acid	9.65	3.60	1.30	0.0074
2-ethylbutyric acid	0.0335	0.00364	0.00582	0.00186
Caproic acid	0.0215	0.0584	0.0400	0.00434
2-ethylcaproic acid	0.221	0.674	0.297	0.116
Caprylic acid		0.0436	0.0859	
2-butylcaproic acid		0.225	0.258	0.0279
Capric acid		0.097	0.137	
Lauric acid		0.069	0.071	
Residue, g	0.021	0.326	0.840	0.052
Efficiency ratio [c]	3.7	6.0	10.3	0.72
Ethylene going to volatile products, percent	94	43	15	

[a] HOAc = Acetic acid.
[b] NaOAc = Sodium acetate, the function of which is to neutralize the sodium bisulfate produced from the sodium persulfate initiator.
[c] Efficiency ratio is defined as the number of moles of ethylene consumed per mole of initiator decomposed. In these runs it is based on the assumption that the nonvolatile residue has an average molecular weight of 500.

Examples 1 through 4 show that butyric acid production falls off rapidly as ethylene pressure is increased. This is also generally true with respect to the production of 2-ethylbutyric acid, the yield of which is of the order of 1/300 the amount of butyric acid formed. This indicates that 2-ethylbutyric acid is a product of secondary attack on butyric acid.

The caproic and 2-ethylcaproic acids have distribution curves that are similar to each other. The continually increasing production of 2-butyl-caproic acid with increasing ethylene pressure indicates that the 2-ethyl-caproic acid precursor radical is further converted to the 2-cutylcaproic acid precursor radical to a greater extent as the ethylene pressure is increased. The 2-butylcaproic acid precursor radical can give the expected acid by chain transfer or it can undergo a backbiting reaction. In view of the ratio of 2-ethylcaproic acid to caproic acid the backbiting reaction is probably heavily favored, even more so since the hydrogen atom involved is tertiary. The resulting radical (a tertiary one) is relatively non-reactive toward ethylene, especially at pressures below about 200 psig, so most of it probably goes into chain-termination products.

The distribution of caprylic, capric and lauric acids indicates that these components are still increasing with pressure in a regular manner. Of the higher molecular weight products obtained, the straight chain acids predominate. The compositions of the residues could not be determined with certainty. They are white, low melting, waxy solids, the infrared spectra of which resemble long chain carboxylic acids. It would be expected that these residues would contain the chain-stopping products, and that these would be mainly branched chain compounds (probably substituted succinic anhydrides). Some infrared evidence was found in support of these views.

Example 4 shows the effect of lowering the concentration of acetic acid in the aqueous phase. Although the most favored product was 2-ethylcaproic acid, as was desired, the efficiency ratio was much lower than usual. One anomaly appearing in the results of Example 4 is that the ratio of 2-ethylbutyric acid to butyric acid is much higher than usual. The reasons for this are not understood, although the reduced availability of acetic acid for chain transfer may be involved. Such reduced acetic acid availability would increase the relative attack on the butyric acid product.

Referring to Table 1 it will be noted that there is a steady increase in the efficiency ratio of the initiator with increasing ethylene pressure. Note Examples 1, 2 and 3 where the respective efficiency ratios were 3.7, 6.0 and 10.3 at ethylene pressures of 30, 100 and 400 psig, respectively. This is due to the fact that any attack on the initial products did not cause any serious chain-stopping reactions. (Parenthetically it may be noted that the initial relatively low value of the efficiency ratio is probably due to the use of stainless steel equipment in carrying out the reaction. Stainless steel is known to exert a retarding effect on the ethylene reaction in an acetic acid system using acetyl peroxide as the initiator. The inhibiting effect when using a persulfate initiator may be even greater.)

In marked contrast the general trend in the efficiency ratios of the initiator is downward with increasing pressure when the reaction products are not extracted as and when they are formed. This indicates that the initial reaction products are reacting further in chain-stopping reactions. Thus, averages of two runs, without extraction, indicate an average efficiency of 10.0 at 0 psig ethylene pressure and 7.8 at 5 1/2 psig, while individual nonextraction runs show an efficiency ratio of 9.8 at 25 psig ethylene pressure and 7.2 at 65 psig. In this case the initial efficiency ratios may be relatively high because the runs were made in glass apparatus.

Examples 5 through 10: Examples 5 through 10 involve the use of octene-1, heptene-3 and a mixture of octene-1 and heptene-3 as the olefinic reactant. The data and results are summarized in Table 2 on the following page. The runs of the examples shown in this table were made by mixing all the reactants (200 ml. volume) except the peroxide initiator in a 3-necked, 50 ml. stirred flask fitted with a thermowell and a reflux condenser. Nitrogen, which had been scrubbed with pyrogallol solution, was continuously sparged into the system. In those runs where the peroxide

Fatty Acids

TABLE 2

Example No.	5	6	7	8	9	10
Olefin	Octene-1	Octene-1	Octene-1	Octene-1 / Heptene-3	Heptene-3	Octene-1
Olefin concentration, M	0.096	0.096	0.096	0.048 / 0.048	0.096	0.096
Ac_2O, vol. percent	---	---	---	5	5	5
Solvent	65% HOAc, 35% H_2O	65% HOAc, 35% H_2O	65% HOAc, 35% H_2O	HOAc	HOAc	HOAc
Peroxide	$K_2S_2O_8$	$K_2S_2O_8$	$K_2S_2O_8$	Ac_2O_2	Ac_2O_2	Ac_2O_2
Peroxide, addition rate	*	**	***	*	*	†
Peroxide, millimoles	1.11	1.11	1.11	1.15	1.15	1.28
Temperature, °C.	80	90	94-103	90	90	118
Run duration, hrs.	>5	>8	>6	>5	>5	>7
Acid produced	Capric	Capric	Capric	Capric and Nonanoic	Capric and Nonanoic	Capric
Acid, mmol/mmol peroxide decomposed	0.56	1.72	4.45	0.8	0.72	5.05

*Batch addition.
**The peroxide (6.1 ml. aqueous solution) was added 1 ml. to start and then 1/2 ml. each 15 min. The temperature was maintained for 2 hrs. after the completion of addition.
***The peroxide (6.1 ml. aqueous solution) was added 1/2 ml. to start and then 1/4 ml. each 15 min. The temperature was maintained for 1 hr. after the completion of addition.
†The peroxide solution (10 ml.) was added 1/2 ml. to start and then 1/4 ml. each 7 1/2 min. The temperature was maintained for 1 hr. after the completion of addition.

was added batchwise, it was added before heating was started. The reaction mass was then rapidly brought to reaction temperature and maintained there for at least five half-lives of the peroxide. In the other runs, the peroxide was added in accordance with the schedules given in the footnotes. In Examples 5 and 6 sodium acetate (2.7 milliequivalents) was also added to neutralize the acid formed by persulfate decomposition. In Example 7 the reaction solution also contained 74 millimols of sodium acetate and 0.7 millimol of silver acetate. The runs made with potassium persulfate were worked up by extracting the organic products with ether. The ether solution was then analyzed by gas chromatography.

Examples 5 and 6 show how, when the initiator, potassium persulfate, is added in increments (Example 6) as compared with introducing it all at once with the initial ingredients (batch addition), the reaction temperature can be increased from 80°C. (Example 5) to 90°C. without a consequent increase in free radical concentration. These changes resulted in a significant improvement in efficiency ratio, viz., from 0.66 to 1.72 millimols acid produced per millimol peroxide decomposed. When the temperature is again increased (to 98°C., the boiling point of the reaction mass) and the rate of incremental addition of the peroxide further reduced, a small (about 20%) additional increase in the efficiency ratio is obtained.

Example 7 is similar to Example 6 with the exception that the incremental addition of the peroxide was at a slower rate and a somewhat higher temperature was used; also, about 25 times as much sodium acetate was present, and silver acetate was also added as a catalyst for the persulfate oxidation of the acetic acid. This resulted in a very substantial and unobvious increase in efficiency ratio (from 1.72 to 4.45), being about equal to that of acetyl peroxide under the best conditions for each.

Example 8 shows the results of a run made with an equimolar mixture of octene-1 and heptene-3, and Example 9 using heptene-3 alone. The initiator was acetyl peroxide, which was introduced by batch addition technique, and the solvent was acetic acid. The ratio of products of Example 8 indicates that about 6 times as much terminal olefin was converted to acid as was the internal olefin. However, the efficiency ratio was appreciably lowered. A similarly low efficiency ratio was noted in the results of the run of Example 9.

The run of Example 10 was made with octene-1, and the peroxide initiator was added in increments instead of batchwise. The latter technique permitted the use of a higher reaction temperature (118° vs. 90°C. for each of Examples 8 and 9). Otherwise the ingredients and procedure were much the same as for Examples 8 and 9. The efficiency ratio was 5.05, which was the highest of any of the runs of the examples of Table 2.

Plotting a graph of the effect of product concentration on the peroxide efficiency ratio, based on the results of the foregoing examples and others, shows that this efficiency ratio drops off rapidly after the concentration of organic acid products reaches about 1 1/2%. In other words, the concentration of organic acid product such as capric acid can be allowed to build up to at least 1 1/2% before objectionable deleterious effects are observed.

PREPARATION FROM OTHER SOURCES

FROM HYDROCARBONS

Step-Wise Process

C.B. Berry; U.S. Patent 3,413,323; November 26, 1968; assigned to Ethyl Corporation has developed a process for the oxidation of hydrocarbons to produce straight chain monofunctional carboxylic acids. In accordance with the process, carboxylic acids are produced by the oxidation of hydrocarbons typically using oxygen from the air at pressures of from about atmospheric to several atmospheres and temperatures from 100° to 160°C. Hydrocarbons are oxidized which preferably contain an average of from 4 to 10 carbon atoms per molecule in excess of the average quantity of carbon atoms desired in the product acids because this optimizes the yield of product acids per pound of hydrocarbon feed.

Oxidation times vary depending upon the conditions employed and in general are controlled so as to obtain an oxidation extent of 30% of the hydrocarbon molecules being converted to molecules containing oxygenated groups. The results will be oxidation times varying from a few hours at the higher temperatures to an oxidation period of the order of one or more days at the lower temperatures. Various catalysts, organic and inorganic, can be used.

In the practice of this process several conversion steps are employed and it is essential that some of them be performed in the proper sequence. As a general proposition it is necessary to perform the conversions in two or more separate reactor vessels because of the fact that some of the reactions appear to require conditions which conflict to some extent with conditions desired for other steps. Typically an early processing step applied to the oxidate is saponification which converts molecules having carboxylic acid groups into metal salts. Following the saponification of the acidic molecules it is preferred to separate the soap molecules from the nonsoap or hydrocarbon molecules which separation is readily accomplished because of the fact that the soaps are soluble in an aqueous system leaving the hydrocarbons to float thereupon as a separate phase. The hydrocarbon phase will normally be removed and returned to the oxidizer for further oxidation.

The soap phase that results after removal of the hydrocarbon is hydrogenated under mild conditions to saturate carbonyl groups converting them into secondary hydroxyl groups. This conversion can be accomplished readily under mild conditions having virtually no adverse effect upon the saponified carboxyl groups. Typical conditions for such a mild carbonyl hydrogenation are temperature from 100° to 200°C., pressure from 100 to 500 psi, Raney nickel catalyst 0.1 to 10%, the aqueous solution of the soaps being approximately 30% by weight. Typical hydrogenation times are from 1 to 5 hours during which virtually complete conversion of carbonyls to hydroxyls is obtained.

The saturation of carbonyl groups in the soaps produces hydroxy acid soaps which, although they have some independent utility and sales potential, must be further treated in instances where pure fatty acids are the only desired product. It has been found that such hydroxyl groups are readily removed from the molecules that contain them by dehydration at elevated temperatures. In general it is preferable to perform the dehydration at temperatures in excess of 200°C.

The dehydration of soaps as described results in the formation of large quantities of unsaturated soaps which must be saturated to produce high purity fatty acids. The conversion of unsaturated soaps to saturated soaps is readily accomplished in a mild hydrogenator operative under substantially the same conditions set forth for the carbonyl hydrogenator which preceded the dehydration step. The treatment of the saturated soap solution thus obtained follows conventional practice of acidification with mineral acid such as sulfuric acid, followed by separation of the mineral salt produced leaving the mixture of organic acids. The organic acids thus obtained are quite pure and need be subjected to minimum cleanup steps.

Example: A mixture of normal hydrocarbons having from 14 to 18 carbon atoms per molecule is oxidized with air at a temperature of 140°C. to a conversion of approximately 30% oxygenated molecules. The oxidate is saponified at a temperature of 125°C. using 25% by weight of NaOH. A mildly hydrogenative environment is maintained in the saponifier to saturate free radicals. The effluent from saponification is separated into aqueous and hydrocarbon phases, and the hydrocarbon phase recovered for return to oxidation. The aqueous soaps are then hydrogenated under mild conditions to saturate carbonyl and olefinic linkages. Temperature 125°C., pressure 400 psi, 10% (weight on basis of anhydrous soaps) Raney nickel catalyst, for 3 hours. The product of the first hydrogenation is filtered to recover the catalyst and dehydrated at 35°C. for 3 hours. Operation is under autogenous pressure with water vapor removed. A pH of 8.0 is maintained during hydrogenation.

The dehydrated soaps are then cooled to 100°C. and boiling water added with mixing to produce an aqueous soap solution which is mildly hydrogenated a second time under conditions similar to the carbonyl hydrogenation. The aqueous soaps are then acidified with H_2SO_4 to spring the acids which are separated and purified by distillation. The acids are saturated free of carbonyl and hydroxyl groups, and of esters, lactones and other such impurities normally present. The acids are of light straw color and free of objectionable odor.

Continuous Withdrawal of Formed Acid

A process developed by J.R. Wechsler; U.S. Patent 3,708,513; Jan. 2, 1973; assigned to Stepan Chemical Company relates to the manufacture of straight chained monobasic fatty acids from essentially linear hydrocarbons of an average molecular weight corresponding to one having 2 to 6 more carbon atoms than the desired range of fatty acids. It consists of substantially uniformly dispersing an organic catalyst with the hydrocarbons so as to obtain a mixture and heating the mixture to a temperature of not more than 160°C. The mixture is simultaneously contacted with an oxygen-containing gas to effect an oxidation of the hydrocarbon so as to not exceed 3% fatty acids by weight content of the reaction mixture.

Thereafter, an alkali solution is added and intermixed with the reaction mixture to effect saponification. The saponified mixture is collected and a phase separation effected where an organic phase is removed and recycled for additional oxidation, while the aqueous phase (i.e., the lower phase) is purified to obtain the desired range of straight chained monobasic fatty acids.

The purification processes include hydrogenation of the recovered crude products, with the removal of the volatile impurities therein so as to obtain a concentrated soap solution and thereafter acidifying such concentrated soap solution with a mineral acid and distilling the resultant product to obtain relatively pure fatty acids. The starting materials are paraffin hydrocarbons containing 14 to 20 carbon atoms. The preferred oxygen-containing gas is air. An organic peroxide catalyst is utilized since such catalyst can be intermixed with the reaction system and allowed to remain therein without the necessity of filtering it or otherwise mechanically removing it from the mixture. Preferred peroxides include benzoyl peroxide, ditertiary-butyl peroxide and mixture thereof.

Raw materials and the catalyst are placed in a reactor of a convenient size and heated to a temperature of not more than 160°C. whereupon oxygen-containing gas, such as air, is pumped through the raw materials at a preset rate. After an initial induction period ranging from several minutes to two hours, depending primarily upon the catalyst employed and the hydrocarbon used as raw material, the reaction between the oxygen and the paraffin materials initiates and maintains itself.

After reaction is self-sustaining, the reaction mixture is withdrawn from the reactor at a preset rate, as determined by the level of fatty acids therein, and directed through a heat exchanger to a saponification chamber wherein it is treated under efficient agitation with an aqueous alkaline solution. The intimate mixture of the oxidation reaction mixture and the alkaline solution is then transferred at a constant rate into a separator, wherein stratification or phase separation occurs. The bottom layer consists of a soap solution, while the top layer consists of unreacted or partially reacted raw materials which can then be transferred into a second separator or a liquid-liquid centrifuge to remove the last traces of the soap solution.

The remainder of the partially reacted or unreacted portion of oxidation materials is then recycled back to the reaction chamber and again passed through the reaction cycle just described. A certain amount of fresh raw materials is continuously fed into the reactor along with the recovered partial reacted materials so that the fresh materials compensate for the removal materials from the system in the soap solution.

The bottom layer of the separator is withdrawn at a relatively constant rate and the soap thus obtained is transformed and purified into the desired range of fatty acids. The rate of withdrawal of the reaction mixture from the reactor is so regulated that no more than 3% of free fatty acids by weight of the total reactants within the reaction chamber have accumulated. This control of withdrawal rate inhibits over-oxidation and thus inhibits formation of multifunctional chemical compounds which make purification difficult.

The acidic portion of the crude oxidation reaction product may be purified in a number of alternative methods. One method of purifying the crude soap solutions obtained from the separator include mixing such soap solutions with a predetermined amount of a hydrogen catalyst, purging the air from around such a mixture and simultaneously introducing pressurized hydrogen gas (i.e., at 350 to 650 psi) and heat to obtain a temperature in the range of 190° to 300°C. for a period of time sufficient so that the pressure within the hydrogenation vessel is in the range of 500 to 2,000 psi.

After this brief digestion period, i.e., 10 to 60 minutes the pressure is slowly released and the volatiles are allowed to escape. This distillation is continued until a relatively concentrated, i.e., at least 50% soap solution is attained. The hydrogenation catalyst is then removed, as by filtration, and the filtrate is then suitably acidified to obtain the desired range of fatty acids. If desired, the filtrate may also be converted to relatively pure alkyl esters of such fatty acids.

Example: The apparatus utilized for this example is shown schematically at Figure 3.1. 6,335 grams of raw materials consisting essentially of a mixture of normal tetradecane, pentadecane and hexadecane, was charged into the system by placing 2,400 grams into the reactor, with the rest of the raw materials being divided between the extractor, the two separators and the reservoir vessel. In order to eliminate any induction period, the initial charge of raw materials was preoxidized in a batch-type reaction to an acid content of 0.15 meq./g. and the free acid removed by extraction with an alkaline solution.

FIGURE 3.1: FLOW SHEET FOR CONTINUOUS PROCESS OF FATTY ACID SYNTHESIS

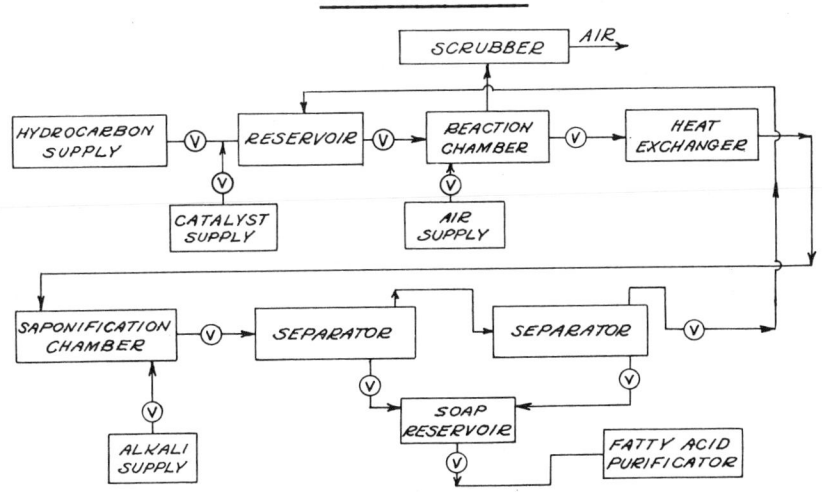

Source: J.R. Wechsler; U.S. Patent 3,708,513; January 2, 1973

One gram of di-tertiary butyl peroxide was placed in the reactor and the material heated to 140°C. Air was sparged through the reactor at a rate of 8 l./min. (corresponding to 3.3 l./kg. oil/min.) and the reaction set in almost at once, as evidenced by formation of water of reaction which was collected in a water trap. When 4 ml. of water was collected, the raw materials were allowed to circulate in the system and the continuous cycle started at a rate adjusted to one hour residence time, which corresponds to a maximum fatty acid formation of 3% by weight of total reactants in the reactor.

The adjustment was by means of adjustable Teflon stop cocks controlling all gravity flows and with conventional pumps. A NaOH solution was charged into the alkali supply vessel at a 2.5% strength and its rate of flow was adjusted to provide enough alkali to neutralize the free acids in the reactants at the saponification chamber.

This cycle was maintained around the clock for 84 hours and at the end of this time period the reaction was stopped. During the reaction time, fresh material (but not additional catalyst, nor any preoxidized material) was constantly fed to the system at a rate which would compensate for the material removed from the system by the alkaline solution and by periodic sampling for analysis. The total charge of raw materials during the cycle was 14,820 grams. At the end of the run, 8,044 grams of oil were accounted for, thus: 6,390 grams in the apparatus, 962 grams removed for sampling and 692 grams recovered from the scrubber system.

Accordingly, the consumed material amounted to 6,776 grams. The soap solution collected in the soap reservoir was acidified with H_2SO_4 to a pH below 3.5, and the obtained layer of crude reaction products, i.e., unpurifed fatty acids, weighed 5,694 grams or about an 84% yield. As will be appreciated, the acidification was performed at this time merely to ascertain the results of the oxidation process and under natural operating conditions it is more practical to continue directly with the purification.

Of this crude product, 5,100 grams was resaponified and the gross impurities removed by repeated extractions with petroleum ether, whereupon the soap solution was acidified and 3,380 grams of fatty acids and 1,465 grams of oil were recoverd. This oil was suitable for use as a recycle material into the oxidation process.

The fatty acids thus obtained had an average molecular weight of 186, generally corresponding to undecanoic acid, and had a molecular distribution as follows: C_6 to C_7 fatty acids, 6.5%; C_8 to C_{10} fatty acids, 26.8%; C_{11} to C_{14} fatty acids, 54.9%; and C_{15} to C_{16} fatty acids, 11.8% as determined by gas chromatography. The water of reaction collected in the trap weighed 2,287 grams and contained 4% H_2O_2 and 9% water-soluble fatty acids and peracids.

ω-Aryl Saturated Acids

E.J. Miller, Jr., A. Mais, and E.S. Hammerberg; U.S. Patent 3,564,030; February 16, 1971; assigned to Armour Industrial Chemical Company have provided a process for monoalkylation of aromatic compounds with unsaturated higher aliphatic compounds such as acids, amines, nitriles, esters, amides, and alcohols, in the presence of hydrofluoric acid to produce a high yield of products having monoalkylation of the aromatic nucleus. The monoalkylated products are useful as plasticizers, emulsifiers, and chemical intermediates.

The process is carried out in liquid hydrofluoric acid. If the reaction is to be conducted at temperatures above the boiling point of hydrofluoric acid, superatmospheric pressure may be used to maintain the hydrofluoric acid as a liquid. As long as the hydrofluoric acid is maintained in the liquid state, it functions both as a catalyst for the reaction and as the reaction medium or solvent.

It is possible to carry out the reaction over a broad range of temperatures from -20° to 100°C., however, 0° to 50°C. is preferable. The monoalkylation process may be carried out on a wide variety of aromatic compounds such as benzene, naphthalene, anthracene compounds which may either be substituted or unsubstituted. Substituted unsaturated aliphatic hydrocarbon compounds useful in the process include those having from 8 to 54 carbon atoms and at least one unsaturated or olefinic linkage.

At least 2 mols of the aromatic compound should be employed per mol of the unsaturated aliphatic compound. Use of from 2 to 10 mols of the aromatic compound per mol of the unsaturated aliphatic compound gives good results, however, it is preferred to use from 2.5 to 6 mols of the aromatic per mol of the unsaturated compound. It has been found that at least 2 mols of hydrofluoric acid should be employed per mol of unsaturated aliphatic compound. It is preferred to use from 3 to 15 mols of hydrofluoric acid per mol of unsaturated aliphatic compound.

The desired reaction proceeds very rapidly, usually complete in less than 4 hours, and in many cases a much shorter time can be used. Under optimal conditions, the reaction proceeds to completion in less than 1 hour after the reactants are introduced into the hydrofluoric acid. For example, reaction times of from 30 seconds to 30 minutes may be used. When the reaction is conducted between benzene and oleic acid, even at temperatures slightly below room temperature, a high yield of phenylstearic acid is formed in 30 seconds, and the reaction is substantially complete in from 2 to 5 minutes. The reactants may be introduced separately or simultaneously into the hydrofluoric acid. For batch reactions, it will usually be most convenient to first introduce the aromatic compound, thereby assuring that a large excess of the aromatic compound is always in contact with the unsaturated compound. Therefore, the oleic acid or other unsaturated aliphatic compound can be gradually introduced while stirring the reaction mixtures.

After completion of the reaction, the monoalkylated compound may be recovered in various ways. For example, the reaction mixture can be added to water, and the monoalkylated product extracted from the water into an organic solvent, such as ethyl ether or benzene. The ether and any excess of the aromatic compound can be stripped off by vacuum distillation, leaving the monoalkylated product. In this process, the hydrofluoric acid and the excess aromatic reactant are removed from the crude reaction product by distillation upon the completion of the reaction. The crude reaction product may be further purified by distillation. Excess aromatic reactant and hydrofluoric acid then can be condensed, and returned to the reaction vessel. This procedure is particularly desirable where a large excess of the aromatic reactant and hydrofluoric acid are employed.

Example 1: A 5 liter polyethylene beaker, equipped with a mechanical stirrer and thermocouple, was charged with 616 grams (30.8 mols) of liquid, anhydrous hydrogen fluoride at 0° to -5°C. About 300 grams (3.25 mols) of toluene were added to the hydrogen fluoride. A solution of oleic acid 800 grams (2.83 mols) in 850 grams (9.25 mols) toluene was then added to the reaction mixture at 5° to 15°C. over a 2 to 3 hour period with vigorous stirring. Stirring was continued for an additional hour; then the reaction mixture was poured into 8 liters of cold water. Four liters of ethyl ether were added, the organic layer separated and washed with 1 liter portions of water until the washings were neutral. The ether and excess toluene were stripped off in vacuo to yield 1,017.4 grams (96.0% of theory) of tolylstearic acid as a viscous amber oil.

Analysis — Neutralization equivalent, 365.0 (calculated 374.6). Iodine value, 3.59. Molecular distillation of the crude acid at 167° to 188°C. at 165 to 190μ afforded a 68% yield of pure tolylstearic acid. A fraction boiling at 199° to 251°C./0.5 to 7μ, amounting to 10 to 12%, was also isolated corresponding to methyl phenylene distearic acid.

Example 2: A 5 liter polyethylene beaker, equipped with a mechanical stirrer and thermocouple, was charged with 826 grams (41.3 mols) of liquid, anhydrous hydrogen fluoride at 0° to -5°C. About 200 grams (2.17 mols) of toluene was added to the hydrogen fluoride. A solution of tallow acid

929 grams (3.36 mols) in toluene 595 grams (6.45 mols) was then added to the reaction mixture at 5° to 15°C. over a period of 1 to 8 hours with vigorous stirring. Stirring was continued for 1 hour; then the reaction mixture was poured into 8 liters of cold water. Four liters of ether were added, the organic layer separated and washed with one liter portions of water until the washings were neutral. The ether and excess toluene were stripped off in vacuo to yield 1,060.7 grams of crude tolyltallow acid as a solid. Analysis — Neutralization equivalent, 317.6 (calculated 332.5). Iodine value, 415.

Example 3: A 2 liter polypropylene beaker, equipped with a mechanical stirrer, thermocouple, and addition funnel, was charged with 492 grams (24.6 mols) of liquid, anhydrous hydrogen fluoride and 82.0 grams (0.64 mol) of naphthalene. The mixture was warmed to 16°C. and a warm solution of oleic acid (137 grams, 0.5 mol) and naphthalene (123 grams, 0.95 mol) was added with stirring over a 45 minute period at 16° to 18°C. The addition funnel was then rinsed with 25 ml. of ether and the ether added to the reaction mixture.

Stirring was continued for one hour at 16° to 18°C. after the addition was completed. The reaction mixture was then poured into 8 liters of cold water. Ether (1.5 to 2 liters) was added and the aqueous phase separated. The organic layer was washed several times with 300 ml. portions of water until the washings were neutral. The ether solution was then dried over anhydrous sodium sulfate and stripped under reduced pressure. Excess naphthalene was removed by sublimation in vacuo. Crude naphthylstearic acid was isolated as a viscous amber oil, 177.7 grams (88.4% mass yield). Analysis — Neutralization equivalent 365.5 (calculated 402). Saponification equivalent 368. Iodine value 6.28.

In related work R.H. Potts, N.D. Gordon, and S.H. Shapiro; U.S. Patent 3,564,031; February 16, 1971; assigned to Armour Industrial Chemical Company has proposed a continuous process for monoalkylation of aromatic carbocyclic compounds with unsaturated higher molecular weight aliphatic compounds wherein the aromatic reactant is used as the stripping gas in the recovery stage.

The process comprises substantially continuously and simultaneously introducing into a continuous reaction zone substantially anhydrous substituted unsaturated aliphatic hydrocarbon reactant, substantially anhydrous aromatic reactant at a molar rate of at least 2 mols per mol of aliphatic reactant, and substantially anhydrous hydrogen fluoride at a molar rate of at least 3 mols per mol of aliphatic reactant; mixing the reactants and hydrogen fluoride for a residence time of from 2 to 60 minutes at a temperature of from 0° to 50°C. to form arylated aliphatic products.

The process goes on continuously passing the products, excess aromatic reactant and hydrogen fluoride into a recovery zone having an upper and lower portion, the lower portion maintained at from 100° to 275°C., freeing the product of excess aromatic reactant and hydrogen fluoride. The product is removed from the lower portion of the recovery zone. Excess aromatic reactant and hydrogen fluoride is removed from the upper portion to a separator zone having an upper and lower portion and maintained at from 20° to 30°C. The hydrogen fluoride removed from the lower portion of the separator zone is returned to the reaction zone in an amount of more than 90% recycle. Excess aromatic reactant from the upper portion of the separator zone is removed to the reaction zone in an amount of more than 90% recycle.

Example: Phenylstearic acid, primarily 9(10)-phenylstearic acid, was continuously produced in high yield by the following described process. A vertical reactor containing four peripheral shelves and a blade type agitator between each shelf was continuously charged at the upper portion of the reactor with distilled commercial grade oleic acid having a typical analysis of oleic acid 79%, linoleic acid 4.0%, palmitoleic acid 6.5%, linolenic acid 1.0%, myristoleic acid 1.5%, and 7 to 8% saturated long chain fatty acids at a feed rate of 890 pounds per hour, benzene at a feed rate of 1,250 pounds per hour, and hydrogen fluoride at a feed rate of 320 pounds per hour, all of the feed stock being substantially anhydrous (containing less than 2% water).

The reactor was maintained at a temperature of 41°C. and a pressure of 15 psig. The residence time in the reactor was 20 minutes. The effluent from the bottom of the reactor was passed through a flasher maintained at a temperature of 22°C. and pressure of 1 psig. The largest portion of excess reactant, benzene, and hydrogen fluoride was removed from the flasher overhead and passed through a water condenser into a separator.

The effluent from the bottom of the flash pot containing the product and remainder of excess benzene and hydrogen fluoride was introduced at the midpoint of a trayed stripping column, the lower portion of which was maintained at 135°C., and a pressure of 1 psig. The remainder of the excess benzene reactant, hydrogen fluoride and water was removed from the stripper overhead, through a water condenser to the separator. The desired product was removed from the bottom of the stripper column at a rate of 1,000 pounds per hour. The crude product had the following analysis expressed in percent.

Gas chromatography (GC):	
Unreacted aliphatic compounds	13
Phenylated acids	87

(continued)

Thin layer chromatography (TLC):
    Primarily monoalkylated acid   80
    Dimers   15
    Higher boilers (pitch)   5
Hydrogen fluoride residue   0.94
Water   Trace

The separator was operated at 25°C. to separate the benzene and hydrogen fluoride, 1,025 pounds per hour of benzene being recycled to the reactor and 305 pounds per hour of hydrogen fluoride being recycled to the reactor.

FROM ALCOHOLS AND KETONES

Oxidation Using Platinum Catalyst

P.H. Williams and E.F. Lutz; U.S. Patent 3,407,220; October 22, 1968; assigned to Shell Oil Company has found that finely divided platinum is a highly effective catalyst for the selective oxidation of straight chain primary alcohols, admixed with branched and highly branched alcohols, to the corresponding straight chain carboxylic acids.

According to the process, straight chain primary alcohols containing from 10 to 20 carbon atoms, in admixture with branched chain primary alcohols of like carbon number, are selectively oxidized to the corresponding carboxylic acids by oxidation with molecular oxygen, e.g., air, in the presence of a platinum catalyst, preferably platinum supported on carbon, using an excess of oxygen and superatmospheric pressures, in liquid phase, at temperatures of between 20° and 80°C. High conversions and yields are obtained in short reaction times under mild conditions.

While no specific amount of the platinum catalyst, either supported on carbon or as the oxide, is required for the proper operation of the process, it is generally economically advantageous to limit the platinum content of the catalyst to less than 10 mol percent, based on the amount of alcohol present. Catalysts containing upwards from 0.5 to 10 mol percent platinum have given good results.

The catalyst may be employed in the form of a stationary bed positioned in a suitable reaction zone providing for intimate contact between reactants and catalyst. Suitable reaction zones may comprise one or more chambers of enlarged cross-sectional area, reaction zones of restricted cross-sectional areas, such as tubular reactors, or combinations thereof. The process further lends itself to being carried out with the catalyst slurried in the liquid. The oxidation may be carried out batchwise, or, preferably, continuously. The rate of alcohol oxidation is a function of the oxygen concentration as well as catalyst concentration, and increases with increasing pressure. It has been found that the Pt/C catalyst is preferential to the oxidation of straight chain primary alcohols over branched and highly branched primary alcohols. The rate of oxidation of pure n-dodecyl alcohol is 4 1/2 times faster than that of a mixture of straight chain, branched and highly branched C_{12} alcohols.

While the reaction time for each oxidation will vary with several parameters such as type and concentration of catalyst, pressure, temperature and the particular alcohol mixture being fed into the reaction zone, and while no fixed time limitation can be set for the general oxidation reactions, it is preferred that the reaction be continued until 90%, of the straight chain alcohols, and until not more than 15%, of the branched and highly branched alcohols have been oxidized. The oxidation, in general, is carried out to obtain a product which contains normal and branched acids in a weight ratio 95:5. This process is particularly useful in the selective oxidation of alcohols to corresponding acids in mixtures having a weight ratio of normal to branched chain alcohols of at least 70:30.

Since, in general, a mixed acid product will result from the oxidation of the mixed alcohol feed, it should be noted that an efficient separation of the straight chain acids from the branched and highly branched acids can be made by a simple esterification of the acids with methyl alcohol over an acid catalyst, followed by distillation of the mixture of methyl esters, taking advantage of the differences in boiling points of the straight chain and branched esters. After fractionation, the separated esters can be hydrolyzed back to the corresponding acids, and recovered in pure form.

Example: A series of oxidations was carried out by placing 0.1 mol of the alcohol, catalyst and solvent in a 300 ml. rocking autoclave. The catalyst was activated by hydrogenation at room temperature and 225 psig until hydrogen uptake was complete. (If 10% by weight Pt/C is used, the hydrogenation step can be omitted without detrimental effects; however, PtO_2 is inactive without hydrogenation). The autoclave was vented and then purged several times with nitrogen. Nitrogen was added, the vessel was pressure-tested, and oxygen added until a composition approximating that of air was obtained (i.e., 20 to 25% O_2).

The autoclave was heated and rocked either for a preset time or until the autoclave pressure dropped to a constant value. After the autoclave was cooled, the contents were transferred to a beaker, the autoclave thoroughly washed with excess solvent, and the catalyst removed by filtration. The reaction solution was dried over anhydrous magnesium sulfate and the solvent vacuum-stripped until the residue (reaction product) reached constant weight. The reaction time was determined as the period between the time at which the autoclave reached the desired reaction temperature and the time at which oxygen uptake was complete. Oxygen uptake was measured by the pressure drop in the system. The products were analyzed by determining their neutral equivalents from which the percentages of acid present were calculated. Where analysis of the neutral compounds was desired, the recovered product mixture was analyzed by gas chromatography. This permitted analysis of all of the neutral compounds formed or recovered. The table sets out the data obtained from a series of runs made under the conditions indicated above. The solvent used was n-heptane and the reaction was run at 60°C.

Alcohol	Pressure, psig	Catalyst mol percent (Alcohol Basis)	Time, hr.	Conversion to Acid, percent	Average % conversion/hr.
Branched $C_{12}H_{27}OH$*	390 air (180 O_2)	PtO_2, 4.76	21	46.5	2.2
2-ethyl-1-hexanol	105 O_2	PtO_2, 2	18.5	11.3	0.61
n-Dodecanol	940 air (190 O_2)	10% by wt. Pt/C, 1.0	1.25	66.4	53.1
Mixed $C_{12}H_{25}OH$**	1,010 air (210 O_2)	10% by wt. Pt/C, 1.0	5.67	63.4	11.2

*Mixture of C_{12} branched and highly branched primary alcohols.
**Mixture of branched and highly branched straight chain $C_{11}H_{23}CH_2OH$ alcohols, containing 71% straight chain alcohol.

Oxidation Using Cobalt-Bromine-Carboxylic Acid Catalyst

A.S. Hay; U.S. Patent 3,173,933; March 16, 1965; assigned to General Electric Company has found a general method whereby alkyl, including cycloalkyl alcohols, and ethers, including acetals, can be readily oxidized with oxygen or air to form carbonyl containing compounds. This process, which occurs under moderate reaction conditions, comprises reacting these compounds in a liquid phase with oxygen in the presence of a catalyst soluble in the reaction mixture and consisting essentially of cobalt, bromine and a carboxylic acid.

In carrying out the process, a solution is made of the alkyl compound in a suitable solvent, which also contains dissolved therein a catalyst consisting essentially of cobalt, bromine, and a carboxylic acid. The solvent preferably is the same compound as at least one of the products of the oxidation reaction, or it may be a carboxylic acid forming part of the catalyst system, such as acetic or propionic acid.

The solution in a suitable reaction vessel is heated to reaction temperature. Oxygen is then passed into the reaction mixture at the desired rate for the desired period of time. After the reaction is completed, the oxygenated products are separated from the reaction mixture by conventional methods. The process can be carried out continuously by adding both alkyl compound and oxygen to a solution of the cobalt-bromine-carboxylic catalyst in a solvent. The combination of components in the catalyst is so unique that the substitution of other elements for one or more component either totally stops or substantially impedes the reaction. The atomic ratio of cobalt to bromine is important for maximum reaction rates. Optimum reaction rates are obtained when cobalt and bromine are present in substantially equiatomic amounts.

The molar ratio of the carboxylic acid-to-cobalt has no upper limit with the result that carboxylic acids can be employed as solvents for the reaction. The cobalt constituent of the catalyst is furnished by cobalt compounds in the divalent or trivalent state. Any cobalt salt which is soluble in the solvent employed, in an amount sufficient to form the catalyst and does not introduce interfering ions, is satisfactory for the process. Because of its availability, the preferred source of cobalt is cobaltous acetate tetrahydrate [$Co(OAc)_2 \cdot 4H_2O$] which may be used in conjunction with cobalt bromide.

The bromine constituent of the catalyst is generally furnished by bromine compounds containing bromine capable of being readily removed from the parent compound, i.e., compounds containing a labile bromine atom. Such compounds are precursors of bromine or hydrogen bromide, which is formed during the oxidation reaction to supply the bromine constituent of the catalyst. Specific compounds include the bromocarboxylic acids, cycloaliphatic carboxylic acids containing removable bromine, acid bromides, for example, bromocarbons containing bromine capable of being readily removed from the parent compound, hydrogen bromide, cobalt bromide, etc. One mole of HBr per mol of cobalt acetate produces an extremely active catalyst. The carboxylic acid constituent of the catalyst is generally furnished by carboxylic acids or salts of carboxylic acids.

From the above discussion it is seen that the catalyst constituents can be selected from a wide variety of starting materials. A single compound which would meet all the requirements of the catalyst would be a cobalt salt of both hydrogen bromide and a carboxylic acid, for example cobalt bromide acetate. However, these compounds are not readily available and offer no advantage over a binary mixture of equimolar amounts of a cobalt salt of a carboxylic acid, for example, cobalt acetate, etc., and a bromine compound, for example, cobalt bromide, hydrogen bromide, bromine, etc. All of these would give a ratio of one atom of bromine to one atom of cobalt, i.e., a bromine-to-cobalt ratio of 1, but by varying the proportions in the binary mixture any desired ratio may be obtained.

Ternary mixtures may be used to form the catalyst. For example, cobalt oxides, hydroxides, or carbonates and a bromine compound, for example, hydrogen bromine, cobalt bromide, etc., may be dissolved in a carboxylic acid to produce the catalyst. The rate of oxygen addition to the reaction is also not critical and may vary within any desired limits. Satisfactory results have been obtained adding oxygen to the reaction mixture at the rate of from 0.01 to 10, and preferably from 0.5 to 5 parts by weight of oxygen per hour per part of the alkyl compound. It should be understood that in addition to employing pure oxygen as the oxidizing agent in the process, it is also possible to employ any oxygen-containing gas in which the ingredient other than oxygen is inert under the conditions of the reaction. Thus, satisfactory results have been obtained employing air instead of pure oxygen in the feed gas to the reaction.

Although the process proceeds at a rapid rate at atmospheric pressure, with certain alkyl compounds, it may be desirable to employ subatmospheric or superatmospheric pressures. Because of the low boiling points of some alkyl compounds, for example the low molecular weight alkyl alcohols and ethers, it may be desirable to increase reaction time and/or temperature by the use of superatmospheric pressure. On the other hand, where products are formed which are capable of further reaction, it may be advantageous to use subatmospheric pressure to remove the products as fast as they are formed. The temperature of the reaction of the process may also vary within fairly wide limits. Satisfactory results are obtained when running the reaction at temperatures from 80°C. up to a temperature of 160°C.

Example 1: This example illustrates the oxidation of an alkyl alcohol, the use of benzene as a solvent during the initial part of the reaction and the product of oxidation as the solvent during the latter part of the oxidation and the use of small amounts of acetic acid. A reaction mixture of 150 parts of n-hexanol-1 and 50 parts of benzene, this mixture being 0.15 molal in respect to cobalt and 0.1 molal in respect to bromine [$CoBr_2 \cdot 6H_2O$ and $Co(OAc)_2 \cdot 4H_2O$] was heated to reflux as oxygen at the rate of 84 parts/hour was passed into the reaction mixture for two hours.

The temperature of the reaction rose during the reaction from 89° to 143°C. as benzene was distilled off. The reaction mixture was cooled, dissolved in ether, and the ether solution was washed first with dilute hydrochloric acid and then with dilute aqueous potassium carbonate. The ether solution was then dried and distilled to yield n-hexyl caproate. The aqueous carbonate layer was acidified with dilute hydrochloric acid, extracted with ether, dried and distilled to give caproic acid. Total yield of caproic acid (as acid and ester based on reacted n-hexanol-1) was 97%.

Example 2: This example illustrates the oxidation of n-octanol-1 using acetic acid as a solvent. A reaction mixture of 20.6 parts of n-octanol-1 and 105 parts of acetic acid, the acetic acid being 0.1 molal in respect to cobalt and 0.075 molal in respect to bromine [$Co(OAc)_2 \cdot 4H_2O$ and

HBr], was heated in a closed system to 38°C. as oxygen was passed into the reaction mixture (for two hours) as fast as it was absorbed to yield n-octanoic acid and its ester.

Example 3: This example illustrates the oxidation of an alkyl ether and the use of benzoic acid and the material to be oxidized as a solvent for the reaction. A reaction mixture of 50 parts of benzoic acid, 140 parts of di-n-butyl ether, this reaction mixture being 0.1 molal in respect to both cobalt and bromine [Co(OAc)$_2 \cdot$4H$_2$O and CoBr$_2 \cdot$6H$_2$O] was heated to reflux 130° to 133°C. as oxygen at the rate of 84 parts/hour was passed into the reaction mixture for two hours. The reaction mixture was distilled to yield a mixture of oxygenated products including about a 50% combined yield of butyric acid and butylbutyrate based on reacted di-n-butyl ether.

Example 4: This example illustrates the oxidation of a longer chain secondary alkyl alcohol in acetic acid. A reaction mixture of 5.6 parts of n-heptanol-3 and 105 parts of acetic acid, the acetic acid being 0.1 molal in respect to cobalt and 0.075 molal in respect to bromine [HBr and Co(OAc)$_2 \cdot$4H$_2$O], was heated to 92°C. as oxygen was passed (for 3.5 hours) into a closed system as fast as it was absorbed to yield n-heptanone-3 and butyric acid.

Example 5: This example illustrates the oxidation of a polyfunctional alkyl compound, alkanediol, in acetic acid. A reaction mixture of 26.15 parts of 1,10-decanediol and 105 parts of acetic acid, the acetic acid being 0.1 molal in respect to cobalt and 0.075 molal in respect to bromine [Co(OAc)$_2 \cdot$4H$_2$O and HBr], was heated to 90°C. as oxygen was passed in for 6 hours. From the reaction mixture was recovered acetoxydecanoic acid, 10-hydroxydecanoic acid and sebacic acid.

Cyclic Secondary Alcohols and Caustic

J.H. Bartlett and S.B. Lippincott; U.S. Patent 3,121,728; February 18, 1964; assigned to Esso Research and Engineering Company have found that cyclic secondary alcohols may be fused with caustic to obtain high yields of the corresponding straight chain monocarboxylic acid salts. Thus, for example, the equation for reacting cyclododecanol with caustic is presented below:

$$\begin{array}{l} CH_2-CH_2-CH_2-CH_2-CH_2-CH_2 \\ | | \\ CH_2-CH_2-CH_2-CH_2-CH_2-COH \\ | \\ H \end{array} \xrightarrow{NaOH} CH_3(CH_2)_{10}COONa + H_2$$

The alcohols used in the process are cyclic secondary alcohols, having the formula given below.

$$\left(\begin{array}{c} R \\ \diagdown \\ C \\ \diagup \\ R' \end{array} \right)_n \hspace{-0.3em} \boxed{CHOH}$$

In this formula n is a number from 2 to 30 and each R and R' is radical selected from the group consisting of C_1 to C_{25} alkyl groups and a hydrogen atom. In general the total number of carbon atoms in the alcohol will be in the range of 4 to 60. Examples of these alicyclic secondary alcohols which may be reacted are the unsubstituted cyclic secondary alcohols such as cyclopentanol, cycloheptanol, cyclohexanol, cyclooctanol, cyclodecanol, cyclododecanol, cyclopentadecanol, cycloeicosanol, cyclotriacontanol, etc. Examples of the substituted monocyclic secondary alcohols are nonylcyclohexanol, 2,3- or 4-methylcyclohexanol, or mixed methylcyclohexanols obtained for example by hydrogenation of mixed cresols, etc.

The process is carried out at temperatures in the range of 320° to 350°C. Atmospheric pressure is satisfactory. The caustic alkali materials which may be used are the alkali metal hydroxides and the free alkali metals themselves. In practice, it is desirable to mix the reactants and to heat the resultant mixture until a substantial evolution of hydrogen occurs, as evidenced either by its escape from the reaction zone or by the rate of increase of pressure if the system is closed. The temperature can be either held at this point or increased somewhat if a more rapid rate of reaction is desired. Completion of the reaction will be apparent from the decrease in the rate of hydrogen evolution, at which time approximately the theoretical quantity of gas will be found to have been given off.

The salt of the acid may be recovered from the reaction zone directly or may be purified of unreacted materials by dissolving it in water, or a water C_2 to C_4 alcohol mixture. Thus, the salt of the acid is dissolved in the aqueous solution and is recovered by evaporation or distillation. Further purification may be obtained if desired by contacting the water layer with a light hydrocarbon such as a petroleum ether to remove unreacted alicyclic alcohols or other oil-soluble products. Where the free acid is desired the water-alcohol solution or the caustic fusion product itself may be acidified with a mineral acid, thus springing the monocarboxylic acid which is then separated, by distillation.

Example: A one gallon nickel reactor, equipped with a stirrer, thermometer, feed line and condenser was charged with 300 grams Primol D solvent (i.e., a highly acid treated naphthenic mineral oil having a boiling range between 395° to 520°C.), 108 grams NaOH pellets and 94 grams KOH pellets. After heating the mixture to 320°C., 91 grams of cyclododecanol dissolved in 600 grams of Primol D was added gradually during 45 minutes with the temperature at 320° to 370°C. For most of this period the temperature was at 350° to 360°C. During the course of the reaction 0.6 ft.^{3} of gas were evolved.

After allowing the reactor to cool to 270°C. the product was removed by suction and dispersed in 4 liters of water to which was added 500 cc isopropyl alcohol. This mixture was given three extractions with petroleum ether. The remaining aqueous layer was acidified with HCl and the acid removed by extraction with petroleum ether. On evaporation a residue of 64 grams of crude acid was obtained. The crude acid mixture was then esterified with methanol using toluene sulfonic acid as a catalyst. The ester was washed with 5% NaOH and then with water and then evaporated on the steam bath. The total ester recovered was 51 grams which was distilled through a spinning band column. In the distillation 36.7 grams of product was obtained having a boiling range of 98°C. at 6.5 mm. to 88°C. at 3.5 mm.

The above methyl ester had a saponification number 261.5 mg. KOH/g. (theory 262). Its mass spectrogram showed it to be the methyl ester of a C_{12} acid. The nuclear magnetic resonance showed that there was only one methyl group in addition to the methyl ester grouping and that all the other hydrogen atoms are very similar. Thus the product is the methyl ester of n-dodecanoic acid.

Dicarboxylic Acid from Cyclic Alcohols and Ketones

According to J.O. White and D.D. Davis; U.S. Patent 3,637,832; January 25, 1972; assigned to E.I. du Pont de Nemours and Company a C_8 to C_{12} dicarboxylic acid which can be readily refined to high purity is produced by conducting the oxidation of an alcohol and a ketone with all of the reactants in the liquid phase, and after substantially all of the alcohol and ketone have been oxidized maintaining the oxidate in the liquid phase under oxidizing conditions at a temperature in the range 90° to 110°C. for a time in the range 3 to 60 minutes.

Referring to Figure 3.2, nitric acid and catalyst are introduced into stirred reactor (1) via line (2). The compounds to be oxidized, usually an alcohol and/or a ketone, are introduced via line (3). The gaseous effluent which consists of carbon oxides, nitrogen oxides, water, ketone and small amounts of alcohol and nitric acid are directed to a suitable recovery system via line (4). The liquid is discharged from the reactor (1) into reactor (5) via

FIGURE 3.2: DICARBOXYLIC ACID FROM CYCLIC ALCOHOLS AND/OR KETONES

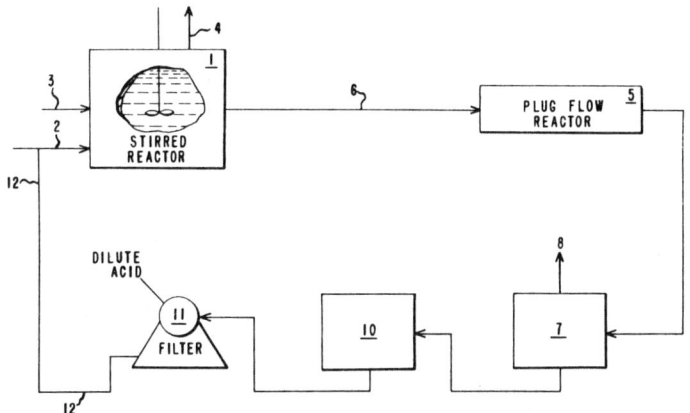

Source: J.O. White and D.D. Davis; U.S. Patent 3,637,832; January 25, 1972

line (6). Reactor (5) is preferably operated under conditions of plug flow. The effluent from reactor (5) is then directed to a gas liquid separator (7) wherein carbon oxides, nitrogen oxides, water and nitric acid are removed via line (8). Liquid is directed towards a crystallizer (10) where most of the acid crystallizes. Solids are removed via filter (11) and the mother liquor is returned to the constant environment reactor (1) via line (12). The nitric acid which is present in the dibasic acid obtained from crystallizer (11) can be removed by washing. The oxidation is conducted at a temperature in the range of 85° to 105°C. and is advantageously operated at pressures of 1 to 2 atmospheres absolute.

Example: To a glass reaction vessel equipped with mechanical agitator, heating and cooling coil, thermometer, reflux condenser and bottom draw-off was charged 10 parts by volume of 55% HNO_3 containing 0.1% vanadium and 0.3% copper by weight. The charge was heated to 98°C. and 1.25 parts by volume of a molten mixture of cyclododecanol-cyclododecanone (approximately 5/1 ratio) was added by dropping funnel at rate of 0.04 part per minute while maintaining the temperature at 98° to 99°C. Upon completion of the addition, the temperature of the mixture was maintained at 98° to 99°C. for two minutes, then the mixture was quickly drained into a crystallization vessel, where the temperature was dropped to 60°C. over a 30 minute period. The resulting slurry was filtered on a suction filter and washed on the filter with 6 parts H$_2$O, followed by slurrying with 10 parts water and refiltering. The final cake was melt extracted twice with 6 parts water per extraction at 120°C., followed by drying at 95° to 100°C. under vacuum. The resulting product was analyzed for color and total nitrogen with the results shown in the table below as Procedure A. The total nitrogen was obtained by known techniques. The color of the acid was determined by reflectance measurements (according to the general procedure of AST D-1925-63T) taken on solid cakes cast from molten acid. This color number can be correlated with the ultimate color of polyamides prepared from the acids.

The preceeding example was repeated with the following modification. Upon completion of addition of the alcohol-ketone, the temperature was immediately raised to 102° to 103°C. and held there for 15 minutes. The product was then treated in exactly the same manner as in Procedure A with the results shown in the table as Procedure B. The cake obtained in Procedure B following water washing on the filter was redissolved in 5.25 parts by volume of 55% nitric acid containing a minor amount of urea, cooled slowly (30 minutes) to 75°C. and filtered. This cake was washed, melt extracted, and dried as in Procedures A and B. The quality is shown in the table as Procedure C.

	Product quality	
	Color	Total nitrogen (p.p.m.)
Procedure:		
A	5.7	469
B	0.96	85.7
C	0	8.3

It should be readily apparent that this process produces an acid which is remarkably superior in color to acid produced by prior art techniques. The acid produced by this process is readily refined to acid of extraordinary high purity especially with respect to color and nitrogenous impurities, two factors which are critical in the manufacture of acceptable polymer from the acid.

Oxidation of Ketene-Ketone Polymers

During the reaction of ketene and carbonyl compounds one can obtain, in the presence of acid or neutral catalysts, low polymeric products of the general formula:

$$\left[\begin{array}{c} R_1 \\ \diagdown \\ \diagup \\ R_2 \end{array} \begin{array}{c} \\ C-CH_2 \\ | | \\ O-CO \end{array} \right]_n$$

In the formula shown on the preceding page R_1 is H, alkyl, cycloalkyl, aryl, aralkyl; R_2 is H, alkyl, cycloalkyl, aryl, aralkyl; and n is 2 to 50.

J. Heckmaier and G. Kunstle; U.S. Patent 3,553,188; January 5, 1971; assigned to Wacker-Chemie GmbH, Germany have found a process for producing saturated carboxylic acids by the catalytic hydrogenation of these low polymeric products. The process is characterized by treating the raw, catalyst-containing low polymeric products, suitably after removal of the excess carbonyl component, under normal pressure and in the liquid phase while continuously increasing the reaction temperature within a range from 50° to 250°C.; with excess, dry hydrogen which is circulated through the reaction zone. A Raney nickel hydrogenation catalyst is used.

According to the process all low polymeric products which are formed during the reaction of ketene with carbonyl compounds, e.g., with formaldehyde, acetaldehyde, propionic aldehyde, n- and isobutyraldehyde, crotonaldehyde, diethylacetaldehyde, capronaldehyde, acetone, methylethylketone, diethylketone, methylisobutylketone, benzaldehyde, n- and p-toluenealdehyde, phenylacetaldehyde, furfurol and acetophenone, can be successfully processed into unsubstituted or substituted propionic acids. For instance, one obtains from: ketene and formaldehyde, propionic acid; ketene and acetaldehyde, n-butyric acid; ketene and propionic aldehyde, n-valerianic acid; and ketene and butyraldehyde, n-capronic acid.

When carrying out the process, the raw low polymeric products are used for hydrogenation after removal of the excess carbonyl compounds, if any. No removal of the catalyst used during the ketene reaction is necessary. Figure 3.3 is a diagrammatic illustration of a system suitable for carrying out the process discontinuously.

Example: The apparatus used consists of a heatable hydrogenation reactor (1) equipped with a stirring mechanism, a condenser (5), a liquid ring pump (7) driven by concentrated sodium hydroxide as the ring liquid, the separator (9) and the drying column (14) which is supplied with sodium hydroxide.

Production of the Low Polymeric Product — 214.2 weight parts of a mixture consisting of 4.2 weight parts tetra-n-butyl titanate and 210 weight parts crotonaldehyde containing 0.1 weight percent of 2,6-di-tert-butyl-p-cresol are reacted with 84 weight parts of gaseous ketene at 90°C. From the resulting reaction product, the excess unconverted crotonaldehyde is withdrawn at 20 torr, and one obtains besides 34 weight parts of crotonaldehyde 264 weight parts of a raw, crotonaldehyde-free and catalyst-containing low polymeric reaction product.

FIGURE 3.3: OXIDATION OF KETENE-KETONE POLYMERS

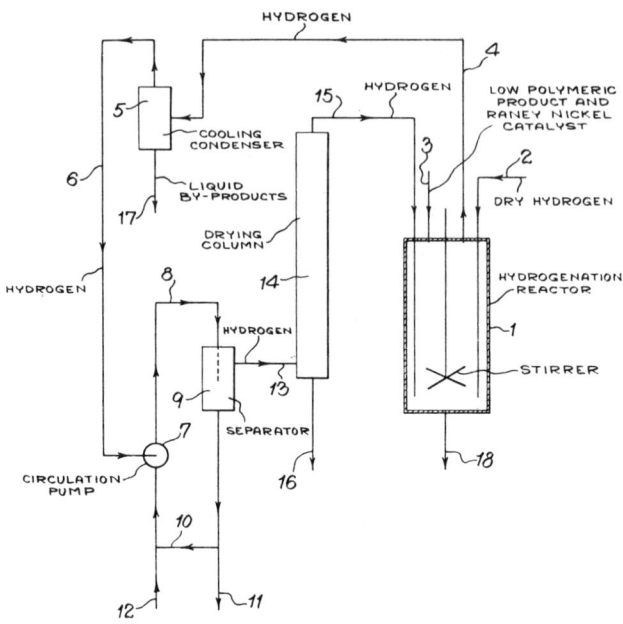

Source: J. Heckmaier and G. Kunstle; U.S. Patent 3,553,188; January 5, 1971

Hydrogenation — 264 weight parts of the reaction product and 6 weight parts of Raney nickel are fed into the hydrogenation reactor (1) through line (3). Under stirring the contents are heated to 80°C. At the same time dry hydrogen in excess quantity is piped in through line (2) and circulated. This is done by means of the liquid ring pump (7) which is driven by a circulating [through line (8), separator (9), and line (10)] concentrated sodium hydroxide as the ring liquid.

By this hydrogen is siphoned in from the hydrogenation reactor (1), piped through line (4) into condenser (5), where the easily volatile, liquid by-products which were created on a small scale in reactor (1) by side reactions, are condensed and sluiced out through line (17). From there the hydrogen is siphoned in through line (6) into the liquid ring pump (7) where carbon dioxide is washed out from the circulating hydrogen gas by concentrated sodium hydroxide. Together with the sodium hydroxide the circulating hydrogen is carried onto the separator (9). In the latter the purified hydrogen can escape from the ring liquid. While the ring liquid is returned through line (10) into the liquid ring pump (7) once more, the hydrogen is first piped to the drying column (14), then through line (15) again into reactor (1). Sodium carbonate-containing sodium hydroxide is sluiced out through line (11). The loss of sodium hydroxide is equalized by adding fresh sodium hydroxide through line (12). Through line (16) one obtains little concentrated sodium hydroxide.

If at a final temperature of 180°C. no more hydrogen is absorbed, the process is shut off and through line (18) first the Raney nickel is withdrawn, and then the hydrogenation product. The latter is subjected to a vacuum fractionation, where one obtains 190.5 weight parts capronic acid (boiling point, 10 torr: 97.0° to 98.5°C., MP: 4.8°C.). The residue remaining after fractionation is hydrogenated again at 160° to 200°C., as described above, and processed. There another 18 weight parts of pure capronic acid are obtained.

FROM DERIVATIVES

Decomposition and Isomerization of Anhydrides

D.M. Fenton; U.S. Patent 3,592,849; July 13, 1971; assigned to Union Oil Company of California has found that when an anhydride, e.g., isobutyric anhydride, is contacted with a Group VIII noble metal in complex with a biphyllic ligand such as triphenylphosphine, the anhydride is decomposed and isomerized to form an alkanoic acid, e.g., normal butyric acid, an olefin and carbon monoxide. In similar fashion, a straight chain anhydride may be converted to a branched chain acid. The reaction proceeds according to the following typical equation:

$$(CH_3)_2CHCOOCOCH(CH_3)_2 \xrightarrow{catalyst} CH_3CH_2CH_2COOH + C_3H_6 + CO$$
isobutyric anhydride → n-butyric acid

or

$$CH_3CH_2CH_2COOCOCH_2CH_2CH_3 \xrightarrow{catalyst} (CH_3)_2CHCOOH + C_3H_6 + CO$$
n-butyric anhydride → isobutyric acid

As is apparent from the above reactions, either the straight chain or the branched chain acid can be formed from the branched chain or straight chain anhydride, respectively. The straight chain acids are the most useful and most valuable products and therefore the process has the greatest utility in decomposing branched chain anhydrides to form the straight chain acid. The catalyst comprises a Group VIII noble metal in complex with a biphyllic ligand. The biphyllic ligand is a compound having at least one atom with a pair of electrons capable of forming a coordinate covalent bond with a metal atom and simultaneously having the ability to accept the electron from the metal, thereby imparting additional stability to the resulting complex. Biphyllic ligands can comprise organic compounds having at least 3 carbons and containing arsenic, antimony, phosphorus or bismuth in a trivalent state. Of these the phosphorus compounds, i.e., the phosphines, are preferred; however, the arsines, stibines and bismuthines can also be employed. In general these biphyllic ligands have the following structure: $E(R)_3$ wherein E is trivalent phosphorus, arsenic, antimony or bismuth; and wherein R is the same or different alkyl, cycloalkyl, or aryl having 1 to 18 carbons. Preferably the ligand is triaryl.

The aryl phosphines and particularly the triarylphosphines (e.g., triphenylphosphine) are preferred because of their greater activity. The Group VIII noble metal may be ruthenium, rhodium, palladium, osmium, iridium or platinum. A catalytic quantity of the metal is added (e.g., 0.002 to 2% of the reaction medium) and the metal may be added as a soluble salt, a carbonyl, a hydride or as a chelate.

The Group VIII metal may be complexed with the above described biphyllic ligand before being introduced into the reaction medium or the complex may be formed in situ by simply adding a compound of the metal and the biphyllic ligand directly into the reaction medium. In either case, it is generally preferable that the quantity of biphyllic ligand be in excess (e.g., 10 to 300%) of that stoichiometrically required to form a complex with the Group VIII metal. The complex has from 1 to 5 mols of biphyllic ligand per atom of the metal and other components such as hydride, or soluble anions such as sulfate, nitrate, C_1 to C_5 carboxylates (e.g., acetate, propionate, isobutyrate, valerate, etc.), halide, etc. may be included in the complex catalyst.

These components may be incorporated in the catalyst by the formation of the catalyst complex from a Group VIII metal salt of the indicated anions. Preferably the complex includes at least one halide, e.g., chloride, iodide or bromide or a carboxylate since these ligands improve the activity of the catalyst. The reaction is performed under liquid phase conditions and can be performed in the presence of a liquid organic solvent having a solvency for the reactants and the catalyst and inert to the reactants and/or products under the reaction conditions. Suitable solvents include for example, hydrocarbons, ketones and ethers.

The reaction is performed at relatively low temperatures from 150° to 250°C.; and at low pressures, e.g., 1 to 10 atmospheres on an absolute basis), sufficient to maintain liquid reaction conditions. The decomposition releases carbon monoxide and therefore pressure will increase with time.

Suitable pressure controlling devices may be used to maintain a constant pressure. The reaction may be carried out in a batch or in a continuous process.

Example: Into a bomb were introduced 50 ml. of isobutyric anhydride, 0.5 gram palladium chloride and 3 grams of triphenylphosphine. The bomb was purged with nitrogen, pressured with carbon monoxide to 8 atmospheres and heated to and maintained at 200°C. for 6 hours. The bomb was then cooled, depressured and opened. The products were analyzed by gas chromatography to reveal that 9.5 grams of n-butyric acid and some isobutyric acid were formed in the process. When the reaction is repeated in the presence of 150 ml. heptane as an inert reaction solvent, similar results are obtained.

3,3-Disubstituted Acids from Lactones

In this process A.J. Lundeen; U.S. Patent 3,308,155; March 7, 1967; assigned to Continental Oil Company relates to a general method for preparing 3,3-disubstituted carboxylic acids in which the 3 position substituents are monovalent hydrocarbon radicals by reaction of a β-lactone with tri(monovalent hydrocarbon radical) aluminum. In another aspect, the process relates to preparation of 3,3-disubstituted valeric acids by reaction of a β,β-disubstituted propiolactone with triethylaluminum. It was found that trialkylaluminum reacts with a 3,3-disubstituted carboxylic acid according to the equation:

$$Al(R_3)_3 + \begin{array}{c} R_1 \\ | \\ R_2-C-O \\ | \\ H_2-C-C=O \end{array} \longrightarrow \begin{array}{c} R_1 \quad O \\ | \quad \| \\ R_3-C-CH_2-C\,O\,Al(R_3)_2 \\ | \\ R_2 \end{array}$$

where R_1 and R_2 are monovalent hydrocarbon radicals of identical or differing structure, and R_3 is alkyl. The aluminum salt reaction product can then be hydrolyzed to the corresponding 3,3-disubstituted carboxylic acid. The reaction has general applicability to 3,3-disubstituted propiolactones where the 3 position substituents are of monovalent hydrocarbon radicals including such groups as alkyl, aryl, alkaryl, alkenyl, cycloalkyl and aralkyl. Use of triethylaluminum will results in formation of the corresponding 3,3-disubstituted valeric acid, while other trialkylaluminum compounds will produce other 3,3-disubstituted acids. Although the triethyl compound is preferred because of its availability, the trialkyl compound can contain up to 10 carbons per alkyl group, and can be either branched or straight chain.

As to the 3,3-disubstituted propiolactone, the only limitations when both R_1 and R_2 are alkyl are availability and ability to find a suitable solvent. However, when either R_1 or R_2 contains a ring structure, i.e., when either of R_1 or R_2 is selected from the group consisting of aryl, alkaryl, aralkyl and cycloalkyl, it is preferred that the total carbons in both substituents be at most 15, and that the other substituents be selected from either alkyl or alkenyl.

The reaction between the lactone and the trialkylaluminum is preferably carried out in an inert solvent or diluent for the reactants, such as, e.g., toluene, xylene, benzene, heptane, hexane, isooctane or kerosene. Reaction pressure need only be sufficient to maintain liquid phase, and atmospheric pressure usually suffices, depending on choice of solvent or diluent. The reactants are preferably maintained under an inert atmosphere such as nitrogen or helium in order to prevent oxidation of the trialkylaluminum.

The reaction is preferably carried out between -80° and 100°C., and more preferably between -80° and 0°C. Although the lactone is preferably added to the trialkylaluminum, the reverse addition is also operable. Rate or addition need be controlled only to maintain reaction temperature within the desired range, since the reaction proceeds rapidly. Stirring of the reactants is preferred in order to ensure intimate contact.

The crude reaction product, which comprises the carboxylic acid aluminum salt together with any unreacted starting material in the solvent or diluent, can be treated in known manner for recovery of the purified acid product. For example, the acid salt can first be hydrolyzed by adding a mineral acid such as hydrochloric or sulfuric acid. The carboxylic acid thus formed can then be extracted from the organic reaction product phase by contact with a solvent for the carboxylic acid which is immiscible with the crude product phase, such as an aqueous alkali metal hydroxide solution, e.g., aqueous NaOH.

After phase separation, the aqueous phase contains the corresponding alkali metal salt of the carboxylic acid. The aqueous salt solution can then be evaporated to dryness, or alternatively, again hydrolyzed to the corresponding carboxylic acid by addition of mineral acid. Extraction of the resulting aqueous carboxylic acid solution with an immiscible solvent for the carboxylic acid, such as ether or a liquid paraffin, results in an organic solution of the desired carboxylic acid.

Example 1: Toluene in the amount of 150 ml. and triethylaluminum in the amount of 15 ml. were placed in a dry 500 ml. flask. The flask was fitted with a dropping funnel containing 10.2 grams of 3-isovalerolactone (3,3-dimethyl propiolactone) and 100 ml. of toluene. The contents of the dropping funnel were added to the flask with stirring over a period of 70 minutes, during which time the reaction mixture was maintained at -24°C.

and ±2°C. At the outset of the reaction, the flask was flushed with dry nitrogen, and all subsequent operations were conducted under an inert atmosphere of dry nitrogen. At the expiration of the 70 minute addition period, the reaction mixture was hydrolyzed by the addition of 100 ml. of 30% sulfuric acid. The organic acid produced upon hydrolysis was isolated from the reaction mixture by extracting the solution with an aqueous potassium hydroxide solution.

The aqueous potassium hydroxide solution was then acidified with dilute sulfuric acid to convert the potassium valerate to the valeric acid. The valeric acid thus obtained was completely removed from the aqueous phases by an ether extraction. The ether extraction was then removed by distillation under reduced pressure to yield 11.3 grams of product. Gas chromatographic analysis of this product, in addition to a neutralization equivalent determination indicated that the product was approximately 80.0% C_7 carboxylic acid. This yield of the C_7 acid amounted to 68% of theory. The C_7 acid was identified as 3,3-dimethyl valeric acid by conversion to its amide derivative (MP, 77° to 78°C.), and to its anilide derivative (MP, 101° to 102°C.).

Example 2: The procedure of Example 1 is followed, except that instead of 3-isovalerolactone, there is used a stoichiometric amount of 3-phenyl-3-isopropyl propiolactone. Dilute hydrochloric acid is used for hydrolysis, and aqueous sodium hydroxide is used for extraction of the carboxylic acid as its salt. Acidification of the sodium salt solution and subsequent ethanol extraction produces 3-phenyl-3-isopropyl valeric acid.

Example 3: The procedure of Example 2 is followed, except that instead of 3-phenyl-3-isopropyl propiolactone there is used, 3-p-tolyl-3-vinyl propiolactone, and in place of triethylaluminum there is used tri-n-heptyl aluminum; 3-p-tolyl-3-vinyl capric acid is recovered.

Example 4: The procedure of Example 2 is followed, except that instead of 3-phenyl-3-isopropyl propiolactone there is used 3-cyclo hexyl-3-benzyl propiolactone; 3-cyclo hexyl-3-benzyl valeric acid is recovered.

Hydrolysis of Nitriles

The hydrolysis of nitriles to carboxylic acids is well-known to readily occur with strong acids such as hydrochloric or sulfuric acid in which the nitrile is partially soluble. When the organic portion of the nitrile is fairly large, about 5 or more carbon atoms, the nitrile becomes only slightly soluble, even at high temperatures. Consequently, the hydrolysis of such long chain nitriles must be conducted at relatively high reaction temperatures (greater than 150°C.) or for long periods of time (24 or more hours).

Under these conditions side reactions occur which lower the purity and yield of the carboxylic acid produced. Hydrolysis of nitriles with aqueous hydrochloric acid is difficult because the nitrile is even less soluble in aqueous hydrochloric acid than in sulfuric acid, and in addition the hydrochloric acid has a tendency to evaporate from the reaction mixture so that the practical operating temperature is only 60° to 70°C. at atmospheric pressure.

C.M. Starks; U.S. Patent 3,542,822; November 24, 1970; assigned to Continental Oil Company has unexpectedly found that the use of an organic soluble strong acid such as a sulfonic acid, a F, Cl or NO_2 substituted carboxylic acid, or a phosphonic acid catalyzes the nitrile hydrolysis such that aqueous hydrochloric acid or aqueous sulfuric acid can be used to hydrolyze nitriles having 5 or more carbon atoms. The nitriles suitable for use as starting materials include:

(a) 1-cyanoalkanes such as RCN, where R has at least 5 carbons. There is essentially no upper limit on the number of carbon atoms; however, the larger the number of carbon atoms the greater the amount of organic acid catalyst required;

(b) branched chain alkyl cyanides,

$$R-\underset{\underset{CN}{|}}{C}H-R'$$

where R + R' total at least 5 carbons;

(c) aryl cyanides and aralkyl cyanides such as phenyl acetonitrile and phenyl acetonitriles substituted in the phenyl group or at the benzyl carbon;

(d) alkoxy propionitriles, $ROCH_2CH_2CN$, such as those prepared by addition of alcohols to acrylonitrile; and

(e) di- and polycyano compounds such as succino nitrile, adiponitrile, o-, m-, and p-di-cyanobenzene, telomers and polymers of acrylonitrile and methacrylonitrile.

The organic acid catalysts found suitable for this process include:

(a) sulfonic acids RSO_3H,
(b) substituted carboxylic acids $R-CX_2CO_2H$ and $R-CHXCO_2H$, where X is F, Cl, NO_2, etc., and
(c) phosphonic acids

$$R\underset{\searrow O}{P(OH)_2}$$

The R groups may be alkyl, aryl, aralkyl or other radicals, just as long as it is of sufficient composition to make the catalyst soluble in the organic phase of the reaction mixture. Sulfonic acids which can be used include alkylbenzene sulfonic acids such as dodecylbenzene sulfonic acid and heavy alkylbenzene sulfonic acids such as those used in the manufacture of oil-soluble detergents.

Substituted carboxylic acids which can be used include those wherein the substituents increase the pKa of the acid. Such substituents may be F, Cl, NO_2, COOH, or other electron withdrawing groups. Specific examples are α,α-dichlorocarboxylic acids, α,α-difluorocarboxylic acids, α-fluorocarboxylic acids, and alkyl substituted succinic or maleic acids. Phosphonic acids which can be used include alkyl or aryl phosphonic acids or polyphosphonic acids where the alkyl group is big enough to make the acid organic soluble.

The aqueous acid concentration range suitable for this process is from 5 to 100% acid. The most desirable concentration will depend on the particular acid used. For example, with hydrochloric acid the higher the concentration the lower the boiling point, the lower the solubility of by-product ammonium chloride will be in the acid and the more corrosive the acid will be.

For hydrochloric acid the most desirable concentration is 20 to 30% HCl in water. For sulfuric acid, the boiling point is high enough that this is not a factor, but corrosiveness is. Moreover, concentrated sulfuric acid, particularly hot sulfuric acid, promotes a number of side reactions which will lower the product yield. For sulfuric acid the most desirable concentration is 5 to 20% H_2SO_4 in water. It is to be noted that the aqueous acid concentration does not affect the rate of hydrolysis of nitriles since the hydrolysis reaction takes place in the organic phase or at the organic aqueous interface.

The organic acid catalyst concentration range is 0.01 to 25%. The most desirable range depends on how fast the reaction needs to be. The higher the catalyst concentration the faster the reaction will proceed. Temperatures can vary between 25° and 200°C., depending on catalyst type and on ease of nitrile hydrolysis. Preferred temperature is typically 100°C. to get rapid rate of reaction but still avoiding unwanted side reactions.

The reaction times can vary over a fairly wide range depending on all the other factors such as organic acid concentration, reaction temperature and on the particular material being hydrolyzed. This reaction time normally ranges between 0.1 to 10 hours. The following example illustrates a typical reaction using the method of this process.

Example: A mixture of 50 grams of 1-cyanodecane and 100 ml. of 37% hydrochloric acid in water was heated under reflux (65°C.) and stirring for a total of 7 hours. During this time samples were withdrawn from the organic layer and examined by infrared spectroscopy. No reduction in the nitrile band absorbance (at 2,250 cm.$^{-1}$) and no appearance of a carbonyl band (expected at 1,700 cm.$^{-1}$) was observed, indicating that no hydrolysis of the nitrile to carboxylic acid had taken place.

Two and one-tenth grams of a sulfonic acid (prepared by alkylation of benzene with C_{12} to C_{14} chloroparaffins, followed by sulfonation to produce an alkylbenzene sulfonic acid) was added to the reaction mixture and refluxing was continued as above. After one hour approximately 50% of the nitrile had been hydrolyzed to undecanoic acid as determined by infrared spectra. After four hours all of the nitrile had been hydrolyzed as determined by the complete disappearance of the CN band at 2,250 cm.$^{-1}$, and the appearance of a large band at 1,705 cm.$^{-1}$, and the broad band at 2,800 to 3,200 cm.$^{-1}$, characteristic of carboxylic acids. Distillation of the product gave undecanoic acid, boiling point 135° to 140°C. at 1 mm. Hg pressure.

Thus, in the example it is shown that refluxing a mixture of 1-cyanodecane and hydrochloric acid for seven hours produces no hydrolysis of the nitrile; however, after the addition of a catalytic amount of nitrile-soluble sulfonic acid, the hydrolysis is complete in four hours.

FROM SULFATES AND SULFONATES

Oxidation of Alkyl Sulfuric Acids

J. Kamlet; U.S. Patent 3,261,856; July 19, 1966; assigned to The Procter & Gamble Company has developed a process for the production of aliphatic monocarboxylic acids from alkyl sulfuric acids and their salts. More particularly, it is a process whereby aliphatic monocarboxylic acids, containing from 2 to 21 carbon atoms, are produced from the sulfation products of relatively inexpensive and plentiful raw materials, for example, the alpha olefins. The process involves the following steps:

(1) Reacting alpha olefins, or mixtures thereof, containing 8 to 22 carbon atoms with sulfuric acid or other sulfating reagent in a conventional manner to result in a reaction product consisting primarily of alkyl sulfuric acids having the sulfuric acid ester group attached to the second carbon atom (2-alkylsulfuric acids).

(2) Treating the alkyl sulfuric acid reaction product of step (1), or the water-soluble salts thereof formed by neutralization with water-soluble hydroxides, with an oxidizing reagent, for example, nitric acid, with or without the addition of oxidizing catalysts, whereby the alkyl sulfuric acids are cleaved and oxidized to result in a mixture of aliphatic monocarboxylic acids together with by-products which may include nitrogenous compounds when HNO_3 is used as the oxidizing reagent.

(3) Recovering the aliphatic monocarboxylic acids, together with any nitrogenous compounds formed in step (2), by conventional distillation or extraction procedures and, if nitrogen containing by-products are produced in step (2) and their removal is desired, removing them by, for example, digesting the crude monocarboxylic acid products with hydrochloric acid or another nonoxidizing mineral acid at advanced temperatures.

Suitable sources for the terminal or alpha olefin raw materials for use in the first step are the cracked products of branched or straight chain paraffins. The olefin raw materials can also be obtained from the polymerization of ethylene in the presence of organo-aluminum catalysts. The isomerization route for the conversion of higher internal olefins to lower terminal olefins via the organoborane route also provides suitable alpha olefin raw materials.

Conventional methods with any convenient sulfating agent can be employed to carry out the sulfation of the terminal olefins. For practical and economic reasons, however, sulfuric acid is preferred as the sulfating agent. Also, a sulfation procedure which maximizes the 2-alkyl sulfuric acid content of the sulfation product is preferable, if an optimum yield of fatty monocarboxylic acids is desired. The second step of the process, the oxidation step, can be carried out by adding the alkyl sulfuric acids to an agitated aqueous solution of nitric acid having a concentration between 25 and 35%, with or without the presence of a water miscible, nonreactive solvent.

Although the oxidation reaction will take place in the absence of catalysts, copper, manganese dioxide, ammonium vanadate, benzoyl peroxide, vanadium pentoxide, cobaltic oxide, and mixtures thereof are effective when employed in amounts between 0.005 and 5.0% based on the weight of the alkyl sulfuric acids entering into the oxidizing reaction. These catalysts increase the yield of monocarboxylic acids, decrease the nitrogen content of the monocarboxylic acid products and render any nitrogen containing by-products more susceptible to removal. Of the catalysts enumerated above, a combination of 0.75% of powdered copper together with 0.25% of ammonium vanadate based on the weight of the alkyl sulfuric acids has particular advantage and 1.2% of vanadium pentoxide on the same basis is most desirable. The alkyl sulfuric acids are added to the agitated nitric acid oxidizing solutions at such a rate that the temperature is 80° to 115°C. After completion of the oxidation, recovery of desired monocarboxylic acids is effected; the liquid reaction mass can be allowed to stratify and separate into:

(1) A lower aqueous layer, containing short chain, water-soluble monocarboxylic acids, any excess oxidizing agent, the catalyst, water-soluble side products, and
(2) an organic layer, containing fatty water-insoluble monocarboxylic acids and water-insoluble by-products. Both of these product layers may contain small and variable amounts of nitrogenous materials.

A water-miscible, nonreactive solvent diluent, for example, dimethyl sulfoxide, can be added to the reaction mass to promote oxidation and to suppress nitration. The use of a solvent diluent can also have the effect of trapping nitrogen-containing by-products in the aqueous layer. Therefore, the addition of water-miscible, nonreactive solvents provides a means of reducing the nitrogen content of the fatty monocarboxylic acid product.

Since the presence of nitrogen compounds in the product monocarboxylic acids may be detrimental to certain properties including the odor and color stability of products in which they are subsequently used, precautions are taken to minimize formation of nitrogen compounds. If the separation of nitrogen compounds from the product monocarboxylic acids is desired, they can be removed by hydrolysis with hydrochloric acid at elevated temperatures. In general the preferred process consists of hydrolyzing the nitrogenous compounds in the crude acids with hydrochloric acid having a concentration of 20 to 40% at temperatures of up to 250°C. for periods of 2 to 8 hours.

Example 1: An aqueous slurry containing approximately 22% by weight of the sodium salts of C_{12} alkyl sulfuric acids derived from C_{12} alpha olefin was added slowly, over a period of 155 minutes, to an aqueous solution containing 30% by weight of nitric acid. The nitric acid solution was preheated to a temperature of 80°C. The initial volume of the nitric acid solution was such that one mol of the alkyl sulfuric acid salts was added per 11.5 mols of nitric acid, and the addition was made at a rate which maintained the oxidation temperature at 80°C. A catalyst, consisting of 0.54% of powdered copper together with 0.18% of ammonium vanadate based on the weight of the alkyl sulfuric acid salts, was added to the aqueous solution of nitric acid prior to adding the alkyl sulfuric acid salts. Mechanical agitation and refluxing were provided during the oxidation and 11.5 mols of additional nitric acid per mol of alkyl sulfuric acid solution were added to the reaction mass as an aqueous solution containing 70% by weight of nitric acid to maintain the nitric acid concentration above 20%. The oxidation was terminated when gas evolution ceased, and the product, recovered as a fatty acid containing water-insoluble upper layer after stratification of the reacted mixture, exhibited an acid value of 226 and a nitrogen content of 1.56%. Water-soluble short chain length monocarboxylic acids were present in the lower aqueous phase. The molar yield of water-insoluble fatty monocarboxylic acid was 54.5% based on the mols of alkyl sulfuric acid salts entering the reaction.

In another run, under substantially the same conditions as those of the process of Example 1 above, with the exception of the oxidation temperature, which was 100°C. and the addition time of the alkyl sulfuric acid salts which was 45 minutes, the fatty acid containing water-insoluble layer had an acid value of 240 and a nitrogen content of 1.53%. The molar yield of the water-insoluble fatty monocarboxylic acids in this run was 62.4% based on the mols of alkyl sulfuric acid salts entering the reaction. The fatty acids produced by the process of Example 1 are useful in the production of soap for detergent purposes.

Example 2: A mixture containing equal parts, by weight, of the sodium salts of C_{14} and C_{16} alpha olefin was added slowly, over a period of approximately 25 minutes, to an aqueous solution of nitric acid having a 30% concentration. The initial volume of the nitric acid solution was such that one mol of the alkyl sulfuric acid salt mixture was added per 7 mols of nitric acid at a rate which maintained the oxidation temperature at 100°C.

During the oxidation, approximately 9 mols of additional 70% nitric acid were added per mol of alkyl sulfuric acid salts. The water-insoluble products recovered as a fatty acid-containing water-insoluble upper layer after termination of the oxidation and stratification of the reacted mixture exhibited an acid value of 176, an hydroxyl value of 58 and a nitrogen content of 1.46%. The substitution of the sodium salts of C_{22} alkyl sulfuric acids derived from C_{22} alpha olefin in the process of this example results in the formation of monocarboxylic acids containing from 2 to 21 carbon atoms.

Hydroxyalkane- and Alkenesulfonates

The process developed by D.N. De Mott; U.S. Patent 3,471,535; Oct. 7, 1969; assigned to The Procter & Gamble Company relates to conversion of hydroxyalkanesulfonates, alkenesulfonates, and mixtures thereof to carboxylates of one less carbon atom than the starting material. More specifically, this process relates to the reaction of a strong base with a sulfonate containing a hydroxyl group or a double carbon-to-carbon bond, to form a carboxylate of one less carbon atom than the sulfonate starting material.

Specific examples of hydroxyalkanesulfonates and alkenesulfonates which can be used in the process include the following: lithium 2-hydroxyoctadecanesulfonate, lithium 4-pentadecenesulfonate, potassium 3-hydroxydodecanesulfonate, and sodium 4-hydroxyeicosanesulfonate. These compounds can be prepared in a variety of ways. The 2-hydroxyalkanesulfonates can be made from sodium sulfite and either 1,2-halohydrins, 2,1-bromohydrins, or 1,2-epoxides.

In addition to hydroxyalkanesulfonate or alkenesulfonate, the process requires a strong base. Strong inorganic bases, such as lithium hydroxide, potassium hydroxide, and sodium hydroxide can be used, and are preferred; but strong organic bases such as potassium tert-butoxide, $KOC(CH_3)_3$, can also be used. The use of an anhydrous base is not required; concentrated aqueous base of 85% or higher concentration can also be used.

According to the process, compounds as described above are heated for 30 minutes to 1 hour to a temperature of 285° to 300°C. The reaction can be carried out under an atmosphere of air or an inert gas such as argon or nitrogen; it is preferred to exclude oxygen, in order to increase the yield. The molar ratio of strong base to hydroxyalkanesulfonate or alkenesulfonate can vary from 1:1 to 20:1, 15:1 to 20:1 is preferred.

The products (carboxylic salts and dienes) can be purified by conventional means to yield pure carboxylic acids. Since the commonest starting materials will be derived from naturally occurring sources, and therefore will have even numbers of carbon atoms, and since this process yields carboxylic acid salts having one less carbon atom than the starting material, the usual product will be a carboxylic acid salt having an odd number of carbon atoms. This process, therefore, represents a novel and convenient route to carboxylic acids having an odd number of carbon atoms.

Example 1: In a mortar and pestle, 5.0 grams of sodium 2-hydroxyhexadecanesulfonate and 15 grams of anhydrous potassium hydroxide pellets were thoroughly ground together. This gave a ratio of 17 mols base per mol of sulfonate. The mixture was then poured into a 50 ml. stainless steel standard taper flask, which was equipped with a distillation head and gas flushing tube. The apparatus was flushed with argon for 5 minutes and immersed in a Woods' metal bath at 300°C. for 30 minutes. During this time a slow stream of argon was passed through the system. After 3 minutes a white vapor appeared in the condenser followed by distillation of two immisicible liquids after 7 minutes. The flask was cooled to room temperature and the contents dissolved in 500 ml. of distilled water. The water layer was extracted twice with 500 ml. portions of pentane, acidified to pH 1 with concentrated hydrogen chloride and reextracted with pentane to yield 1.83 grams (50% yield) of crude pentadecanoic acid, identified by gas-liquid chromatography comparison of the methyl ester with an authentic sample of methyl pentadecanoate. 1.30 grams of a diene of the formula $C_{16}H_{30}$ were also obtained. The product, purified and obtained in the form of a carboxylic acid, can be converted back into a pure salt, useful as a soap or emulsifier, as described above; or into acyl chloride, esters, amides, alcohols, etc.

Example 2: A mixture of alkenesulfonates and hydroxyalkanesulfonates was prepared according to the method of Lambert et al, reported in J. Chem. Soc. (London) 1949, 46. This mixture contained 85% alkenesulfonates, of which most comprised potassium 2-hexadecenesulfonate, and 15% hydroxyalkanesulfonates, which was mostly a mixture of potassium 2-, 3-, and 4-hydroxyhexadecanesulfonates. Twenty-five grams of this mixture and 9 grams of potassium tert-butoxide (molar ratio of base to sulfonate 1.2:1), together with 50 ml. of tert-butyl alcohol were combined in a glass autoclave liner. The components were placed in an autoclave under a nitrogen atmosphere for 6 hours at 150°C.

After cooling, the reaction mixture was dissolved in 500 ml. of water, and the water solution was extracted with three 250 ml. portions of diethyl ether. Water and ether were evaporated on a steam bath, and the solution was then extracted with acetone and filtered. The soluble portion of the solids left upon evaporation of acetone was then dissolved in a 20% ethanol-80% water solution. This ethanol-water solution was then acidified to pH 3 with HCl, causing a precipitate to form. The precipitate was then washed into a flask with acetone, and the acetone was evaporated to yield 3.8 grams of pentadecanoic acid, identified (1) by methyl esterification and gas-liquid chromatographic comparison with known methyl pentadecanoate, and (2) by elemental analysis.

FROM NATURAL SOURCES

Seed Oils

K.L. Mikolajczak; U.S. Patent 3,217,046; November 9, 1965; assigned to the U.S. Secretary of Agriculture has found the presence of large amounts of an industrially attractive fatty acid constituent, namely cis-11-eicosenoic acid, in heretofore uncultivated or rarely cultivated plants. It is present in the seed oils of two unique members of the Cruciferae family, namely Alyssum maritimum (also known as Lobularia maritima) and in Selenia grandis and in the seed oil of an entirely unique member of the family Compositae, namely Marshallia caespitosa. By oxidatively cleaving cis-11-eicosenoic acid per se or the methyl ester of cis-11-eicosenoic acid, each obtained from the seed oils it is possible to prepare undecanedioic acid as well as nonanoic (pelargonic) acid and the corresponding methyl esters in advantageous yields.

Example: Isolation of cis-11-Eicosenoic Acid from Marshallia Seed — Ground Marshallia seed (52.6 grams) was Soxhlet-extracted overnight with petroleum ether (BP 30° to 60°C.). The solvent was removed in vacuo with a rotary evaporator, yielding 11.99 grams of Marshallia seed oil. A portion of the oil (8.90 grams) was saponified by refluxing with 1 N ethanolic potassium hydroxide under nitrogen for 1 1/2 hours. The saponification mixture was extracted with ethyl ether, yielding 0.48 gram of unsaponifiable material. The alkaline liquor was acidified and reextracted with ethyl ether, yielding 7.70 grams of mixed fatty acids. A large aliquot of the mixed fatty acids (6.8 grams) was esterified by refluxing for 2 hours with methanol containing 1% sulfuric acid; 6.4 grams of mixed methyl esters (94.1% yield) was obtained.

The mixed methyl esters were fractionally distilled through a spinning band column. Distillation conditions and the weights of collected fractions are shown in the table below. The vacuum in the spinning band apparatus was released each time a fraction was removed from the collector, but the column was operated at total reflux for some time before each collection. The head temperatures given in the table were obtained at total reflux and at the end of the collection.

Distillation of Mixed Methyl Esters

Fraction	Marshallia Caespitosa		
	Head Temp., °C.	Pressure, mm. Hg	Weight, grams
1	131 to 135	0.35	1.630
2	135	0.35	0.750
3	135 to 137	0.30	0.180
4	138 to 140	0.30	0.200
5	140 to 141	0.30	0.190
6	141 to 142	0.30	0.140
7	143 to 144	0.30	0.150
8	144	0.30	0.410
9	144	0.30	0.370
10	144 to 145	0.30	0.230
11	145 to 147	0.30	0.225
12	147 to 148	0.20	0.440
13	148 to 153	0.20	0.470
14	153 to 157	0.20	0.650

GLC analysis of selected fractions showed that fractions 9, 10, and 11 were substantially pure and could be combined for identification. Accordingly, a 0.13 gram portion of combined fractions 9 to 11 was saponified, acidified, and then extracted with ethyl ether. Upon removal of the solvent there remained 0.12 gram of a viscous colorless liquid. After three recrystallizations from freshly redistilled acetone at -18°C., cis-11-eicosenoic acid melting at 21.0° to 22.5°C. was obtained.

Steam Hydrolysis of Fats

There exist numerous processes for the hydrolyzing of fats and oils. For example, one of the oldest processes is an alkali saponification to make soap. Subsequently, other processes were developed involving the catalytic hydrolysis of fats to fatty acids using certain chemicals or reagents such as the Twitchell reagent. However, in all of these processes, liquid water, usually under great pressures to maintain it in a liquid state is reacted with the fat at high temperatures.

One recognized commercial process requires pressures of approximately 800 psi, a temperature of 300°C. and a two hour residence time in a countercurrent reactor tower in order to carry out the hydrolysis reaction. This process gives glycerine-water effluent and fat effluent streams. Because of the relatively high pressures required in such processes, the apparatus required for carrying out such processes is relatively expensive to fabricate and maintain. Also, as can be seen from the above, such processes require relatively long residence times which limits the production from the apparatus. The high pressures, long residence times and high temperatures all contribute to excessive operational costs.

K.E. Lunde; U.S. Patent 3,253,007; May 24, 1966; assigned to Carad Corporation have provided a process and apparatus for the hydrolysis of fats and oils which will overcome the above named disadvantages. The fat or oil to be hydrolyzed is introduced into a reactor in either solid or liquid form. The solid or liquid fat is then heated to a temperature ranging from 150° to 350°C. so that it is in a liquid phase. The liquid phase is then perturbed with a gaseous phase which can be in the form of superheated steam.

The gaseous phase, while passing through the reactor, perturbs the liquid phase or phases and thereby induces extreme turbulence in the liquid phase which is also passing through the tubular reactor to provide a greatly increased rate of molecular collisions within the liquid phase and also to greatly increase the interfacial area between the liquid and gaseous phases, allowing reactions to proceed rapidly. This process can be carried out at relatively low pressures and is preferably carried out at or near atmospheric

166 Fatty Acids

pressure or in vacuo. The liquid fat phase is maintained at a temperature ranging from 150° to 350°C. so that the reaction, e.g., hydrolysis, occurs at a very rapid rate. At or near atmospheric pressure, the reaction product, e.g., the fatty acid and glycerine, is volatilized into the vapor phase from which it can be readily isolated in purified form.

The apparatus shown in Figure 3.4a consists of a reactor (10) which is in the form of a relatively long tube (11) of a suitable material such as stainless steel. The tube (11) is covered with a heating jacket (12) of a conventional type and which is heated by suitable means. Suitable feeding means (16), such as a T, is provided on the inlet end of the reactor (10). A continuous flow of fat at a controlled rate is supplied through a pipe (17) to the T (16) and to the reactor (10). A continuous flow of steam at a controlled rate is supplied through a pipe (18) to the T (16) and the reactor (10). Alternatively, water and a gas may be supplied to the pipe (18).

FIGURE 3.4: STEAM HYDROLYSIS OF FATS

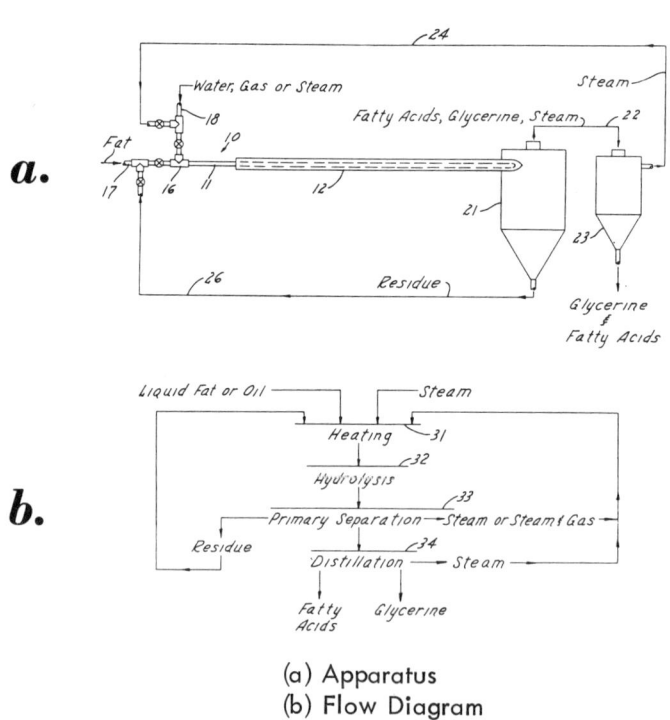

(a) Apparatus
(b) Flow Diagram

Source: K.E. Lunde; U.S. Patent 3,253,007; May 24, 1966

Preparation from Other Sources

The outlet or effluent end of the reactor (10) is connected to a cyclone separator (21) of a conventional type which separates the vapor phase from the liquid phase. The vapor phase, as hereinafter described, contains the products of the hydrolysis, i.e., fatty acids and glycerine of distillation quality, which are fed by a pipe (22) into a recovery unit (23). The glycerine and the fatty acids are separated from the steam in the recovery unit (23) as indicated and the steam is recirculated through a pipe (24) into the reactor (10). The unreacted fat or partially hydrolyzed fat in the residue of the separator (21) is recirculated through a pipe (26) and fed into the reactor (10) for reuse. Figure 3.4b is a flow diagram illustrating the process.

Example 1: Animal fat (tallow) containing 1% zinc oxide as the oleate was melted and metered into a fat preheating section where it was preheated to a temperature of approximately 100°C. The fat was then metered into the reactor at a continuous rate where it was contacted with a metered liquid water. The fat was introduced into the reactor at the rate of 100 grams per minute and the water was introduced at a rate of 70 grams per minute.

Approximately the first part of the reactor was used as a preheater and steam generator, whereas the last 20 feet of the reactor was operated at a temperature of approximately 160°C. with a pressure ranging from 80 to 90 psig. An unexpectedly high degree of hydrolysis occurred within the reactor. With a single pass through the reactor, the hydrolysis was 15% of the possible hydrolysis which theoretically could occur. This high degree of hydrolysis was greater by more than ten times that which should have been obtained in accordance with results calculated from rate constants in the literature.

Example 2: Four kilograms of commercial tallow was charged into a feed tank with zinc oleate and potassium acetate where it was melted. This fat mixture was pumped at the rate of 100 grams per minute into a preheat section and heated to 200°C. and then metered into the reactor. Live steam, equivalent to 30 grams of water per minute, was charged through a steam preheater and heated to a temperature of 200°C. This live steam was contacted to the preheated fat stream as the fat stream entered the reactor. The reactor was maintained at a temperature ranging from 200° to 280°C. The effluent was discharged into a fat recovery cyclone. The steam phase was discharged to a second cyclone to recover the fatty acids and glycerine. The excess steam was condensed in an effluent condenser.

On the first pass of the liquid fat, hydrolysis was 16% complete. When the glycerized mixture from the fat cyclone was recycled, the total conversion rose to 70% with no apparent limitation on the degree of hydrolysis.

Essentially pure distilled grade fatty acids were readily recovered from the fatty acid recovery system. No attempt was made to isolate the glycerine. The steam phase had a linear velocity of 180,000 feet per hour and the fat phase had a linear velocity of 3,500 feet per hour. The residence time per pass for the fat was from 10 to 30 seconds and the residence time for the steam was from 1/3 to 1 second. Substantially all of the fatty acids were in the vapor phase. The reactor was operated at atmospheric pressure.

Example 3: A single pass run was carried out in accordance with Example 2 but utilizing the steam equivalent to 15 grams of water per minute. The percent of hydrolysis was 16%. In the foregoing Examples 1, 2 and 3, the linear velocity of the liquid phase and the linear velocity of the gas phase were within the limits hereinbefore set forth. By comparison of Examples 2 and 3, it can be seen that the hydrolysis can be carried out with a great excess of steam. As pointed out, this is advantageous in that it facilitates the formation of the fatty acids and glycerine in the vapor phase which subsequently facilitates separation of the glycerine and fatty acids in relatively pure form in a simple inexpensive distillation operation. Examples 2 and 3 also show that the process is not limited by liquid phase equilibrium considerations.

Hydrolysis and Acidification of Cocoa Butter

Cocoa butter is known to be essentially a large number of triglycerides in varying amounts. It is also known that it is very difficult to obtain all the triglycerides by ordinary methods of saponification. It is known, however, that cocoa butter and cocoa butter fatty acids solidify to difficultly manageable hard masses even at ordinary temperature and must be heated and held hot if they are to be transported by pipe or tank car or truck. The triglyceride materials recovered from cocoa butter by standard saponification techniques seldom have an iodine number above 25.

The free fatty acids produced by the method of C.S. Castner; U.S. Patent 3,654,327; April 4, 1972; assigned to Schuyler Development Corporation not only have a higher iodine number than those prepared by ordinary saponification techniques but in addition appear to have the unique property of carrying a great variety of medicinal agents through or at least deep into the epidermal and subdermal tissues. For example aspirin can be dissolved or at least completely dispersed in this material and when applied to the surface of the skin appears to be carried into the skin surface. Similarly germicidal agents are readily dissolved and act as highly effective skin cleansing and purifying agents.

Melted cocoa butter and hot sodium hydroxide or similar caustic are reacted in the presence of hot water at a temperature in the range of 160° to 212°F.

This mixture is held at elevated temperature and stirred continuously until hydrolysis is completed. When hydrolysis is completed, the mass is acidified by slow addition of hydrochloric acid accompanied by vigorous stirring to a pH in the range 6.6 to 6.8. The resulting mass is then washed with water to remove soluble salts, excess hydrochloric acid and glycerine. It is essential that the free acids be formed in the range of pH 6.6 and 6.8. Above pH 6.8 the product is a hard lumpy mass. Below pH 6.6 the product is another hard mass which is virtually unusable because of the difficulty in handling it.

Example 1: 29.7 pounds of cocoa butter was melted and it together with 8.0 pounds hot (160° to 212°F.) sodium hydroxide, was added to a reactor vessel containing 75 pounds of hot water (160° to 212°F.). The reaction mixture was stirred constantly and was checked for completion of hydrolysis after 30 minutes of stirring. Successive checks for completion of hydrolysis were made every 15 minutes until hydrolysis was completed. The process of hydrolysis was monitored by removing a small portion of reaction mixture to a beaker of water and observing the result. When hydrolysis is complete the material is completely dissolved. If incomplete the unreacted butter is readily seen on the surface of the beaker.

When hydrolysis was completed, the mass was blended with sufficient hydrochloric acid to provide and maintain a pH of 6.6 to 6.8 with constant agitation. The resulting product was then washed with distilled water to remove NaCl and any other salts in the solution. The resulting product was a milk white creamy paste, soft to the touch and easily handled.

Example 2: A similar amount of cocoa butter and sodium hydroxide were added to hot water in a reactor as in Example 1. As the reaction progressed solids accumulated on the surface and were removed to another vessel. At the same time an amount of melted cocoa butter and sodium hydroxide was added to the reactor equivalent to that present in the removed solids. The removed surface solids were treated with hydrochloric acid to maintain a pH of 6.6 to 6.8 and agitated to convert the hydrolyzed cocoa butter to free fatty acids. The fatty acids were removed as a white, soft, creamy mass. This run was operated in a continuous fashion as distinguished from the batch operation of Example 1. The results were the same as both cases.

MISCELLANEOUS STARTING MATERIALS

Nitroalkane and Sulfuric Acid

A.F. Ellis; U.S. Patent 3,586,704; June 22, 1971; assigned to Gulf Research & Development Company has proposed a process for the conversion of selected 1-nitroalkanes to a reaction product containing at least one of a fatty acid, a fatty acid amide or an alkyl nitrile. A fatty acid having from 2 to 24 carbon atoms is prepared by contacting either 1-nitro-2-nitrosoalkane having a hydrogen atom on the beta carbon atom or a 1-nitroalkanone-2 oxime with a reaction medium comprising an aqueous mineral acid to form a first reaction product at a temperature of between 60° and 160°C. for a time between one second and 120 minutes.

The anhydrous mineral acid concentration of the aqueous mineral acid is at least 65 weight percent. Thereafter a sufficient amount of water is added to the reaction mixture to decrease the anhydrous mineral acid content of the aqueous mineral acid to less than 65 weight percent. The resulting reaction mixture is heated at a temperature and for a time sufficient to convert the first reaction product to the desired fatty acid. The charge stock can be any 1-nitroalkane selected from the group consisting of a 1-nitro-2-nitrosoalkane having a hydrogen atom on the beta carbon atom or a 1-nitroalkanone-2 oxime. The 1-nitroalkane suitably has from 3 to 25 carbon atoms and preferably has from 4 to 18 carbon atoms.

Suitable charge stocks include the monomeric forms of the 1-nitroalkane charge stocks, namely the monomeric 1-nitro-2-nitrosoalkanes and the 1-nitroalkanone-2 oximes in addition to the dimeric 1-nitro-2-nitrosoalkanes known in the art as the bis(1-nitro-2-nitrosoalkanes).

The dimeric form of the 1-nitro-2-nitrosoalkanes is a solid, while the monomeric and oxime forms tend to be liquid and are thus easier to disperse in the reaction medium. This feature is important since the reaction is highly exothermic and gas is evolved. Thus, ease of dispersion of the charge stock in the reaction medium area aids in temperature control and overall smoothness of the reaction. However, the 1-nitro-2-nitrosoalkane is usually added in the form of the dimer which is believed to form the monomeric 1-nitro-2-nitrosoalkane before it reacts with the mineral acid.

In the presence of aqueous sulfuric acid having the proper concentration, the reaction product has been found to comprise at least one of the compounds selected from the group consisting of fatty acids, fatty acid amides and alkyl nitriles, the amount depending on the particular charge stock and mineral acid concentration employed, the reaction conditions and on the reaction procedure.

It is believed the initial reaction product is the fatty acid amide which then hydrolyzes to the fatty acid or dehydrates in the presence of concentrated sulfuric acid to the nitrile. Thus, it has been found that the higher sulfuric acid concentrations, lower temperatures and shorter contact times favor the recovery of the fatty acid amide. The formation of the fatty acid amide is believed to be so fast as to be a substantially instantaneous reaction under the temperatures of this reaction. The formation of the alkyl nitrile and fatty acid are secondary reactions and are somewhat slower. Further, it has been found that if the 1-nitroalkane charge stock and sulfuric acid are mixed at room temperature and heated to reaction temperature, increased amounts of nitrile are produced relative to fatty acid at lower mineral acid concentrations compared to a reaction procedure wherein the 1-nitroalkane is added slowly to a reaction medium comprising the sulfuric acid heated to reaction temperature.

On the other hand, the fatty acid forms in increasing amounts as the concentration of anhydrous mineral acid is decreased and as the reaction temperature and time are increased. The minimum H_2SO_4 concentration for the aqueous sulfuric acid should be that concentration which is sufficient to result in a one phase reaction medium with the 1-nitroalkane at 60°C. This minimum concentration is 65 weight percent or a molar ratio of anhydrous H_2SO_4 to water of at least 0.33:1.

It has been observed that when the weight percent H_2SO_4 content of the aqueous sulfuric acid is below 65, the product of the reaction between the 1-nitroalkanes defined above and the sulfuric acid is primarily an alpha nitro-ketone, which alpha nitro-ketone is somewhat resistant to further hydrolysis in acid medium to an organic acid having one less carbon atom than the alpha nitro-ketone.

Thus, it appears that a different mechanism is occurring depending upon the anhydrous H_2SO_4 concentration of the aqueous sulfuric acid. It has also been observed that when the concentration of the H_2SO_4 is above 65 weight percent, the 1-nitroalkane charge stock appears to form a one phase reacton mixture with the strong mineral acid whereas at concentrations below 65 weight percent, a two phase reaction mixture results. The difference in reaction products may, at least in part, be due to the difference in the solubility of the 1-nitroalkanes in the dilute or concentrated sulfuric acids.

It has also been found that aqueous phosphoric acid produces results similar to those obtained using aqueous sulfuric acid under the same concentration conditions except an alkyl nitrile product has not been observed. This is probably because the phosphoric acid is not as good a dehydration medium. It was found, however, quite unexpectedly, that aqueous phosphoric acid appears to be a much better hydrolysis medium than sulfuric acid for the subject reaction. Thus, aqueous phosphoric acid having an anhydrous H_3PO_4 content of 85 weight percent resulted in the conversion of 1-nitrodecanone-2 oxime to substantially only pelargonic acid with no amide or nitrile being detected, while the use of sulfuric acid in a similar concentration range resulted in nitrile plus fatty acid. The use of anhydrous phosphoric acid results in substantially only amide product. The process will be further described with reference to the following experimental work. The nitroalkane charge stock was either a C_6 or C_8 nitro-nitroso dimer which was prepared by the reaction of N_2O_3 with either hexene-1 or octene-1 as described below, or the charge stock was the oxime form of the monomeric form of the dimer.

A typical example for the preparation of the dimer charge stock is as follows. Gaseous N_2O_3 was bubbled through 4 mols of octene-1 held at 36°C. for one hour, at which time 0.66 mol of N_2O_3 had been added. The stoichiometric ratio of effective nitrogen oxides to olefin was 0.66:4 or 0.165. The weight of solid dimer isolated by filtration was 89 grams. The N_2O_3 was completely consumed and the mol percent conversion of octene-1 based on the N_2O_3 was 16.5%. The efficiency of the reaction to the formation of dimer is therefore 72%, that is, 0.66 mol or 124 grams of monomer (in the form of dimer) was expected and 89 grams were isolated.

Analysis showed the dimer to have the empirical formula $C_8H_{15}N_2O_3$. On melting, the dimer formed a greenish-blue liquid which is characteristic of a 1-nitro-2-nitrosoalkane monomer. The melting point of the dimer was 94.5°C. The infrared band spectra were the same as those published by J.F. Brown, Jr., in JACS, 77, 6341, 1955, for an octene-1 nitro-nitroso dimer. The oxime forms of the bis(1-nitro-2-nitroso hexane) and bis(1-nitro-2-nitroso octane) were prepared by heating the bis compounds in excess glacial acetic acid for 20 minutes at 100°C. until the characteristic yellow color of the oxime is observed and subsequently isolating the oxime by diluting the reaction medium with water.

Example 1: In the run for this example, 5 grams (0.03 mol) of the octene-1 nitro-nitroso dimer described above were added to 50 grams of sulfuric acid having an H_2SO_4 content of 80 weight percent, and the temperature was raised to 95°C. and maintained at that temperature for one minute. The molar ratio of anhydrous sulfuric acid to the nitro-nitroso compound was 13.

The dimer melted and went into solution in the sulfuric acid at 95°C. The reaction mixture, after one minute, was cooled quickly to 40°C. to prevent charring. The mixture was then diluted with water and analysis of the organic phase showed that 33% of the dimer had been converted to 1-heptanitrile and 33% of the dimer had been converted to heptanoic acid. No dimer charge material was recovered. The remainder of the product was a brownish tar which was not further analyzed.

Example 2: In the run for this example, 28 mmol. of bis(1-nitro-2-nitroso hexane) was added with stirring slowly (5 to 10 minutes) to 30 grams of sulfuric acid having an H_2SO_4 content of 80% while the sulfuric acid was maintained at a temperature of 100°C. After the addition of the charge stock the temperature was maintained for an additional 5 minutes at reaction temperature followed by cooling of the reaction mixture to 40°C. The cooled reaction mixture was poured into 115 ml. of water and ice at 0°C. The organic products were isolated, and analysis showed the organic products were composed of 50% valeric acid and 50% valeramide by gas-liquid chromatography (GLC).

Magnesium Dialkyls and Carbon Dioxide

K. Ziegler, R. Koster and W. Grimme; U.S. Patent 3,217,020; Nov. 9, 1965 have found that almost quantitative yields of carboxylic acids may readily be obtained by treating saturated magnesium dialkyls with carbon dioxide.

They have developed a process for the transalkylation of magnesium alkyl compounds, in particular for the production of magnesium alkyl compounds of relatively high carbon number from those having a lower carbon number, in which the higher alkyl radicals may originate from lower olefins. The process thus makes it possible for olefins to be employed for the synthesis of magnesium alkyl compounds in particular of high carbon number which may then be converted to carboxylic acids.

In the transalkylation of magnesium alkyl compounds, organic magnesium compounds are reacted with boron alkyl compounds. In this process, it is advantageous to use free boron trialkyls as one of the components of the reaction mixture. Magnesium dialkyl compounds with lower alkyl radicals, are reacted with free boron trialkyls having higher alkyl radicals. If the magnesium alkyls and boron alkyls are reacted according to the process an equilibrium is set up as shown in the following equation provided that the alkyl radicals were initially different in the two reactants:

$$3MgR_2 + 2BR'_3 \rightleftharpoons 3MgR'_2 + 2BR_3$$

The most favorable results are obtained by using magnesium diethyl and magnesium dipropyl. Establishment of the exchange equilibria proceeds very quickly. It is sufficient for this purpose for the reaction components to be stirred together at room temperature. The boron trialkyls can be obtained by various known methods, which ultimately in general start with olefins. They can for example be obtained from trialkyl borazanes or from diborane. The volatile boron alkyl compounds which form in the reaction can be removed in various ways from the reaction mixture. For example, the reaction mixture can be directly heated to a maximum of 140°C. By carrying out the process in this manner the boron triethyl (BP 95°C.) which forms, distills off. It is possible for the low-boiling boron trialkyl separated from the transalkylation mixture, for example the boron triethyl, to be reconverted into higher boron trialkyls and thus into the starting materials for the transalkylation. The conversion of the magnesium dialkyl compounds with carbon dioxide proceeds in a surprisingly complete manner and leads to practically quantitative conversions to the carboxylic acids.

Example 1: Seventy-three grams (0.434 mol) of dodecene-1 are heated to 150°C. in a three necked flask comprising a dropping funnel, stirrer device and distillation head and 16.0 grams (0.14 mol) of triethyl borazane are added dropwise while stirring. Triethylamine immediately distills off. A residue is extracted at 10 mm. Hg. 17.8 grams (0.217 mol) of magnesium diethyl is then dissolved at room temperature with stirring in the boron tridodecyl which is formed. The solution is heated in a bath under reduced pressure (10 mm. Hg) to 50°C., 13.5 grams of boron triethyl distilling off.

Eighty-two grams of magnesium didodecyl remain as a crystal-clear viscous oil with the correct magnesium content (6.6%). The presence of magnesium didodecyl was proved as follows. 18.1 grams of the substance are dissolved in the absence of air in 100 cc of dry and air-free ether and this mixture is poured into 20 to 30 grams of solid carbon dioxide, again with exclusion of air. After complete evaporation of the carbon dioxide, the reaction mixture is decomposed with 10% sulfuric acid, the ether layer is extracted with caustic alkali solution and the carboxylic acid which has formed is recovered in the usual way from the soap solution. Nineteen grams (89% of the theoretical) of tridecyl acid with the melting point 41°C. are obtained.

Example 2: Thirty-five grams of boric acid trimethyl ester are added to 118 grams of aluminum trialkyl, prepared in known manner from 1-vinyl-3-cyclohexene and aluminum triisobutyl, in the absence of air and after the reaction, which gives rise to violent spontaneous heating, has subsided, the substance is heated for another 2 hours to 100°C. The reaction mixture is then carefully introduced in the absence of air into 250 cc of 5% sulfuric acid plus 250 grams of finely crushed ice, the oil which precipitates is separated out as quickly as possible, it is washed with iced water and cold bicarbonate solution and finally dried (always in the absence of air) over anhydrous calcium chloride.

The boron tri-β-(cyclohex-3-ene-1-yl) ethyl finally obtained in this way is dissolved in 300 cc of dry and anhydrous toluene, 41 grams of magnesium diethyl are added (always in the absence of air), the mixture is heated under a small column and the temperature is so adjusted that boron triethyl preferentially distills over between 90° and 105°C. The magnesium diethyl dissolves. The experiment is completed when no more boron triethyl appears in the distillate. If necessary, toluene is also added during the distillation. If the toluene is extracted in vacuo, a magnesium compound of the formula:

$$\left[\begin{array}{c} CH-CH_2 \\ CH \diagdown \\ \diagup CH-CH_2-CH_2 \\ CH_2-CH_2 \end{array} \right]_2 Mg$$

is left behind as a thick colorless oil with a magnesium content 9.9%. If a sample is carboxylated as described in Example 1 (or even directly in the original toluene solution), the β(1-cyclohexen-3-yl) propionic acid (melting point 33°C.) is obtained with a yield higher than 90% of the theoretical.

PREPARATION OF UNSATURATED ACIDS

C$_{18}$ Cyclic Acid

M.O. Bagby and K.L. Mikolajczak; U.S. Patent 3,356,699; Dec. 5, 1967; assigned to the U.S. Secretary of Agriculture have described a process for obtaining very high yields of isomeric C$_{18}$ vicinally disubstituted cyclohexadiene type monocarboxylic acids from an acetylenic acid, namely cis-9-octadecen-12-ynoic acid (crepenynic acid) which is a major constituent of the vegetable oils present in the seeds of Crepis foetida and to a smaller extent in the oil of Helichrysum bracteatum (strawflower). The acetylenic acid has the formula

$$CH_3(CH_2)_4-C\equiv C-CH_2-CH=CH(CH_2)_7COOH$$

The process is based on the discovery that crepenynic acid even under extremely mild conditions rapidly isomerizes first to a conjugated ene-allenic acid at room temperature and then at 100°C. to a recoverable approximately 2:1 mixture of trans-8, cis-10, trans-12-octadecatrienoic acid and trans-8, cis-10, cis-12-octadecatrienoic acid, which mixture then with only a slight further increase in temperature undergoes cyclization to the C$_{18}$ cyclic acids in very high yields.

Example 1: Ground seeds of Crepis foetida were Soxhlet extracted overnight with petroleum ether (BP 30° to 60°C.). Removal of the solvent provided a 22.0% yield of oil. Mixed methyl esters were prepared by refluxing 141 grams of the oil with 1,100 ml. of about 4% HCl in methanol and 800 ml. benzene under nitrogen for 3 hours. The reaction mixture was concentrated, diluted with 4 volumes of water, extracted with ethyl ether, and the extract of mixed esters dried over anhydrous sodium sulfate: yield 137 grams, analyzing 59.8% methyl crepenynate by gas-liquid chromatography. By countercurrent distribution using acetonitrile as the lower phase and n-hexane as the upper phase, there was obtained 67.5 grams of methyl crepenynate having a purity by gas-liquid chromatography of 99.7%.

Potassium t-butoxide reagent was prepared by gradually adding an excess of metallic sodium to absolute t-butyl alcohol, refluxing for 1 hour, distilling the t-butyl alcohol, slowly adding 4.33 grams of potassium to 100 ml. of the dry alcohol, and permitting the stoppered flask to stand at room temperature overnight.

The potassium t-butoxide in t-butyl alcohol reagent (90 ml.) was added to a 0.50 gram sample of methyl crepenynate and the solution then stored at 1°C. overnight. The solidified reaction mixture was warmed to room temperature and allowed to isomerize for 4 hours before diluting with water, acidifying with dilute hydrochloric acid, extracting with ethyl ether, drying the extract, and removing the solvent. These also obtained an ene-allenic conjugated triene product, i.e., cis-9,11,12-octadecatrienoic acid

$$CH_3(CH_2)_4-CH=C=CH-CH=CH-(CH_2)_7COOH$$

The alkali-free ene-allenic conjugated triene was heated at 100°C. under nitrogen, and infrared spectra determined periodically. The bands at 1,935 and 874 cm.$^{-1}$ had completely disappeared at 100 minutes of heating on the bath coinciding with the complete conversion to the conjugated trans,cis,trans- and trans,cis,cis-8,10,12-octadecatrienoic acids. The temperature was increased to 180°C. for 40 minutes to permit cyclization to take place. Yield of C_{18} cyclic acids: 0.45 gram having a purity of 70%. The product displayed infrared absorption at 14.2μ.

Example 2: A 1.29 gram sample of pure methyl crepenynate was added to 250 ml. of a 10% solution of potassium hydroxide in the ethylene glycol at 185°C. in a reaction vessel equipped with ebullition means for the admission of a stream of nitrogen. At the end of 5 hours the reaction was stopped by diluting with water and acidifying with dilute hydrochloric acid. The acidified solution was extracted with diethyl ether, washed to neutrality with water, and the solvent removed to provide 1.16 grams of product whose infrared bands at 10.1μ and 14.2μ respectively indicated conjugated triene and cyclic acids. To permit separation and analysis, the product was then methylated by reaction with diazomethane and a 1.15 gram sample of the esterified material subjected to fractionation by urea adduct formation. Infrared analysis of the 0.20 gram of material thusly obtained from the urea adduct crystals indicated it to consist entirely of trans, trans, trans conjugated triene. The isolated nonadduct-forming component, 0.95 gram, was shown by infrared and by gas-liquid chromatography to consist almost exclusively of the esterified cyclic acids with only a trace of conjugated triene.

Hydrolysis of 2-Substituted-2-Oxazolines

H.L. Wehrmeister; U.S. Patent 3,466,308; September 9, 1969; assigned to Commercial Solvents Corporation has developed a method for preparing unsaturated aromatic acids and unsaturated aliphatic acids, useful as intermediates in the preparation of perfumes, cosmetics, polymers and plant growth modifiers, by the acid-catalyzed hydrolysis of 2-substituted-2-oxazolines. An object of the process is the provision of a method for the production of compounds having the formula

$$E''-CH=\underset{\underset{E'}{|}}{C}-COOH$$

wherein E'' can be hydrogen, alkyl of from 1 to 14 carbon atoms, aryl (including halogen, hydroxy-, dialkylamino-, and nitro-substituted aryl); and E' can be hydrogen, alkyl of from 1 to 20 carbon atoms, alkenyl of from 2 to 20 carbon atoms, or aryl. Compounds corresponding to the above formula are advantageously prepared by the hydrolysis of 2-substituted-2-oxazolines, corresponding to the formula

$$\begin{array}{c} A' \\ | \\ CH_2-C-A' \\ | \quad\quad | \\ O \quad\quad N \\ \diagdown\; \diagup\!\!\!/ \\ C \\ | \\ E'-C-CH-E''' \end{array}$$

wherein A' can be hydrogen, alkyl or hydroxyalkyl; and E' and E''' as defined above. These compounds include phenylethenyloxazolines and aliphatic ethenyloxazolines. The hydrolysis is advantageously acid catalyzed with mineral acids.

Preparation of Phenylethenyloxazolines: The phenylethenyloxazolines are employed in the preparation of cinnamic acids. They were prepared generally by the iodine-catalyzed condensation of oxazolines with aromatic aldehydes by the following general procedure. Alkylethenyloxazolines useful for the preparation of unsaturated aliphatic acids are prepared in the same manner except that an aliphatic aldehyde, e.g., formaldehyde, is employed instead of an aromatic aldehyde. The aldehyde (1 mol), oxazoline (1 mol), and toluene (100 ml.) or in some cases benzene were charged to a 500 ml. flask equipped with a sealed stirrer, thermometer, Vigreux column (18"), water separator (20 ml.), and reflux condenser.

The mixtures were then heated under reflux for several hours with azeotropic removal of water. If after several hours it was evident that the reaction was not proceeding at an appreciable rate, there was added 1 gram of iodine. The water evolution would start almost immediately. The heating was continued until water evolution was essentially completed. Part of the toluene was removed by distillation if a high pot temperature was desired. Occasionally a second or third 1 gram portion of iodine was added in an attempt to speed up the reaction.

Reactions using materials other than iodine as a catalyst were conducted similarly except that the materials were added from the start of the run rather than after several hours of heating. Five grams each of xylenesulfonic acid, zinc chloride and sodium bisulfate were used. After the water of reaction was removed the mixtures were distilled at reduced pressure through an 18" Vigreux column, except that the p-hydroxy derivative was isolated by crystallization rather than distillation. Some properties of the products obtained are summarized in the table below. The phenylethenyloxazoline compounds produced in the following examples are of the formula

$$Z\text{−}\langle\text{C}_6\text{H}_4\rangle\text{−CH=C−C} \begin{array}{c} \text{E}'\text{N−C(CH}_3\text{)−A}' \\ | \quad\quad\quad\quad | \\ \text{O−−−−CH}_2 \end{array}$$

wherein the values for A', Z and E' are set forth in the table below.

	Product		B.P., °C. (mn.)	Caled.		Found	
Z	E'	A'		N	Neut. equiv.	N	Neut. equiv.
H	CH₃	CH₃	117(0.9) 120(0.6)	------	215.3	------	219.5
p-Cl	CH₃	CH₃	133(1.0) 151(1.5)	5.61	249.7	5.49	251.6
o-Cl	CH₃	CH₃	133(0.5)	5.61	249.7	5.50	261
p-HO	CH₃	CH₃	[1] 176-177	6.06	231.3	5.93	240
p-Me₂N	CH₃	CH₃	155(0.6) 163(0.3)	10.84	129.2	11.47	136.3
m-NO₂	CH₃	CH₃	155(0.6) 159(0.4)	10.76	260.3	10.80	[2] 261.3
p-Cl	CH₃	CH₂OH	168(0.3) 182(0.6)	------	265.7	------	[3] 272
H	H	CH₃	112(0.4) 120(0.5)	6.96	201.3	6.88	206.1
p-Cl	C₁₆H₃₁	CH₃	209(0.9) 248(0.7)	3.06	458	3.93	[4] 1,360
p-Cl	H	CH₃	140-160 (0.9)	5.90	235.7	6.09	[5] 238.8

[1] Recrystallized.
[2] Redistilled.
[3] Calcd: Cl, 13.34. Found: Cl, 12.38, 12.70.
[4] Calcd.: Cl, 7.74. Found: Cl, 7.66.
[5] Calcd.: Cl, 14.61. Found: Cl, 15.04.

Hydrolysis of Phenylethenyloxazolines to Cinnamic Acids: The phenylethenyloxazolines were hydrolyzed to the cinnamic acids by the following general procedure, used with but minor modifications for every example given. The phenylethenyloxazoline (0.1 mol) was dissolved in 200 ml. of dilute hydrochloric acid (1 part concentrated HCl to 3 parts H_2O) and heated at reflux for 3 hours.

The precipitated solid was collected by filtration, washed twice with 50 ml. of water and dried. This crude product (used as a basic for the reported yields) was recrystallized, generally from ethanol to give a product with a melting point usually in close agreement with the literature values. The products were recrystallized until no change in melting point occurred. These products were then submitted for analysis by titration. In the case of the p-dimethylamino derivative the pH of the mixture after hydrolysis was adjusted to 4 by the addition of aqueous sodium hydroxide solution. The precipitated solid was then collected, washed, dried and recrystallized. The compounds produced are of the formula:

$$Z\text{-}C_6H_4\text{-}CH=C(E')\text{-}COOH$$

wherein the values for Z and E' correspond to the values for Z and E' in the starting material.

Acetylenic Acids by Grignard Synthesis

The process developed by J.M. Osbond, P.G. Philpott and J.C. Wickens; U.S. Patent 3,033,884; May 8, 1962; assigned to Hoffmann-La Roche Incorporated comprises condensing a halogeno compound having the general formula

$$CH_3-(CH_2)_4-(C\equiv C-CH_2)_s-X$$

with a compound having the general formula

$$CH\equiv C-CH_2-(C\equiv C-CH_2)_t-(CH_2)_b-Y$$

wherein s and t stand for integers each ranging from 0 to 4 but totalling 1 to 4, b stands for an integer of from 0 to 8, X represents a chlorine, bromine or iodine atom, and Y represents a carboxyl or a hindered orthoester group, in a Grignard reaction in the presence of copper or a cuprous salt. The condensation of the halogeno compounds and the acids used as initial materials by means of a Grignard reaction is suitably carried out using tetrahydrofuran as a solvent. Two molecular proportions of the Grignard reagent are utilized in order to form the acid complex required in the condensation. The hydrolysis, where required, of the condensation product is suitably carried out using aqueous sulfuric acid.

The acetylenic halogeno compounds used as initial materials may all be prepared from pentyl bromide and propargyl alcohol. Thus, 1-bromo-octyne-2 can be prepared by heating pentyl bromide with a dimagnesium bromide derivative of propargyl alcohol in the presence of cuprous chloride and brominating the resulting octyn-2-ol-1 with phosphorus tribromide. The acetylenic acids used as initial materials may be prepared by the condensation of an acid of the general formula:

$$CH \equiv C-CH_2-(CH_2)_b-COOH$$

with a propargyl halide (preferably propargyl bromide) in a Grignard reaction in the presence of copper or of a cuprous salt and then, if necessary, similarly and repeatedly condensing the produced acid until the desired chain length is obtained.

Example: To a standard ethereal solution of 116.6 ml. (0.11 mol) of 0.9435 N ethyl magnesium bromide were added 80 ml. of dry peroxide free tetrahydrofuran. Ether was distilled off until the temperature reached 46°C. The mixture was cooled to 0°C. and 8.4 grams (0.05 mol) of decyn-9-oic-1 acid in tetrahydrofuran added over 1/2 hour. The mixture was stirred at room temperature for 3 hours when evolution of ethane appeared complete. 0.7 gram of cuprous chloride was added and the mixture stirred for 1/2 hour. 9.45 grams (0.05 mol) of 1-bromo-octyne-2 was added dropwise over 1/2 hour, the mixture stirred at room temperature for 2 hours, and then heated under reflux in an atmosphere of nitrogen for 24 hours. A further amount of cuprous chloride (0.3 gram) was added and the heating under reflux continued for a further 16 hours.

The reaction mixture was poured into a mixture of ice and dilute hydrochloric acid and extracted three times with ether. The ether solution were extracted four times with 2 N potassium carbonate solution and the aqueous extracts acidified with concentrated hydrochloric acid (with the addition of ice) and extracted twice with ether. The ether extracts were washed with water and dried over sulfuric acid. Evaporation of the ether gave 12.34 grams of a brown oil. To this crude octadecadiyne-9, 12-oic acid was added a solution of absolute ethanol and 5 ml. of concentrated sulfuric acid at 0°C. The solution was set aside at room temperature for 45 hours, under nitrogen. The ethanolic ester solution was poured into water and extracted three times with petrol (40° to 60°C.), washed twice with

2 N sodium carbonate solution and twice with water, then dried over sodium sulfate. Evaporation of the ether, followed by distillation of the residue gave 7.23 grams of octadecadiyne-9,12-oic-1 acid ethylester; yield 47.5%; BP 124° to 126°C./0.00014 mm. Redistillation gave a sample which boiled at 106° to 108°C./0.00021 mm.; $n_D^{20} = 1.4692$. 6.29 grams of the product thus obtained were dissolved in 100 ml. of petrol [40° to 60°C. (purified)]. 0.5 gram of Lindlar catalyst was added and the ester hydrogenated at room temperature and atmospheric pressure until the hydrogen uptake began to subside. The catalyst was filtered off, the petroleum evaporated and the residue distilled, yielding 5.4 grams (84.8%) of ethyl linoleate; BP 150° to 154°C./0.05 mm.; $n_D^{20} = 1.4582$.

5.02 grams of ethyl linoleate were added to aqueous ethanolic sodium hydroxide (2.8 grams sodium hydroxide, 7 ml. water and 63 ml. ethanol) and set aside overnight at room temperature under a nitrogen atmosphere. Aqueous sulfuric acid (1:1) was added, the mixture diluted with water and extracted three times with petrol (40° to 60°C.). The extract was dried and the petrol evaporated under nitrogen. The residue was crystallized from 100 ml. of petrol (40° to 60°C.) at -20°C. to remove traces of saturated acid. On further cooling to -60°C. in a carbon dioxide/ethanol bath, the crystalline acid separated and was filtered off. First crop: 1.73 grams, MP -10° to -8°C. Distillation of this first crop gave 1.26 grams of an oily product, linoleic acid; BP 148° to 152°C./0.0011 mm.; $n_D^{22} = 1.4660$, MP -6° to -5°C.

Reduction of Polyacetylenes

The process developed by B.F. Adams and J.H. Wotiz; U.S. Patent 3,299,111; January 17, 1967; assigned to Diamond Alkali Company relates to compounds represented by the following formula

$$R'\underset{H}{\overset{H}{C}}=\underset{H}{\overset{}{C}}\left[-(CH_2)_x\underset{H}{\overset{H}{C}}=\underset{}{\overset{}{C}}-\right]_n R''$$

wherein R' and R" are selected from the group consisting of hydrogen, carboxy, $(CH_2)_xNH_2$, $(CH_2)_xNHCOOH$ and x is a number from 1 to 20, inclusive; and n is a number from 1 to 100, inclusive. Specific illustrative examples of compounds of this process include trans-2-trans-8-trans-14,20-heneicosatetraene-1-oic acid

$$CH_2=CH\left[-(CH_2)_4\underset{H}{\overset{H}{C}}=\overset{}{C}-\right]_3 COOH$$

These compounds may be prepared from polyacetylenic compounds of the formula

$$R^1C\equiv C[R^3C\equiv C(R^4C\equiv C)_m]_nR^2$$

by chemical reduction with metallic sodium dissolved in liquid ammonia. In the above formula R^1 and R^2 are selected from the group consisting of hydrogen, alkyl, aminoalkyl, carbamato-alkyl, $COOR^5$ and

$$R^3NHCOO^-NH_3^+R^5\left[\left(\underset{H}{\overset{H}{C}}=\underset{H}{\overset{H}{C}}-R^4\right)_m\underset{H}{\overset{H}{C}}=\underset{H}{\overset{H}{C}}-R^3\right]_n\underset{H}{\overset{H}{C}}=\underset{H}{\overset{H}{C}}-R^1$$

wherein R^3 and R^4 are divalent hydrocarbon radicals containing straight chains of at least one carbon atom; R^5 is selected from the group consisting of hydrogen, alkyl, aryl and aralkyl; m is a number from 0 to 1, inclusive; and n is a number from 1 to 100, inclusive.

Example 1: The preparation of 1,7,13,19-eicosatetrayne is as follows. A 5 liter, three necked flask, equipped with a stirrer, Dry Ice condenser and gas inlet tube, is charged with 3 liters of liquid ammonia and 234 grams (6 mols) of sodamide. 4.5 mols of acetylene is measured into the stirred suspension at which point the mixture begins to clear, and then the gas inlet tube is replaced by an addition funnel and 648 grams (3 mols) of 1,4-dibromobutane is added slowly as stirring is continued.

The ammonia is allowed to evaporate overnight and the residual mixture is hydrolyzed by cautious addition of 300 ml. of water. The aqueous and organic layers are separated and the aqueous layer is extracted several times with 100 ml. portions of ether. The ether extracts and organic layer are combined, washed with 5% aqueous solutions of hydrochloric acid and sodium carbonate and dried over calcium sulfate. After removal of the ether by evaporation, the residue is distilled under reduced pressure. The desired 1,7,13,19-eicosatetrayne boils at 165° to 170°C. at 0.3 mm. Hg.

Example 2: The preparation of 2,8,14,20-heneicosatetrayne-1-oic acid is as follows. Three mols of 1,7,13,19-eicosatetrayne disodium salt is prepared from 798 grams (3 mols) of 1,7,13,19-eicosatetrayne and 7 mols of $NaNH_2$ in 3.5 liters of anhydrous ammonia. The ammonia is replaced by 6 gallons of a 1:1:1 (by volume) mixture of benzene, ethyl ether and tetrahydrofuran and the suspended salt is pressurized with CO_2 at 25°C. and 500 psi in a 10 gallon autoclave for 60 hours. After venting, the mixture is hydrolyzed with 1 gallon of water. The organic layer is separated and dried and the solvent is evaporated; there is recovered 354 grams of impure unreacted 1,7,13,19-eicosatetrayne. The aqueous solution is acidified with hydrochloric acid and the precipitated solid is extracted with ether. After evaporation of the ether the residue is treated with pentane in a Soxhlet extractor, yielding 133 grams (26% conversion) of soluble white product, MP 54° to 55°C. which is identified as 2,8,14,20-heneicosatetrayne-1-oic acid. The results of the chemical analysis indicate the formation of the desired $C_{21}H_{26}O_2$, and are as follows:

Element	Actual Percent by Weight	Calculated Percent by Weight
Carbon	80.9	81.3
Hydrogen	8.4	8.4

The actual neutralization equivalent found is 313, while the calculated value is 310. The infrared spectrum is consistent with the assigned structure.

Preparation of Queen Substance

Although activity attributable to the existence of a queen substance has been in alcoholic extracts of queen bees, attempts to isolate a definite active single substance (which it was considered would be a steroid, a wax or a paraffin) in a pure state had been unsuccessful because of difficulties produced by the royal jelly acid (10-hydroxy-dec-3-enoic acid) contained in the crude material.

The process developed by R.K. Callow, C.G. Butler and N.C. Johnston; U.S. Patent 3,162,659; December 22, 1964; assigned to National Research Development Corporation is based upon the discovery that the activity can be concentrated by subjecting crude material, containing it, to a solvent fractionation process wherein an aqueous solution containing water-soluble impurities is rejected at one state (conveniently by partitioning the crude material between ether and water) and impurities soluble in petroleum are rejected at another state. Subsequently the remaining active material may be extracted into alkali, recovered at pH 8.5 to 9.0 and further purified to yield anhydrous waxy crystals of substantial purity melting at 45° to 50°C. which are recrystallizable from aqueous methanol.

The recrystallizable substance has been found to be trans-9-oxo-dec-2-enoic acid. In a method of preparing a 1-alkyl trans-9-oxo-dec-2-enoate by synthesis, a 1-monoalkyl trans-non-2-enedioate acid halide of the general formula $XOC-(CH_2)_5CH=CH-COOR$ in which X represents a halogen atom, preferably chlorine, and R represents an alkyl group, is reacted with a dialkyl cadmium or other metal alkyl to yield a complex which is decomposed with water. The acid itself may be obtained from the ester by acid hydrolysis. Attempts to obtain the acid by hydrolysis with alkali hydroxides have been unsuccessful. As the hydrolysis of the ester presents difficulties, it is preferred to employ the ester itself as the final active material. In a preferred form of the method the 1-monoalkyl trans-non-2-enedioate acid halide is prepared from a 1-alkyl hydrogen trans-non-2-enedioate (by reaction with thionyl chloride or other acid halide-forming agent, e.g., phosphorus trichloride) which may, be produced from a monoalkyl azelate acid halide by selective halogenation, preferably selective bromination to yield a 9-alkyl 2-haloazelate-1 acid halide which is then subjected to the steps of esterification, dehydrohalogenation (for which purpose 2,4,6 collidine is a convenient base) and partial hydrolysis.

Example: Preparation of Dialkylbromoazelates from Alkyl Hydrogen Azelates — Methyl hydrogen azelate (90.3 grams) was mixed with 140 ml. of thionyl chloride and the mixture heated under reflux on a water-bath for 2 hours. At the end of this time the formation of the acid chloride was complete, and bromination was carried out by addition of 1.05 mols of bromine (78.5 grams) over a period of 4 hours to the gently boiling solution. After allowing to cool and stand overnight the mixture was poured into an excess (300 ml.) of methanol. A vigorous reaction took place, with evolution of sulfur dioxide and hydrogen chloride.

After 2 hours, during which the mixture was shaken at intervals, the product was poured into water, the organic layer, which is denser than water, was separated, and the aqueous layer was extracted with ether twice, the ether extracts being added to the organic layer first separated. The ethereal mixture was dried over sodium sulfate, the ether removed by evaporation, and the residue distilled under reduced pressure. Dimethyl bromoazelate is a liquid distilling at 105° to 112°C. 0.1 mm. or 134° to 140°C. 1.5 mm. Yield, 72 grams. Analysis: found, C, 44.6; H, 6.26; Br, 26.5%. $C_{22}H_{19}O_4Br$ requires C, 44.8; H, 6.51; Br, 27.1%.

Dialkyl Esters of Trans-Non-2-Enedioic Acid — Dimethyl bromoazelate (72 grams) was mixed with 2 volumes of 2,4,6-collidine and the mixture was boiled gently under reflux for 1 hour. The product, after cooling, was poured into water. The heavy oil was separated and the aqueous layer extracted twice with ether. The ether extracts were added to the oil and the mixture treated with dilute hydrochloric acid until the reaction to test paper was acid. The organic layer was then dried over sodium sulfate and, after removal of the ether, was distilled under reduced pressure. The product distilled in one main fraction, BP 117° to 126°C./0.3 mm. yield 13.5 grams (Found, C, 60.4 H, 8.3%. $C_{11}H_{18}O_4$ requires C, 61.6; H, 8.5%.) The infrared absorption spectrum of the liquid dimethyl trans-non-2-enedioate shows a peak at 1,647 cm.$^{-1}$ characteristic of an ethylenic linkage.

Mono-Alkyl Esters of Trans-Non-2-Enedioic Acid — Dimethyl trans-non-2-enedioate (13.5 grams) was treated at 20°C. with a mixture of 35 ml. of 10% by weight aqueous potassium hydroxide solution and 70 ml. of methanol. After standing overnight the mixture was diluted with water and unchanged ester extracted with ether. The aqueous solution was then acidified with hydrochloric acid and again extracted with ether several times. The combined ethereal extracts were dried over sodium sulfate, the ether removed and the residue distilled under reduced pressure. After a small amount of low-boiling material had passed over, the desired half ester came over at 152° to 153°C./0.3 mm. Yield 4.7 grams. The isopropyl ester, BP 142° to 148°C./1.5 mm. or 130° to 132°C./0.8 mm. was prepared similarily from the methyl isopropyl and ethyl isopropyl diesters.

Monoalkyl Trans-Non-2-Enedioate Acid Chloride — The monomethyl trans-non-2-enedioate obtained as described (5.6 grams) was mixed with 12 ml. of thionyl chloride and a piece of porous pot added to assist the evolution of gas. After keeping overnight at room temperature the reaction mixture was heated for half an hour on the steam bath, the excess of thionyl chloride was removed at the water pump, and the residue was distilled under reduced pressure. The acid chloride distilled at 114° to 116°C./0.6 mm. Yield 5.1 grams.

Methyl Trans-9-Oxodec-2-Enoate — A Grignard reagent was prepared from 1.23 grams magnesium and an excess of methyl bromide in ether. To this was added 4.4 grams of cadmium chloride while the reaction vessel was immersed in ice water. After refluxing until reaction was complete, the ether was distilled off, benzene was added, and then partly distilled off, and finally 5.12 grams of monomethyl trans-non-2-enedioate acid chloride.

A vigorous reaction took place, and after heating on the steam bath for 10 minutes the mixture was cooled, decomposed with ice and dilute sulfuric acid, and the product extracted with benzene. The benzene extracts were washed with water, 5% sodium carbonate solution, again with water and finally dried, the benzene removed, and the residue distilled under reduced pressure. There was obtained 2.22 grams of methyl trans-9-oxodec-2-enoate, BP 116° to 120°C./1.5 mm. Isopropyl trans-9-oxodec-2-enoate, BP 120° to 130°C./1 mm. was obtained by a similar reaction. Both of the esters were found to possess biological activity in the test for queen substance (inhibition of building of queen cells).

Trans-9-Oxodec-2-Enoic Acid — This acid was obtained from the isopropyl ester as follows. The ester (0.25 gram) was dissolved in acetone (4 ml.) and concentrated hydrochloric acid (1 ml.) was added. The mixture was kept at room temperature for 5 days. It was then diluted with water and extracted with ether. The ether solution was extracted with aqueous 5% sodium carbonate solution. The alkaline solution was acidified with hydrochloric acid and the trans-9-oxodec-2-enoic acid which separated as an oily product was extracted with ether. The ethereal solution was dried and evaporated. The residue 0.1 gram deposited crystals when kept at 2°C. These crystals separated from the adherent oil, melted at 45° to 52°C. and showed the characteristic infrared absorption of queen substance obtained from queen bees. It also had the same rate of travel on a paper chromatogram as the natural material and within the limits of error of the bioassay, had quantitatively the same biological activity in inhibiting construction of queen cells.

Another preparation of queen substance is described by K. Eiter; U.S. Patent 3,288,826; November 29, 1966; assigned to Farbenfabriken Bayer AG, Germany. According to this procedure, dec-2-en-9-one-1-acid and more particularly trans-dec-2-en-9-one-1-acid having the structural formula:

$$CH_3-CO-(CH_2)_5-\overset{H}{\underset{H}{C}}=C-COOH$$
(1)

can be readily produced by the process that involves the reaction of glutaric dialdehyde (2) with the known compound, triphenyl phosphoric carbomethoxy methylene (3), in which reaction only one of the two formyl moieties present in the dialdehyde is actually reacted with the organophosphorus compound, to yield the hept-2-en-7-al-1-acid methyl ester (4).

The resulting heptenal acid methyl ester (4) is condensed with acetone (5) according to Knoevenagel reaction with piperidine, piperidine acetate, potassium hydroxide, barium hydroxide or ammonium acetate, to yield deca-2,7-dien-9-one-1-acid methyl ester (6). The activated Δ^7-double bond of this latter molecule is then partially hydrogenated with a lead or quinoline poisoned palladium catalyst to yield dec-2-en-9-one-1-acid methyl ester [(7) and (7a)]. If desired, the cis-components (7a) of this ester present in the latter reaction product mixture can be readily isomerized with catalytic amounts of iodine, whereupon the saponification of the resulting trans-dec-2-en-9-one-1-acid methyl ester (7) with sodium carbonate (e.g., a 2 N sodium thereof) yields the desired trans-dec-2-en-9-one-1-acid (1) (MP of 52° to 54°C.). The reaction sequence thus described can be represented structurally as follows:

$$OHC-(CH_2)_3-CHO + (C_6H_5)_3P=CH-COOR \longrightarrow$$
(2) (3)
$$OHC-(CH_2)_3-CH=CH-COOR + (C_6H_5)_3P=O$$
(4)

$$\text{ROOC-CH=CH-(CH}_2\text{)}_3\text{-CH=O} + \text{CH}_3\text{-C-CH}_3 \xrightarrow[\text{Conditions}]{\text{Knoevenagel Reaction}}$$
$$\underset{(4)}{} \quad \underset{(5)}{\overset{\text{O}}{\|}}$$

$$\text{ROOC-CH=CH-(CH}_2\text{)}_3\text{-CH=CH-}\underset{\overset{\|}{\text{O}}}{\text{C}}\text{-CH}_3$$
$$(6)$$

$$\text{H}_2 \Big| \begin{array}{l}\text{Pd catalyst poisoned}\\ \text{with quinoline or lead}\end{array}$$

$$\text{ROOC-CH=CH-(CH}_2\text{)}_5\text{-}\underset{\overset{\|}{\text{O}}}{\text{C}}\text{-CH}_3$$
$$(7) \text{ and } (7a)$$

$$\text{I}_2 \Big|$$

$$\text{CH}_3\text{-}\underset{\overset{\|}{\text{O}}}{\text{C}}\text{-(CH}_2\text{)}_5\text{-}\underset{\overset{|}{\text{H}}}{\overset{\text{H}}{\text{C}}}\text{=C-COOR} \xrightarrow{2\text{NNa}_2\text{CO}_3}$$

$$\text{CH}_3\text{-}\underset{\overset{\|}{\text{O}}}{\text{C}}\text{-(CH}_2\text{)}_5\text{-}\underset{\overset{|}{\text{H}}}{\overset{\text{H}}{\text{C}}}\text{=C-}\underset{\overset{|}{\text{H}}}{\text{C}}\overset{\overset{\text{O}}{\diagup}}{\diagdown_{\text{OH}}}$$
$$(1)$$

wherein R is an alkyl radical containing 1 to 2 carbon atoms, i.e., methyl or ethyl. The glutaric dialdehyde (2) used as starting material is known from the literature and is technically easily accessible. The triphenyl phosphoric carbomethoxy methylene (3) used in the first step of the reaction is also readily obtainable, for example, from bromoacetic ester and triphenyl phosphine and treatment of the salt formed with an aqueous lye.

Example: (A) Preparation of Hept-2-en-7-al-1-Acid Methyl Ester, of the Formula

$$\text{CH}_3\text{-O-}\overset{\overset{\text{O}}{\|}}{\text{C}}\text{-CH=CH-(CH}_2\text{)}_3\text{-}\overset{\overset{\text{O}}{\|}}{\text{C}}\text{H}$$

A mixture of 60.9 parts by weight of freshly distilled glutaric dialdehyde and 101.7 parts by weight of triphenyl phosphoric carbomethoxy methylene warms up when the two components are mixed together and is then stirred for 90 minutes at 80° to 90°C. Fifty parts by volume of ether are then added thereto, the mixture cooled to -20°C. and the separated triphenyl phosphine oxide removed by filtering off with suction and subsequent washing with a small amount of a cold mixture of ether and petroleum ether.

The filtrate is freed from solvent in a vacuum and the remaining residue distilled at 0.12 mm. Hg. 47.7 parts by weight of crude heptenal acid methyl ester distill over at 54° to 75°C. and are again distilled. 39.1 parts by weight of hept-2-en-7-al acid methyl ester distill over at 58° to 60°C. at 0.07 mm. Hg; $n_D^{20} = 1.4590$.

(B) Preparation of Deca-2,7-Dien-9-one-1-Acid Methyl Esters, of the Formula

$$CH_3-O-\overset{O}{\underset{\|}{C}}-CH=CH-(CH_2)_3-CH=CH-\overset{O}{\underset{\|}{C}}-CH_3$$

A mixture of 50 parts by weight of the hept-2-en-7-al-1-acid methyl ester and 100 parts by volume of dry acetone are mixed with 8 parts by weight of glacial acetic acid and 10 parts by weight of piperidine. The reaction mixture is then boiled under reflux for one hour, cooled, the excess acetone distilled off in a vacuum, the residue taken up in ether and the ether solution shaken out with water, dilute sulfuric acid, water, sodium bicarbonate solution and water until neutral, dried with sodium sulfate and, after evaporation of the ether, 40 parts by weight of substance remain. The distillation of this crude substance in a high vacuum gives a colorless distillate which goes over at 100° to 150°C. (air bath temperature) and is again distilled; BP 120° to 130°C./0.1 mm. Hg; $n_D^{20} = 1.4908$; yield: 20 parts by weight.

(C) Preparation of Dec-2-en-9-one-1-Acid Methyl Ester, of the Formula

$$CH_3-O-\overset{O}{\underset{\|}{C}}-CH=CH-(CH_2)_5-\overset{}{\underset{\|}{C}}-CH_3$$
$$\overset{}{\underset{O}{}}$$

0.3 parts by weight of Lindlar catalyst are charged with hydrogen in 20 parts by volume of methanol and 10.55 parts by weight of the deca-2,7-dien-9-one-1-acid methyl ester in 20 parts by volume of methanol added thereto. After the calculated amount of hydrogen has been taken up, the hydrogenation is stopped, the catalyst filtered off, the filtrate freed from methanol in a vacuum and the residue distilled in a high vacuum at 0.001 mm. Hg and 80° to 100°C. air bath temperature. The yield is quantitative: $n_D^{20} = 1.4590$.

(D) Preparation of Dec-2-en-9-one-1-Acid, of the Formula

$$CH_3-\overset{O}{\underset{\|}{C}}-(CH_2)_5-\overset{H}{\underset{H}{\overset{|}{C}}}=C-\overset{O}{\underset{\|}{C}}-OH$$

8.5 parts by weight of the dec-2-en-9-one acid methyl ester are dissolved in 20 parts by volume of petroleum ether and mixed with a solution of small iodine crystals in 5 ml. of petroleum ether and left to stand overnight. In the morning, the petroleum ether solution is shaken out with a N/10 sodium thiosulfate solution and water and the solvent driven off in a vacuum. The residue is boiled under reflux for 3 hours with 20 parts by volume of a 2 N sodium carbonate solution and 20 parts by volume of dioxane, whereafter a clear reaction solution is observed.

Thereupon, the dioxane and some water are driven off under water pump vacuum, the mixture cooled and the aqueous alkaline solution shaken out with ether. The aqueous phase is acidified with 95 parts by volume of 2 N hydrochloric acid, saturated with sodium chloride and shaken out with ether. There are obtained in quantitative yield 7.9 parts by weight of rapidly crystallizing acid which distills as a colorless, thickish oil at 0.001 mm. Hg and 100° to 130°C. air bath temperature. When recrystallized from ether-petroleum ether, the acid melts at 53° to 55°C. It shows an infrared spectrum which is identical with the spectrum published in the literature for the queen substance.

α-Substituted Unsaturated Acids

L.S. Bondar and R.A. Okunev; U.S. Patent 3,530,156; September 22, 1970 describe a method for the production of α-substituted unsaturated acids which comprises reacting an alkyl or cycloalkyl malonic ester with α,β-unsaturated aliphatic alcohols, such as terpene alcohols, at a temperature above the boiling point of the alcohol and saponifying the resultant ester. The products are useful as detergents, wetting agents, flotation agents, foaming agents, solvents and plasticizers for rubbers and plastics, emulsion or suspension stabilizers, special-purpose detergents, disinfectants, preservatives, and also as pharmaceutrical preparations.

Alkyl or cycloalkyl-substituted malonic esters are used as the monosubstituted malonic esters, while any terpene alcohol, such as linalool or nerolidol, may be used as the α,β-unsaturated aliphatic alcohol. The method has been employed for the synthesis of the α-hexyl- and α-cyclohexyl-5,9,13-trimethyl-4,8,12-tetradecatrienoic acids which may find commercial applications analogous to those indicated above.

The method has been accomplished in the following manner. The reactants, viz, an alkyl- or cycloalkyl-substituted malonic ester and a terpene alcohol taken in equimolar amounts (or the substituted malonic ester is taken in excess) are charged into a reaction vessel and heated to a temperature above the boiling point of the alcohol. The reaction mass is then subjected to fractionation or the volatile components are stripped off, followed by saponifying the ester fractions corresponding to the target product or the residue after stripping off the volatile components. The process is assumed to be complete when the rate of carbon dioxide evolution from the reaction mixture diminishes sharply. The method is advantageous in that it can be effected in a single stage, involves a minimum of auxiliary process steps, calls for the employment of a limited range of starting materials, and presents practically no fire or explosion hazards.

Example 1: Synthesis of α-Butyl-5,9-Dimethyl-4,8-Decadienoic Acid — A mixture of 108.2 grams of butylmalonic ester and 77.1 grams of linalool (BP 196°C.) is placed in a reaction vessel connected to a condenser, a receiver and a gasometer flask (measuring cylinder) and maintained at a temperature of 210° to 230°C. for a period of 1.0 to 1.5 hours. Upon termination of the reaction, as evidenced by a sharp drop of the rate of carbon dioxide evolution (from 40 to 45 ml./min. down to 7 to 10 ml./min.), the reaction mixture is fractionated in vacuum to separate ethyl α-butyl-5,9-dimethyl-4,8-decadienoate. The ester is then saponified with an alcoholic solution of potassium hydroxide and fractionated in vacuum to yield 50 grams of α-butyl-5,9-dimethyl-4,8-decadienoic acid (40% of the theoretical amount).

Example 2: Synthesis of α-Undecyl-5,9-Dimethyl-4,8-Decadienoic Acid — Into a reaction vessel are charged 76.8 grams of undecylmalonic ester and 38.5 grams of linalool and the reaction mixture is maintained at a temperature of 210° to 250°C. for a period of 1.5 to 2.0 hours. The end of the reaction is noted as disclosed in Example 1. Then the reaction mixture is fractionated to separate ethyl α-undecyl-4,9-dimethyl,4,8-decadienoate, which is subjected to saponification with twice the theoretical amount of 4 N alcoholic potassium hydroxide and thereafter fractionated in vacuum. The yield of α-undecyl-5,9-dimethyl-4,8-decadienoic acid is 52 grams (60% of the theoretical amount).

Trienoic Acids

P.J.A. Chabardes; U.S. Patent 3,493,590; February 3, 1970; assigned to Rhone-Poulenc SA, France provides a process for preparation of a triethylenically unsaturated carboxylic acid ester which comprises reacting together at least two molecular proportions of a conjugated diolefin and one molecular proportion of an acrylic or methacrylic ester in the presence of, as catalyst, an organometallic complex of zero-valent nickel.

When butadiene is reacted with an acrylic ester, a mixture of isomeric undecatrienoic acid esters is obtained having the 3 double bonds in the 2,5,10- and 3,5,10-positions. A proportion of by-products is obtained, chiefly homo- and cooligomers of the starting olefins, and Diels-Alder adducts of the diolefin and the acrylic or methacrylic ester. The separation of the triethylenic esters from the by-products may be effected by any appropriate conventional purifying method, for example fractional distillation. The triethylenic esters obtained by the process may be converted into trienoic acids by saponification, using any usual method. When the ester is a mixture of isomers, this saponification is accompanied by conversion of the less stable into the more stable form, so that a single trienoic acid is obtained. For example, the saponification of a mixture of 2,5,10-alkatrienoic and 3,5,10-alkatrienoic esters leads to a 3,5,10-alkatrienoic acid.

These esters and acids produced with the process are compounds useful as intermediate agents in organic synthesis. On hydrogenation, they give the corresponding saturated esters and acids. By reaction via their double bonds they are useful in the preparation of bifunctional products which are useful in the manufacture of polycondensates. They may also be employed in the manufacture of drying oil compositions.

Example: Butadiene 15 grams, triphenylphosphine 2.4 grams, nickel acetylacetonate 2.2 grams, and anhydrous benzene 30 cc are introduced under a nitrogen atmosphere into a 500 cc autoclave. When the solid compounds have dissolved in the benzene, the solution is cooled to 0°C., the autoclave is purged with nitrogen, and a solution of diethylethoxyaluminum 2.5 grams in benzene 10 cc is added. An orange-red solution is thus obtained.

Methyl acrylate (30 cc, 0.33 mol) and butadiene (95 grams, 1.76 mol) are then added. The product is then heated at 100°C. for 3 hours, 45 minutes under autogenous pressure while stirring is continued. When the pressure becomes constant, the reaction product is cooled and, by distillation under 20 mm. Hg with gradual heating until the temperature of the reaction mass reaches 60°C., the unreacted butadiene is eliminated, followed by the light fractions. The heavy fractions distilling up to 150°C. under 0.3 mm. Hg are then rapidly distilled, leaving a residue of 36 grams. On fractional redistillation, these heavy fractions give: 8.6 grams of a fraction BP 30° to 50°C./0.3 mm. Hg, n_D^{25} = 1.4589, which is methyl cyclohexene carboxylate; 25 grams of a fraction BP 80° to 86°C./0.3 mm. Hg, n_D^{25} = 1.4745; and 5.8 grams of heavy products.

The intermediate fraction is identified by infrared spectrography and nuclear magnetic resonance as methyl 2,5,10-undecatrienoate. Saponification of this ester with sodium hydroxide followed by acidification gives 3,5,10-undecatrienoic acid, BP 119° to 120°C./0.5 mm. Hg, n_D^{25} = 1.500. Hydrogenation of methyl 2,5,10-undecatrienoate over Adams platinum, followed by saponification, gives undecanoic acid. If butadiene and methyl acrylate are reacted together under the same conditions but replacing the nickel acetylacetonate by cobalt(III) acetylacetonate, methyl undecatrienoate is not formed, and, apart from resinous materials, the only isolatable products are methyl cyclohexene-carboxylate and a methyl heptadienoate.

BIOLOGICAL SYNTHESES

CONJUGATED UNSATURATED ACIDS

Octadecatrienoic Acid Using Tung Nut Enzymes

T.J. Jacks and L.Y. Yatsu; U.S. Patent 3,661,710; May 9, 1972; assigned to The U.S. Secretary of Agriculture found that acetone-insoluble powders prepared from developing tung nuts catalyze the formation of conjugated octadecatrienoic acid from fatty acids of castor oil. The preferred synthesis required reduced coenzyme A (CoASH), reduced nicotinamide-adenine dinucleotide (NADH), enzyme from tung nuts, and either adenosine-$5'$-diphosphate (ADP) or adenosine-$5'$-triphosphate (ATP) for best results.

Developing tung nuts were collected before, during, and after the period of active oil accumulation in the endosperm (M.R. Easterling and L.Y. Yatsu, Plant Physiol, 39:1017, 1964). Thinly sliced tissue was macerated in liquid nitrogen with a mortar and pestle. The small, frozen pieces were added to an equal weight of sand and homogenized at -78°C. with sufficient acetone to ensure fluidity of the homogenate. The insoluble residue was washed by vacuum filtration with acetone at -78°C. until the filtrate appeared colorless and then with sufficient ether to displace residual acetone.

Ether was removed by immediately fluffing the powder at room temperature in an exhaust hood. The powder was further dried over P_2O_5 in a vacuum of 0.05 torr and then stored in sealed ampules at -20°C. Enzyme was prepared by triturating the powder in 0.1 M tris-HCl buffer (pH 7.2), filtering the suspension through glass wool, and centrifuging the filtrate at 1,100 g for 10 min. Dithiothreitol was added to the supernatant to a concentration of 4×10^{-3}M. This enzyme preparation, containing 49 mg of protein, (mostly storage protein of the seed), 120 μmols of tris-HCl buffer (pH 7.2) and 4.8 μmols of dithiothreitol was homogenized with 5 μmols of CoASH, 11 μmols of NADH, 10 μmols of ATP, 1.2 μmols of $MgSO_4$, 230 μmols of castor oil fatty acid, and sufficient 0.5 N KOH to neutralize the mixture. The mixture was allowed to incubate for 45 minutes at 30°C. with continual homogenization. At various time intervals portions of 0.6 ml. were removed and added to 0.4 ml. of 0.5 N HCl. Fatty acids were extracted from each acidified reaction mixture into 3.0 ml. of hexane (spectrophotometric grade) and the content of conjugated trienoic fatty acid was determined spectrophotometrically (A.O.C.S. Official Method Cd 7-58, Revised 1959; J.S. Hoffman, R.T. O'Connor, D.C. Heinzelman, and W.G. Bickford, J. Am. Oil Chem. Soc. 34:338, 1957).

Example 1: The reaction described above was repeated except that CoASH was omitted. After 45 min. 12.4 mμmols of conjugated trienoic fatty acid was produced.

Example 2: The reaction was again repeated except that NADH was omitted. After 45 min. 12.3 mμmols of conjugated trienoic fatty acid was produced.

Example 3: In this example NADH was omitted and 11 μmols of oxidized nicotinamide-adenine dinucleotide, NAD, was present. After 45 min. 29.9 mμmols of conjugated trienoic fatty acid was produced.

Example 4: NADH was absent in this run and 11 μmols of oxidized nicotinamide-adenine dinucleotide phosphate, NADP, was present. After 45 min. 9.2 mμmols of conjugated trienoic fatty acid was produced.

Example 5: The reaction was repeated once more except that ATP was omitted. After 45 min. 1.5 mμmols of conjugated trienoic fatty acid was produced.

Example 6: This time ATP was omitted and 10 μmols of ADP were present. After 45 min. 31.0 μmols of conjugated trienoic fatty acid was produced.

Isolinoleic Acid Using Bacteria

W.D. Butt; U.S. Patent 3,455,785; July 15, 1969; assigned to Lever Brothers Company provides a method for the preparation of octadeca-11,15-dienoic acid, which comprises partially hydrogenating a polyunsaturated fatty compound containing at least three olefinic double bonds with bacteria of the genus Clostridium or Lactobacillus. Particularly suitable polyunsaturated fatty compounds from which octadeca-11,15-dienoic acid may be produced by partial bacterial hydrogenation are polyunsaturated

Biological Syntheses

trienoic fatty compounds containing the grouping:

—CH$_2$—CH$_2$—CH=CH—CH$_2$—CH=CH—CH$_2$—CH=CH—CH$_2$—CH$_2$—

Such compounds may be linolenic acid, its glycerides, esters and soaps; mixtures of these with other fatty acids such as can be obtained by hydrolysis of oils; and also mixtures with fatty glycerides, esters and soaps. The preferred compound is an oil containing linolenyl glycerides, e.g., linseed or soyabean oil. Free linolenic acid may be used dispersed in a suitable carrier, such as paraffin or olive oil.

The micro-organisms are preferably of the species Clostridium sporogenes or Lactobacillus helveticus. Actively growing cells of the selected organism are first cultured in a suitable nutrient medium for a time insufficient to attain maximum growth but sufficient to ensure that the bacteria are reproducing logarithmically. The cells may then be washed by centrifugation, suspended in water, and then introduced into a medium suitable for supporting further active growth and containing the polyunsaturated fatty compound. Cells of either organism may also be introduced directly into the medium containing the polyunsaturated fatty compound.

Microbiological hydrogenation is usually carried out under anaerobic conditions. Preferably the medium is stirred and blanketed with an inert gas, such as nitrogen. The polyunsaturated fatty compound is preferably introduced as an emulsion which is first prepared with water or a portion of liquid medium, plus a small proportion of any suitable emulsifying agent. The emulsion is then added, together with cells of the chosen organism, to the bulk of the medium. The medium is agitated throughout the period of incubation so that the polyunsaturated fatty compound is adequately dispersed.

The process may be a batch or continuous process. When the process is carried out batch-wise the time of incubation is preferably one to seven days. When incubation times shorter than 12 hours are employed very little yield is obtained. Prolonged incubation beyond seven days adds little to the yield. The temperature range within which the microbial hydrogenation normally occurs depends on the organism used. A temperature of 25° to 40°C. may be applied when using Clostridia. With the Lactobacilli the incubation temperature may be from 35° to 40°C.

The pH of the medium containing the fatty compound should preferably be about pH 7.0. Lactobacilli will, in general, tolerate a lower pH than Clostridia. The recovery of free isolinoleic acid can be achieved by acid-ether extraction. The oil emulsion is first broken by shaking with methanol and then the reaction mixture may be acidified with sulfuric acid to a pH of 1 to 2, and the lipid material extracted with ether. The free fatty acids may then conveniently be further separated as their soaps, from other liquid materials by extraction with an alkali, such as sodium hydroxide. Further acidification and ether extraction is then necessary to obtain the free fatty acids. The isolinoleic acid may be separated from the other free fatty acids by preparative gas-liquid chromatography or counter-current distribution. Octadeca-11,15-dienoic acid is of particular use in the flavoring of food, in particular for imparting a cream or butter-like flavor.

Example 1: This example describes the production of isolinoleic acid from linseed oil using Clostridium sporogenes. Cells of Clostridium sporogenes 1365 were grown in 3% peptone at pH 7.4 under nitrogen for 48 hours at 37°C. with stirring. Linseed oil was added to the culture at a level of 1% and the culture was regassed with nitrogen. Incubation was continued under these conditions for 6 days. At the end of this period the culture was acidified with dilute hydrochloric acid and extracted with about one-tenth of its volume of diethyl ether using a little methanol to break the emulsion. The free fatty acids were extracted from the ether layer by washing twice with equal volumes of 1.5 N potassium hydroxide.

After acidification of the combined alkali washings, the fatty acids were extracted into ether. The ether solution was dried and the solvent evaporated to give a mixture of fatty acids containing about 30% of isolinoleic acid. This isomer was separated from other fatty acids present by preparative gas-liquid chromatography.

Example 2: This example follows that of Example 1, except that the linseed oil was added to the medium before inoculation with Clostridium sporogenes. After inoculation, incubation was carried out for 6 days at 37°C. under nitrogen with stirring. The yield of isolinoleic acid was again about 30% but there was a greater proportion of short chain fatty acids also present than was found in the preparation described in Example 1.

DIBASIC ACID

Using Yeast Fermentation

In the process described by G.W. Elson, R. Howe, and D.F. Jones; U.S. Patent 3,483,083; December 9, 1969; assigned to Imperial Chemical Industries Limited, England α-ω-alkylenedioic acids and esters of these acids are prepared by fermenting a compound of the formula: CH_3AR^1 in which R^1 is an ester group; and A is either a group of the formula $-(CH_2)_y-$, y being an integer from 15 to 25, or an unsaturated straight chain aliphatic group containing 15 to 25 carbon atoms, with certain strains of Torulopsis. Typically the compound to be converted is n-hexadecyl bromide and the ester produced is dimethyl 1,16-hexadecanedioate. The corresponding dicarboxylic acid may be produced by hydrolysis of the diester. The product of the fermentation may be reacted with a compound of the formula R^2OH, in which R^2 stands for an alkyl or aryl radical of not more than 10 carbon atoms, under acidic or alkaline conditions, after which, if desired, the diester obtained is converted into the corresponding dicarboxylic acid by hydrolysis. Alternatively, the product of the fermentation may be hydrolyzed under acidic or alkaline conditions to give the dicarboxylic acid directly.

The active microorganism used here signifies the Torulopsis strain NCYC 675 [which has been deposited under this number, and typed as a strain of Torulopsis gropengiesseri, in the National Collection of Yeast Cultures (Brewing Industry Research Foundation, Nutfield, Redhill, Surrey, England)]. The compounds CH_3AR^1 may be added to the culture medium in a single portion or in several portions at intervals.

The fermentation may be carried out in an aqueous medium containing a carbon source (glucose at 5 to 20% w./v.); a nitrogen source, (urea at 0.05 to 0.5% w./v. and/or yeast extract at 0.1 to 1.5% w./v.); a magnesium source (magnesium sulfate heptahydrate at 0.05 to 0.7% w./v.); a sulfur source, (the sulfate referred to above); a phosphorus source, (potassium dihydrogen phosphate at 0.001 to 0.5% w./v.); and a potassium source (the phosphate referred to above). Traces of salts containing metals, for example: salts of iron up to 10 ppm; copper, up to 5 ppm; zinc, up to 10 ppm; manganese, up to 5 ppm; and molybdenum, up to 5 ppm may also be present in the aqueous medium.

The fermentation may conveniently be carried out at a temperature between 18° and 32°C. The product of the fermentation may be hydrolyzed directly to the appropriate dicarboxylic acid under acidic conditions by the use of acetic acid, or under alkaline conditions by the use of an alkali metal hydroxide such as sodium hydroxide. The hydrolysis is carried out in the presence of water. An organic solvent, such as methanol may also be present. Suitable acidic conditions for use in the interaction involving a compound of the formula R^2OH, are provided, by the use of an inorganic acid such as sulfuric or hydrochloric acid, or an organic acid such as p-toluenesulfonic acid.

This interaction may be accelerated or completed by the application of heat. Suitable alkaline conditions for use in this interaction are provided by the use of a compound of the formula R^2OM, in which R^2 has the meaning stated above and M stands for an alkali metal. The dicarboxylic acids may alternatively be obtained from the corresponding diesters by hydrolysis with an alkali metal hydroxide, for example sodium or potassium hydroxide, in the presence of water or in the presence of an organic diluent or solvent such as methanol. In those cases of the process where the main chain of A contains 15 or 16 carbon atoms, the process involves no loss of carbon atoms from the main chain and therefore fermentation of n-hexadecyl bromide [A standing for $(CH_2)_{15}$] affords 1,16-hexadecanedioic acid and derivatives thereof. Specific products of the process are, for example: dimethyl 1,16-hexadecanedioate; dimethyl 1,17-heptadecanedioate; dimethyl 1,18-octadecanedioate, etc.

These esters and acids are useful as intermediates, for example in the manufacture of synthetic lubricants, plasticizers, thermoplastic resins, adhesives, elastomers, antioxidants, synthetic fibers, and perfumes. In particular, the dialkyl esters, for example dimethyl 1,16-hexadecanedioate, can be converted by conventional means into the corresponding diamides and then into the corresponding diamines, (hexadecane-1,16-diamine,) which can then be reacted with terephthalic acid to form salts which can be polymerized to form fiber-forming polymers.

Example 1: A nutrient solution having the following composition is prepared by dissolving the constituents in one liter of distilled water.

Glucose	100 g.
Yeast extract	5.0 g.
Urea	1.0 g.
KH_2PO_4	1.0 g.
$MgSO_4 \cdot 7H_2O$	3.0 g.
$FeSO_4 \cdot 7H_2O$	1.0 mg.
$CuSO_4 \cdot 5H_2O$	0.15 mg.
$ZnSO_4 \cdot 7H_2O$	1.0 mg.
$MnSO_4 \cdot 4H_2O$	0.1 mg.
K_2MoO_4	0.1 mg.

The resulting solution is adjusted to pH 6.5 by the addition of 3.3 ml. of 1 N sodium hydroxide solution. 1,500 parts of the nutrient solution are sterilized by heating in an autoclave at 120°C. for 20 minutes. The sterile nutrient solution is cooled, and is then inoculated with a distilled water suspension of cells prepared from a stock agar culture of the abovementioned strain No. NCYC 675 of Torulopsis. This mixture is incubated at 25°C. on a rotary shaker. At or near the completion of the logarithmic growth phase, that is, from 24 to 36 hours after inoculation, there is added an aqueous emulsion of n-hexadecyl bromide (prepared by stirring 15 parts of n-hexadecyl bromide together with 15 parts of a 3% w./w. aqueous solution of starch, 0.3 part of Tween 55 and 0.03 part of Span 80.

Incubation is continued for 5 days after the addition of n-hexadecyl bromide.

The mixture is culture fluid and cells are extracted with 1,500 parts of ethyl acetate in three equal portions. The ethyl acetate extract is dried, and then the ethyl acetate is evaporated. The residual gum is stirred together with 5 parts of ethyl acetate, and 100 parts of light petroleum (BP 40° to 60°C.) are added to the resulting solution. When the separation of gummy solid is complete, the supernatant liquid is decanted. The gummy solid is dissolved in 250 parts of a 5% w./w. solution of sulfuric acid in methanol, and the solution is kept at 25°C. for 4 hours and then heated under reflux for 5 hours.

The methanol is evaporated under reduced pressure. The residual gum is shaken together with 150 parts of ether and 50 parts of water. The ether layer is washed with 10% w./v. soldium carbonate, and then with water, and is then dried. The ether is evaporated and the solid residue is crystallized from methanol. There is thus obtained dimethyl 1,16-hexadecanedioate, MP 50° to 51°C. 0.1 part of dimethyl 1,16-hexadecanedioate is heated under reflux with a solution of 0.5 part of potassium hydroxide in 5 parts of methanol for 4 hours.

The methanol is evaporated and the residue is shaken together with 5 parts of 2 N hydrochloric acid and 40 parts of ether. The ethereal layer is separated from the mixture, dried, and the solvent is evaporated. The residue is crystallized from acetone and there is thus obtained 1,16-hexadecanedioic acid, MP 123° to 124°C.

ACIDS AND ESTERS

Microbial Production

The process described by N.J. Stevens, J.W. Frankenfeld, and J.D. Douros, Jr.; U.S. Patent 3,409,506; November 5, 1968; assigned to Esso Research and Engineering Company relates to the biosynthesis of waxy-esters from hydrocarbons by aerobically subjecting a hydrocarbon to the metabolic action of a gram negative bacteria in the presence of an aqueous mineral salts solution containing a limited concentration of mineral nutrients selected from the group consisting of magnesium, calcium, and a combination of these. Furthermore, the process uses azelaic acid to stimulate this microbiological production of esters.

If this aqueous mineral salts solution in which a microorganism is aerobically cultivated contains a limited concentration, i.e., below that amount needed for maximum growth of the microorganism, of the specified mineral nutrients, by-product formation of esters is favored at the expense of microorganism cell growth. It has been found that if the concentration of the divalent magnesium cation in the aqueous mineral salts solution is restricted to not more than 0.02 wt. percent, based on the total amount of the aqueous growth medium and/or if the concentration of the divalent calcium cation is restricted to not more than 0.01 wt. percent, based on total amount of the aqueous growth medium, the amount of ester by-product is significantly increased at the expense of cellular growth. It has further been found that the use of small amounts, e.g., between 1 and 75 ppm of azelaic acid, together with the stated restricted magnesium and/or calcium cation concentrations stimulates the biosynthetic production of fatty acid esters.

Hydrocarbon feeds which can be utilized for the process are C_1-C_{30} petroleum hydrocarbon feeds, preferably gas oils boiling in the range of 190° to 320°C. Other suitable feeds are C_1-C_{30} normal and isoparaffins, cycloparaffins, monoolefins, diolefins, aromatics and mixtures of these. Feeds available in large quantities and those particularly suitable are $C_{10}-C_{30}$ normal paraffins from gas oils, light naphthas, and normally gaseous feeds such as methane, ethane, propane, butane and mixtures thereof, e.g., natural gas.

A further preferred feed is one which contains a substantial weight percentage, e.g., 70+ wt. percent, of normal paraffin hydrocarbons having from 10 to 30 carbon atoms. While the presence of branched, non-aromatic hydrocarbons in amounts of up to 30% by weight in the hydrocarbon feed can be tolerated, concentrations in excess of 10 wt. percent of non-normal, non-aromatic hydrocarbons are usually avoided since the preferred microorganisms employed in the process are selective to normal hydrocarbons, especially intermediate range ($C_{12}-C_{20}$) n-paraffins.

A most preferred hydrocarbon feed is a C_6-C_{30} feed stock which has been purified to reduce the level of aromatics, both polynuclear and mononuclear, to below about 100 ppm. This is necessary since organisms which attack aromatics do not usually attack paraffins. A preferred process for purifying the hydrocarbon feed is to adsorb the normal hydrocarbons, preferably paraffins, by 5 A. molecular sieves followed by desorption and a clean-up of the desorbed normal hydrocarbons with 13X sieves or silica gel to adsorb remaining impurities, particularly aromatics.

By preloading the molecular sieve with the displacing medium (preferably ammonia) and by introducing a displacing medium along with the feed, the rate of adsorption is increased and subsequent desorption greatly eased, particularly with high molecular weight materials. The preferred purified hydrocarbon feed contains about 95+ wt. percent of $C_{11}-C_{30}$ n-paraffins and up to about 5 wt. percent normal olefins containing from 11 to 30 carbon atoms. The $C_{11}-C_{30}$ n-paraffins feed can be petroleum feeds, e.g., gas oils boiling in the range of 190° and 320°C. The amount of hydrocarbon feed supplied to the fermentation reactor (including the recycle), based on total aqueous growth medium supplied, is between 0.5 and 2 wt. percent when straight air is used as the oxygen carrying medium. When using oxygen-enriched gases, e.g., gases having 70+ wt. percent oxygen, a preferred amount of hydrocarbon supplied to the reactor is between 0.5 and 5.0 wt. percent, based on the total aqueous growth medium. The weight percent of, for example, C_{11}—C_{30} normal hydrocarbons actually existing in the slurry zone of the continuous reactor during by-product formation can range from 0.01 to 0.05 wt. percent.

Preferred microorganisms are gram negative bacteria which assimilate paraffinic hydrocarbons. There are nine microorganisms especially suitable for hydrocarbon assimilation. These are as follows.

	ATCC Number
Micrococcus cerificans	14987
Pseudomonas ligustri	15522
Pseudomonas pseudomallei	15523
Pseudomonas orvilla	15524
Alcaligenes sp.	15525
Cellumonas galba	15526
Brevibacterium insectiphilium	15528
Corynebacterium sp.	15529
Corynebacterium pourometabolum	15530

The particular class and subclass of bacteria utilized is determined by the particular feed employed. For example, when the microorganisms assimilate methane or other gaseous paraffin feeds, the preferred class of microorganisms is Pseudomonadaceae, such as Pseudomonas methanica. When fermentation is performed using a light naphtha feed, the preferred classes of microorganisms are Pseudomonadaceae and Arthrobacter, such as Pseudomonas fluorescens, Pseudomonas desmolyticum, Pseudomonas aeruginosa and Arthrobacter globiforme. In a preferred method, the biosynthesis is conducted using a bacteria inoculant, especially gram negative coccus bacteria.

Oxygen is supplied to the fermentation reactor in any form capable of being assimilated readily by the inoculant microorganism. Oxygen-containing compounds can be used as long as they do not adversely affect ester production. Conveniently, oxygen is supplied as an oxygen-containing gas, e.g., air, which contains between 19 and 22 mol percent oxygen. Between 0.8 and 2.5 volumes per minute of air are supplied to the reactor per volume of reactor liquid. Nitrogen is also supplied to the fermentation reactor. The source of nitrogen can be any organic or inorganic nitrogen-containing compound capable of releasing nitrogen in a form suitable for assimilation by the microorganism. In the organic category, proteins, acid-hydrolyzed proteins, enzyme-digested proteins, amino acid, yeast extract, etc. can be listed as examples. Economically, it is preferable to employ an inorganic compound such as ammonia, ammonium hydroxide, or salts of these.

A very convenient and satisfactory method of supplying nitrogen is to employ ammonium hydroxide, ammonium phosphate or ammonium acid phosphate, which can be added as the salt per se or can be produced in situ in the aqueous fermentation media by bubbling ammonia through the broth to which phosphoric acid was previously added, thereby forming ammonium acid phosphate. In this way the pH range of 5.5-7.5 is maintained and the requisite nitrogen is supplied.

Ammonium hydroxide can be supplied to the reactor in amounts between 0.1 and 0.15 wt. percent, nitrogen. In addition to the energy and nitrogen sources, it is also necessary to supply requisite amounts of selected mineral nutrients to the fermentation reactor. Thus, potassium, sodium, iron, magnesium, calcium, manganese, phosphorus and other nutrients are included in the aqueous growth medium. These necessary materials can be supplied in the form of their salts, and preferably their water-soluble salts. When either ammonium phosphate or ammonium acid phosphate is used, it can serve as a combined source of nitrogen and phosphorus.

In this process, it has been found that by limiting the concentration of selected nutrient mineral ions in the aqueous nutrient medium to below that required for maximum microorganism growth, the metabolic action of the microorganism can be harnessed to produce esters from the hydrocarbon feed in preference to microorganism cell growth. By altering the composition of the aqueous mineral salts solution by limiting the concentration of selected mineral ions, by-products of the biosynthesis cultivation, such as fatty acid esters, can be selectively produced as the expense of cellular growth.

The magnesium and calcium mineral nutrient concentrations can be restricted independently or at the same time. However, the concentration of the magnesium mineral nutrient has been found to be more critical than that of calcium for the selective production of esters. In general, the concentration of the divalent calcium ion in the fermentation reactor, preferably, will range between 0.005 and 0.01 wt. percent (0.05-0.10 grams/liter). The concentration of the divalent magnesium ion in the fermentation reactor should preferably range between 0.005 and 0.02 wt. percent (0.05 to

0.20 grams/liter). It has been found that the use of minor amounts, e.g., between 1 and 75 ppm of azelaic acid in the aqueous fermentation medium stimulates ester formation. The temperature at which the fermentation reaction is carried out can vary between 20° and 55°C. The exact temperature depends upon the specific microorganism being utilized; but, preferably, the fermentation is conducted at temperatures between 25° and 40°C. The pH of the biosynthesis bath is generally held between 5.5 and 7.5. At the start up of the fermentation, the growth medium is inoculated with a vegetative microbial inoculum.

The initial concentration at the outset of fermentation can vary widely, from 0.1 to 1.0 gram per liter of total fermentation media. The fermentation reactor can be stirred during biosynthesis by any conventional means. The liquid residence time in continuous operations for a bacteria such as Micrococcus cerificans (Arthrobacter ureafaciens), i.e., the volume of liquid in the reactor divided by the amount of the material supplied (and products removed so as to maintain a constant liquid level in the reactor) per hour, is, preferably 1.5 to 2.5 hours. The process can be carried out by batch or continuous means.

The products produced are primarily acids and esters. The specific acids and esters will depend to a large extent on the hydrocarbon feed stock employed. Thus, for example, if a C16 hydrocarbon is employed as the feed, the principal acid and ester produced will be palmitic acid and cetyl palmitate. Mixed hydrocarbon feeds will produce a spectrum of acids and esters. The esters produced are essentially present in the aqueous fermentation media (extracellular). However, some of the esters formed are held within the microorganism cell itself. Esters produced can be extracted using solvents such as acetone or acetone-water-hexane mixtures.

Example: A 4-liter cylindrical reactor was thoroughly sterilized with steam. The reactor was equipped with a stirrer having a power rating of 40-60 horsepower per 1,000 gallons and with various equipment for operating the reactor continuously. The sterilized reactor was charged with 4 liters of an aqueous salt feed having the composition set forth in Run 1 of the table below. Sufficient normal hexadecane was then charged to the reactor so that about 1 wt. percent, based on salt solution feed, was present.

Thereafter, Micrococcus cerificans in the form of an inoculum was added to the reactor so that the microorganism was present in an initial concentration of about 0.5 gram/liter. The temperature of the reactor was adjusted to 95°F. and the pH regulated to about 7.0. Air was introduced into the reactor at a rate between 1.0 and 3.0 liters/minute. The aqueous mineral salts solution was added at the rate of 2 liters/hour. Normal hexadecane was introduced at a rate of 20 g./hr. A material balance was made at steady state conditions and the average percent carbon, unaccounted for as carbon dioxide and cells, calculated. This figure indicates the amount of carbon present in the ester and acid. In general, greater than 85% of the total acid and ester product is present as ester and usually greater than 90% of said total product is ester.

Run 2 was performed in the same manner as Run 1 as was Run 3 with the exception that the concentration of magnesium and calcium salts were changed. Results are tabulated below.

Effect of Cation Feed Concentrations on Acid-Ester Formation

Run	85% H_3PO_4 (g./l.)	KCl (g./l.)	Na_2SO_4 (g./l.)	$FeSO_4 \cdot 7H_2O$ (g./l.)	$MgSO_4$ (g./l.)	$MnSO_4 \cdot H_2O$ (g./l.)	$CaCl_2$ (g./l.)	Average % Carbon Unaccounted for as CO_2 and Cells	Average % Hydrocarbon Converted
1	2.5	1.0	0.5	0.04	0.25	0.04	0.5	9.7	91.0
2	2.5	1.0	0.5	0.04	0.25	0.04	0.5	9.4	94.8
3	2.5	1.0	0.5	0.04	0.2	0.04	0.2	19.7	97.2

The data demonstrates that when the concentration of the magnesium and calcium salts was reduced to about 0.2 g./l., the amount of ester and acid produced was significantly increased.

SYNTHESIS OF HYDROXY ACIDS

CATALYTIC PROCESSES

Cation Exchange Resin Catalyst

The process of A.A. D'Addieco; U.S. Patent 3,169,139; February 9, 1965; assigned to E.I. du Pont de Nemours and Company relates to an improved method for carrying out oxidation reactions with hydrogen peroxide, particularly hydroxylation reactions involving olefinically unsaturated compounds. Hydrogen peroxide has been used as an oxidizing agent in reactions involving a large variety of olefinically unsaturated compounds. Perhaps the most important of such reactions are those involving the hydroxylation or epoxidation of such compounds. The hydroxylation reactions are usually effected in an excess of an organic acid and in the presence of a strong, soluble mineral acid.

Frequently hydroxylation preparation results in the formation of undesirable by-products with accompanying low yields of the polyhydroxy compounds. This process provides a commercially applicable process which results in high yields of the desired hydroxylated products. Recent developments in effecting oxidation reactions with hydrogen peroxide have led to the use of solid resin catalysis. Epoxidation has been carried out with virtual exclusion of by-products, such as hydroxylated products, using polystyrene sulfonic acid exchange resins of medium or low porosity.

High yields of hydroxylated products to the virtual exclusion of by-products, such as epoxides and ethers, can be effected using a lower aliphatic acid, hydrogen peroxide and a sulfonated monovinyl aromatic exchange resin of high porosity. In the hydroxylation of higher fatty esters, the ester linkage remains intact unlike other hydroxylation procedures. It is generally known that a wide variety of olefinically unsaturated compounds can be hydroxylated by reactions with peraliphatic acids. The olefinically unsaturated compounds generally hydroxylated for commercial purposes are those whose structures contain at least five carbon atoms and at least one olefinic double bond. Generally, the materials hydroxylated are animal fats and vegetable oils, especially esters of fatty acids and these, therefore, constitute a preferred group of reactants.

Fatty acids and esters thereof having at least one double bond which can be hydroxylated to 60 to 80% according to the process (based on double bonds removed) are those which have five or more carbon atoms, such as tall oils and soybean oil. Specifically methyl oleate, 2-ethylhexyl tallate and N-butyl tallate are hydroxylated to more than 60%. The hydroxylated products are useful in a variety of applications, such as emulsifiers, greases and plasticizers. Lecithin containing oleic, stearic, palmitic and other fatty acids can be hydroxylated to a useful emulsifier in the manufacture of candies.

According to the process the hydroxylation of olefinic linkages to form dihydroxy compounds is catalyzed by a cation exchange resin in the hydrogen form. These resins are sulfonated copolymers of comparatively little cross-linking having 1 to 6% of polyvinyl aromatic hydrocarbon. Preferred resins are sulfonated copolymers of mixtures of a monovinyl benzene such as styrene with about 4% of a polyvinyl benzene such as divinyl benzene. Such products as Dowex 50-X-4 and Amberlite XE-100 are commercial examples of these resins.

These resins are of the sulfonic acid type in which the active sulfonic acid groups are attached directly to an aromatic ring of a hydrocarbon resin structure and are active catalysts; they are stable under reaction conditions and remain insoluble during extended use. The cation-exchange resins will usually be employed in granular or bead form and should be present in the reaction mixture in an amount sufficient to catalyze the overall reaction at a practical rate. Particle size of the resin does not appear to be critical, commercially available sizes ranging from about 20 to 200 mesh being generally suitable.

A worth-while effect will usually result from the use of as little as 0.5% of the resin based upon the total weight of the reactants. The most preferred amounts, particularly when the reaction is carried out batchwise are usually in two ranges: from about 1 to 4% and from about 10 to 50%, but much larger amounts can be used. The lower range is used to facilitate filtration in the work-up of the product and to allow discard of the resin catalyst at the end of each reaction. The operations can be carried out continuously, e.g., by passing a mixture of the reactants through a column of the cation-exchange resin. In such cases, the resin content of the reaction mixture at any given instant may be quite high, e.g., upwards of 100% or more based on the weight of the reactants. The method can be practiced at temperatures over a wide range, the optimum temperature in any given case depending upon several factors including the particular reaction involved, the particular resin catalyst used, and the stability of the product under the reaction conditions to be employed.

Hydroxylation is carried out at a temperature within the range of about 40° to 90°C. or more, the preferred range being 60° to 80°C., depending on the reaction time. The hydrogen peroxide reactant can be supplied conveniently as an aqueous solution. Aqueous solutions containing at least 25% H_2O_2 by weight will generally be used. Commercial 35%, 50% and 70% solutions are suitable and solutions containing around 35% or more H_2O_2 are preferred.

Hydrogen peroxide equivalent to around 0.9 to 1.1 mols of H_2O_2 for each oxidizable olefinic linkage in the molecule of the compund being hydroxylated will most generally be used. Larger or smaller amounts can be employed depending upon the results desired. In the preferred embodiment of the process an aliphatic acid is also added to the reaction mixture and substantial benefit can be achieved by the addition to the mixture of as little as 0.01 mol of a lower aliphatic acid per mol of hydrogen peroxide employed. Preferably, between about 0.2 to 1.0 mol of the acid per mol of hydrogen peroxide will be added.

Much larger quantities, e.g., up to ten mols or more, can be used but are best avoided because of the costly recovery problem imposed. Aliphatic acids having 1 to 5 carbon atoms are suitable; acetic acid is preferred, although formic, butyric and propionic acids can also be used. Hydroxylation can be carried out in ten or more minutes up to several hours depending on the reaction temperature. If the reaction is carried out for more than ten hours at about 80°C. or above, appreciable amounts of polyethers are formed.

If the reaction temperature is about 60°C., significant polyether formation occurs only after 24 hours or longer. In general, reaction times of more than ten hours should be avoided when the temperature is about 80°C. or above.

Example 1: A mixture of 29.2 g. (0.10 mol) of technical methyl oleate (iodine number 87.1), 7.5 g. of resin (sulfonated copolymer of styrene and 4% divinyl benzene, 4% cross-linkage) containing 1.33 g. acetic acid and 1.97 g. of glacial acetic (0.055 mol total acetic acid) was prepared in a

100-ml. vessel equipped with a mechanical stirrer, thermometer and dropping funnel. While the mixture was being stirred vigorously, 7.45 g. (0.11 mol) of 50% hydrogen peroxide was added so that the temperature reached 60°C. in 15 minutes. The temperature was maintained at about 85°C. for two hours, first with intermittent cooling by ice water until the exothermic reaction subsided and then by warming in a water bath. At the end of this time the mixture was kept warm and the resin was removed by vacuum filtration. The filtrate containing the product was collected in 100 ml. of warm 1% NaCl solution.

The oily product layer was separated and then washed with 100-ml. portions of hot water. After drying in a vacuum at 100°C. for 1 hour, followed by cooling, a light-colored solid with an iodine value of 4.8 and a hydroxyl value of 6.44% was obtained. Recrystallization of the product three times from hot cyclohexane yielded a white powder, melting point 67° to 67.7°C. Analysis for methyl 9,10-dihydroxystearate was C 69.04%; H 11.40%. Calculated value: C 69.04%; H 11.59%. Yields of methyl 9,10-dihydroxystearate of about 75% were obtained in accordance with the above method.

Example 2: A mixture of 40 g. of alkali-refined soybean oil (iodine number 129.5), 11.8 g. of polystyrene sulfonic acid resin (4% cross-linkage) containing approximately 1.8 g. (18%) of acetic acid and about 6.0 g. of glacial acetic acid is prepared in a vessel equipped with a high speed stirrer, thermometer, and dropping funnel. While the mixture is being stirred vigorously, 15.2 g. of 50% hydrogen peroxide is added. Hydroxylation is carried out at 60°C. for three hours. The product is isolated as in the previous example and analyzes as follows: hydroxyl value, 9.6%; iodine value, 6.8; epoxy-oxygen value, 0.8%.

The one-step feature of the method is obviously highly advantageous over the prior multi-step procedures for effecting hydroxylations. An advantage of the method is that it can be operated continuously and at substantially higher temperatures than are generally practical with prior methods. Yet another advantage is the fact that the problem of recovering carboxylic acid is greatly minimized or may even be eliminated. The process is particularly valuable as commercially attractive means of upgrading natural fats and oils since there is a mounting surplus of animal fats and oils.

Lewis Acid Catalyst

Base catalyzed reactions for the conversion of α-keto compounds into their corresponding α-hydroxy compounds are known in the art. Acid catalyzed processes have decided advantages over the base catalyzed reactions. For example, they can be carried out under relatively mild reaction conditions whereas the base catalyzed reactions require strong alkaline conditions and excess heat. Because of this ability to be carried out under relatively mild reaction conditions, the acid catalyzed process is advantageous in the synthesis of α-hydroxy acids and esters which are sensitive to decomposition under strongly alkaline conditions.

The process of J.E. Thompson; U.S. Patent 3,492,325; January 27, 1970; assigned to The Procter & Gamble Company is one in which α-keto acetals are converted into α-hydroxy acids and esters in the presence of a Lewis acid catalyst and an inert solvent and water to form a reaction mixture. The reaction mixture is heated with provision for reflux until the conversion is complete. α-Hydroxy acids and esters are recovered from the reaction mixture by conventional methods. The starting material is an α-keto acetal having the general formula:

$$R-\underset{}{\overset{O}{\underset{\|}{C}}}-\underset{\underset{OR'}{|}}{\overset{\overset{OR'}{|}}{C}}-R''$$

wherein R is selected from the group consisting of straight chain alkyl, branched chain alkyl, alkenyl, aryl and aralkyl hydrocarbon groups having 1 to about 22 carbon atoms; each R' is selected from the group consisting of straight chain alkyl, aryl and aralkyl hydrocarbon groups having 1 to about 6 carbon atoms and R" is selected from the group consisting of hydrogen and straight chain alkyl, branched chain alkyl and aryl hydrocarbon groups having 1 to about 22 carbon atoms.

The reaction is carried out by heating the reaction mixture comprised of the α-keto acetal starting material, the Lewis acid catalyst, the inert solvent and the water to a temperature of about 0° to about 200°C.

Provision for reflux in the form of a condenser to return escaping vapors is provided; otherwise the reaction conditions would cause solvent loss by evaporation during the reaction. Preferably, the reaction is carried out at a temperature of about 60° to about 100°C.

The reaction can be carried out during a period of about 1 hour to about 24 hours until the reaction is complete. In general, the reaction proceeds fairly rapidly, and reaction times of about 1 to about 2 hours are preferred.

The reaction is normally carried out at atmospheric pressure; however, should a reaction appear to be sluggish, higher pressures can be used in order to raise the temperature and allow the reaction to proceed. The general reaction is illustrated by the equation shown on the following page.

$$\text{R}-\underset{\underset{\text{OR}'}{|}}{\overset{\overset{\text{O}}{\|}}{\text{C}}}-\underset{\underset{\text{OR}'}{|}}{\overset{\overset{\text{OR}'}{|}}{\text{C}}}-\text{R}'' + \text{H}_2\text{O} \xrightarrow[\Delta]{\text{Lewis acid solvent}}$$

$$\underset{1}{\text{R}\overset{\overset{\text{OH}}{|}}{\text{C}}\text{HCO}_2\text{R}'} + \underset{2}{\text{R}\overset{\overset{\text{OH}}{|}}{\text{C}}\text{HCO}_2\text{H}} + \underset{3}{\begin{array}{c}\text{R} \quad \text{O} \\ \diagup\text{CH}-\text{C}\diagdown \\ \text{O} \qquad\qquad \text{O} \\ \diagdown\text{C}-\text{CH}\diagup \\ \overset{\|}{\text{O}} \;\; \text{R}\end{array}}$$

The principal products are the α-hydroxy ester (1), the α-hydroxy acid (2) and the lactide (3) corresponding to the α-keto acetal starting material. Either the α-hydroxy ester (1) product or the α-hydroxy acid (2) product can be recovered by conventional means from the reaction mixture illustrated in the above general equation. When R is an alkyl group, the ester and acid products can be utilized as oil soluble metal complexing agents, as emulsifier agents in cake batters, as plasticizers for vinyl polymers, as lubricant additives and as intermediates in the synthesis of oil thickeners for use as ointment bases.

As an example of a general procedure for recovering the ester product subsequent to reaction, 10 volumes of methanol containing 1% by weight of a mineral acid such as sulfuric acid can be added to dissolve the reaction mixture. The resulting solution is heated with provision for reflux for one hour to effect methanolysis. The substitution of other alcohols, for example propyl alcohol, butyl alcohol and ethyl alcohol, results in the recovery of their corresponding ester. The solution is then cooled and poured into an equal volume of water and thereafter extracted with a suitable solvent. Suitable solvents for such an extraction include ether, chloroform, benzene, hexane and carbon tetrachloride.

The solvent extract is then neutralized with a weak base, for example, sodium bicarbonate or sodium carbonate and dried over anhydrous magnesium sulfate. Evaporation of the solvent leads to recovery of the α-hydroxy ester (1) as a residue. If the α-hydroxy acid (2) product is desired, the procedure is the same as for the recovery of the α-hydroxy ester above with the two exceptions that water is substituted for the alcohol and the solvent extract is not neutralized with a weak base prior to solvent evaporation for product recovery.

The α-keto acetal, the Lewis acid catalyst and water are combined in the presence of an inert and, preferably, a polar, water miscible solvent, for example dioxane, to form a reaction mixture. Other suitable polar, water miscible solvents are ethylene glycol dimethyl ether, diethylene glycol dimethyl ether, dimethylformamide, N,N-dimethylacetamide, acetonitrile and acetone. The use of a polar, water immiscible solvent, for example diether ether, or a nonpolar, water immiscible solvent, for example hexane, is also possible. The use of water immiscible solvents will, however, result in decreased product yields. The same process and recovery procedures are involved whether the solvent is water miscible or immiscible; however, longer reaction times are necessary when water immiscible solvents are employed. Examples of Lewis acids which can be utilized as the catalyst in the process of this method include $SnCl_4$, $AlCl_3$, $FeCl_3$, $TiCl_4$, $BF_3 \cdot (C_2H_5)_2O$ and H_2SO_4.

The Lewis acid catalysts, $SnCl_4$ for example, are employed in amounts ranging from catalytic amounts up to equimolar amounts with regard to the mols of α-keto acetal starting material. With small amounts of catalyst, increased reaction times will improve the yield. With large amounts of catalyst, however, the yield decreases as the reaction time increases beyond two hours. The use of greater than equimolar amounts of Lewis acid catalyst on the basis of the mols of α-keto acetal starting material results in a waste of the catalyst. When anhydrous $SnCl_4$, instead of hydrated $SnCl_4$, is used as the catalyst, improved yields are obtained.

Yields are improved by the addition of water subsequent to the combining of an anhydrous catalyst, particularly an anhydrous $SnCl_4$ catalyst, with an α-keto acetal starting material to form a reaction mixture. The addition of water subsequent to the addition of a hydrated catalyst tends to decrease yields. Although the amount of water added to the reaction can be varied, the mechanism of the reaction requires at least one mol of water for every mol of α-keto acetal that is converted into the corresponding α-hydroxy acid or ester.

The reaction has been carried out with about 1 mol of water to about 18 mols of water per mol of α-keto acetal starting material present, and the necessary water for the reaction can be supplied by a hydrated catalyst. The reaction will proceed with only trace amounts of water present, but in such a case α-keto acetal starting material will be wasted because the reaction will cease after the water is consumed. Preferable amounts of water for use in the process have been found to be about 4 to about 10, and preferably about 7, mols of water per mol of α-keto acetal starting material.

Additional water present, over the 1 mol of water per mol of α-keto acetal starting material necessary to satisfy stoichiometric requirements and up to about 17 additional mols of water per mol of α-keto acetal starting material, serves to limit the formation of degradation products during the reaction.

<u>Example:</u> A one liter, three necked flask equipped with a stirrer, a reflux

condenser and a rubber serum cap was used as a reactor. Prior to the addition of water by hypodermic syringe injection through the serum cap, the flask was protected from atmospheric moisture by means of a drying tube filled with anhydrous calcium sulfate. A solution of 30.0 g. (0.13 mol) of 1,1-dimethoxy-2-oxoundecane in 600 ml. of dried dioxane, as a polar, water miscible solvent, was prepared in the one liter, three necked flask, and to this solution were added rapidly and in succession 34.0 g. (0.13 mol) of anhydrous stannic chloride and 16.4 g. (0.91 mol — 7 mol per mol of 1,1-dimethoxy-2-oxoundecane) of water to form a reaction mixture.

The resulting reaction mixture was heated to and maintained at about 100°C., with provision for reflux by means of the reflux condenser, during a two hour period to effect the conversion reaction. The reaction mixture was then cooled and poured into an equal volume of water, and the resulting reaction mixture-water solution was extracted three times with ether.

After the ether extractions and a final extraction with chloroform, the combined chloroform and ether extracts were dried over anhydrous magnesium sulfate prior to evaporating the solvents, and the desolventized extract was neutralized with a sodium carbonate solution. A methanolysis process was then carried out on the neutralized extract and 23.3 g. of methyl 2-hydroxyundecanoate were recovered.

Cobalt Catalyst

In the process of S. Ishimoto, H. Togawa, Y. Honda and N. Saiki; U.S. Patent 3,708,534; January 2, 1973; assigned to Teijin Limited, Japan a ω-hydroxy saturated aliphatic monocarboxylic acid of 4 to 12 carbons can be prepared with high yield and high selectivity. The process comprises contacting a saturated, aliphatic dicarboxylic acid of 4-12 carbons, together with 0.3 to 20 weight times thereof of a saturated aliphatic glycol containing the same number of carbons as of the dicarboxylic acid, with hydrogen, in the presence of a cobalt catalyst which has been sintered at 1000° to 1750°C. and thereafter subjected to a reducing treatment, at a temperature within the range of 180° to 300°C., and a pressure as will provide a partial pressure of hydrogen of 10 to 80 kg./cm.^{2}.

The sintering temperature significantly affects the conversion of starting dicarboxylic acid. When the cobalt catalyst sintered at temperatures below 1000°C. is used in the hydrogenation reaction, conversion of the dicarboxylic acid drops abruptly. Whereas, if the sintering temperature exceeds 1750°C., a part of the cobalt oxide is melted, and the catalyst shows reduced level of activity. Incidentally, the cobalt oxide obtained as the result of sintering is believed to be composed chiefly of $CoO \cdot Co_2O_3$. When the sintering temperature is selected from the range of 1100° to

1600°C., cobalt catalyst of higher activity can be obtained, and starting dicarboxylic acids can be advantageously converted to the corresponding hydroxy acids at higher conversions. The sintered, reduced cobalt catalyst employed can be prepared by compression molding, for example, cobalt oxide, or a cobalt compound which can form cobalt oxide at the above-specified sintering temperatures, such as cobalt nitrate, hydroxide, carbonate, etc., into cylindrical or granular form, for example; sintering the molded product in an oxygen-containing gas such as air, at temperatures ranging from 1000° to 1750°C., preferably 1100° to 1600°C.; and thereafter reducing the cobalt oxide in hydrogen gas-containing atmosphere.

The effectiveness of the reducing treatment can be confirmed by formation of water upon the reduction of the cobalt oxide resulting from the sintering. It is advantageous to carry out the reducing treatment as thoroughly as possible, until the formation of water completely terminates. Preferably, the reducing treatment is performed under heating, at temperatures ranging, e.g., 280° to 500°C. Such sintered, reduced cobalt catalyst can be satisfactorily used in so far as it is composed mainly of cobalt. The catalytic activity of the catalyst can be maintained at approximately the same level with that of the catalyst which is 100% cobalt, when it contains no more than 20% by weight, particularly no more than 10% by weight, of other metallic component, such as manganese, copper, chromium, etc.

The sintered, reduced cobalt catalyst may be bound onto an inert carrier such as, for example, alumina, silica, diatomaceous earth, pumice, etc. In order to form such carrier-bound catalyst, for example, powdered cobalt oxide may be mixed with powdered alumina, compression molded as aforesaid, sintered, and reduced with hydrogen. Or, the carrier may be immersed in an aqueous solution of water-soluble cobalt compound such as cobalt nitrate, followed by drying, sintering, and reduction with hydrogen.

In the process, if the quantity of glycol is less than 0.5 weight times particularly less than 0.3 weight times, of the starting dicarboxylic acid, the selectivity for the ω-hydroxymonocarboxylic acid is lowered, and side-formation of corresponding glycol is increased. Whereas, if the quantity of glycol exceeds 5 weight times, particularly 20 weight times, of the dicarboxylic acid, it becomes difficult to maintain high conversion of the dicarboxylic acid, i.e., the yield of the corresponding ω-hydroxymonocarboxylic acid is reduced.

In the preparation of ω-hydroxymonocarboxylic acid the reaction temperature and partial pressure of hydrogen within the reaction system are also important factors. At the reaction temperatures below 200°C., conversion of the dicarboxylic acid is lowered. Whereas, when it exceeds 270°C., side reactions such as hydrogenolysis are promoted. Consequently, side-formation of, for example, monohydric alcohols containing less number of carbons than the ω-hydroxymonocarboxylic acids is increased, and selectivity for the product is lowered. Again, when the partial pressure of hydrogen in the reaction system at the specified reaction temperature range is below 20 kg./cm.^{2}, conversion of the dicarboxylic acid is lowered. Whereas, if the partial pressure of hydrogen exceeds 60 kg./cm.^{2}, selectivity for the ω-hydroxymonocarboxylic acid is lowered, and side-production of corresponding glycol is increased.

Furthermore, the conversion of starting dicarboxylic acid can be improved by the concurrent presence of water in the described reaction system, in an amount not exceeding 10 molar times, particularly 0.5 to 3 molar times, the dicarboxylic acid. When the water amounts to 10 molar times or more to the dicarboxylic acid, conversion of the dicarboxylic acid can be further improved, but with reduced selectivity for the object ω-hydroxymonocarboxylic acid. Therefore, presence of excessive amount of water should be avoided.

It has been confirmed that under the above-specified reaction conditions, dehydrogenation reaction of saturated aliphatic glycols of 4 to 12 carbons (alkanediols) to form corresponding ω-hydroxymonocarboxylic acids is also actively promoted. Therefore, under the reaction conditions employed in the process, not only the hydrogenation of starting dicarboxylic acid to form corresponding ω-hydroxymonocarboxylic acid progresses, but also the further hydrogenation of the ω-hydroxymonocarboxylic acid to form corresponding glycol, taking place as an objectionable side reaction, is very effectively inhibited.

Furthermore, in certain cases a part of the glycol which is initially added to the reaction system together with the dicarboxylic acid is also converted to the ω-hydroxymonocarboxylic acid. Thus it is possible to obtain the ω-hydroxymonocarboxylic acid at a yield higher than the maximum yield theoretically calculated from the quantity of dicarboxylic acid converted during the reaction.

Various methods are available for separating ω-hydroxymonocarboxylic acids. For example, an alkali such as caustic soda, caustic potash, etc. may be added to the reaction product, to hydrolyze the oligomer of ω-hydroxymonocarboxylic acid and the esters of monocarboxylic acid and oligomer thereof under normally employed saponifying conditions, and thereafter the saturated, aliphatic glycol is removed from the hydrolyzed liquid by distillation or extraction. ω-Hydroxymonocarboxylic acid can be separated from the resulting aqueous solution of alkali salts of the aliphatic dicarboxylic acid and ω-hydroxymonocarboxylic acid, by the steps of adding a mineral acid such as hydrochloric or sulfuric acid to said aqueous solution of alkali salts to adjust the latter's pH to 4.5 to 6.5, selectively extracting ω-hydroxy-monocarboxylic acid therefrom with an extracting agent such as cyclohexanol, and removing the extracting agent from the extract.

Example 1: Cobalt oxide was compression molded, heated in air at 1050°C. for an hour, and the resulting sintered cobalt oxide was reduced in hydrogen current at 320°C. until generation of water substantially terminated. Thus sintered and reduced cobalt was used as the catalyst in the synthesis described below.

Thirty g. of adipic acid, 50 g. of 1,6-hexanediol, 5 g. of water, and the sintered and reduced cobalt obtained through the procedures described above, of the amount corresponding to 70 g. of the sintered cobalt oxide before the reduction, were charged in a vertical agitation type, stainless steel autoclave of 500 cc in capacity. Further hydrogen gas was fed into the autoclave to an elevated pressure of 50 kg./cm.^{2}G., and then the reactants were heated and reacted at 210°C. for 2.5 hours. The partial pressure of hydrogen after the reaction was 52 kg./cm.^{2}G. Upon analysis, the resulting reaction mixture was found to contain 7.55 g. of adipic acid and 18.4 g. of ε-hydroxycaproic acid.

The conversion of adipic acid was 75 mol percent, and the selectivity for ε-hydroxycaproic acid was 92 mol percent. The reaction mixture also contained 49.8 g. of 1,6-hexanediol. Thus the amount of 1,6-hexanediol showed very little change before and after the reaction.

Example 2: Above Example 1 was repeated, except that the hydrogen gas was fed at an elevated pressure of 25 kg./cm.^{2}G., and the reaction was performed at 220°C. for 3 hours. As the result, the conversion of adipic acid was 57 mol percent and the selectivity for ε-hydroxycaproic acid was 100 mol percent. The reaction mixture contained 48.0 g. of 1,6-hexanediol.

Example 3: The reaction of Example 1 was repeated 40 times. Thereafter the activity of the catalyst was observed to be somewhat reduced. Then 30 g. of adipic acid and 50 g. of 1,6-hexanediol were charged into the autoclave, and reacted under the identical conditions with those of Example 1 except that the reaction temperature was 270°C. and reaction time was 45 minutes. As the result, the conversion of adipic acid was 54 mol percent and the selectivity for ε-hydroxycaproic acid was 86 mol percent. The reaction mixture contained 47.5 g. of 1,6-hexanediol.

Neo-Acids Using Acid Catalyst

Neo-acids are compounds having a completely substituted α-carbon atom (i.e. the carbon atom adjacent to the carboxyl radical), and are so named because of their structural resemblance to neopentane (2,2-dimethyl propane). Neo-acids have a variety of uses. They react with acetylene to form vinyl derivatives which can be polymerized to form plastics. The cadmium and barium salts are stabilizers for vinyl resins, and the peroxyesters are catalysts for polymerization reactions. These acids and their derivatives also find utility in the preparation of cosmetics, perfumes, insect repellents, as well as a number of other products.

H.L. Wehrmeister; U.S. Patent 3,466,309; September 9, 1969; assigned to Commercial Solvents Corporation provides a process for the production of neo-acids, i.e., organic acids having a completely substituted α-carbon atom, by the hydrolysis of 2-substituted-2-oxazolines in the presence of an acid. Neo-acids correspond to the following general formula:

$$R_2-\underset{\underset{OH}{|}}{\overset{\overset{H}{|}}{C}}-\underset{\underset{R_1}{|}}{\overset{\overset{R_3}{|}}{C}}-COOH$$

wherein R_1 can be alkyl of from 1 to about 16 carbon atoms, alkenyl of from 2 to about 16 carbon atoms, hydroxymethyl or aryl; R_2 can be hydrogen, alkyl of from 1 to about 15 carbon atoms, or phenyl; R_3 can be alkyl of from 1 to about 15 carbon atoms, or hydroxyalkyl of from 1 to 15 carbon atoms, or phenyl. These neo-acids are produced by the hydrolysis of a group of 2-oxazolines (the Group 1 oxazolines) corresponding to the formula:

$$R_2-\underset{\underset{OH}{|}}{\overset{\overset{H}{|}}{C}}-\underset{\underset{R_1}{|}}{\overset{\overset{R_3}{|}}{C}}-C\underset{O-CH_2}{\overset{N=\underset{\underset{}{|}}{\overset{\overset{R}{|}}{C}}-R}{\diagup}}$$

wherein R can be hydrogen, alkyl of from 1 to 3 carbon atoms, or hydroxymethyl, and R_1, R_2 and R_3 are defined above. The hydrolysis reaction is conducted in the presence of water and a mineral acid catalyst. Hydrolysis conditions include a reaction temperature of from 20°C. to reflux conditions, 100°C. or above. The reaction is conducted for a period of time sufficient to effect the hydrolysis, for instance 1 to 15 hours. After the heating period, the reaction, if incomplete, can be advantageously allowed to continue at room temperature for a period of 24 to 36 hours, preferably with agitation.

The mineral acids are preferably diluted to 10% to 50% by weight, and when desired, additional water is added to provide fluidity to the reaction mixture. The reaction can also be conducted in the presence of a suitable solvent for the oxazoline. Suitable solvents include the lower alkanols, e.g. methanol, ethanol, isopropyl alcohol, and butanol. The neo-acid produced can be separated from the reaction mixture, if desired, by cooling the mixture and allowing the neo-acid to crystallize. In some cases it is advantageous to reduce the volume of the reaction mixture to approximately one-half or less by evaporation of some of the water and solvent. After separation, the neo-acid can be recrystallized from water or other suitable solvent.

An alternate procedure for separating the neo-acid from the reaction mixture is by solvent extraction with a suitable solvent, such as ethyl ether. The amount of acid catalyst employed will depend upon the particular catalyst; however, these amounts will generally range from 10 to 200% by weight of the catalyst, preferably 50 to 100%, based on the weight of the oxazoline. Suitable acid catalysts include organic and inorganic catalysts and include inorganic mineral acids such as sulfuric and hydrochloric acids, preferably hydrochloric acid.

Example 1: Preparation of 2,2-Bis(Hydroxymethyl)-Propionic Acid — 2-[1,1-bis(hydroxymethyl) ethyl]-4,4-dimethyl-2-oxazoline, 40 g., was charged to an acid resistant reaction vessel equipped with a reflux condenser. Hydrochloric acid, 100 ml. concentrated acid diluted with 100 ml. water was added and the mixture was heated for 3 hours at reflux temperature. Following the heating period the solution was extracted continuously for 37 hours with 500 ml. of ethyl ether. The neo-acid extracted by the ether crystallized and was separated by filtration. It was recrystallized from water and dried under vacuum. The melting point found was 192° to 193°C., lit. 181° to 185°C. The neutral equivalent (acid) was 136.1, theoretical 134.1. Equivalent weight by hydroxy determination (acetylation method) was 135.1.

General procedure for hydrolysis of 2-substituted-2-oxazolines to neo-acids is as follows. The oxazoline (0.1 mol) is dispersed in 200 ml. of dilute hydrochloric acid (1 part conc. HCl to 1 part water) in a reaction vessel equipped with a reflux condenser and heated at reflux for at least 3 hours. The mixture is allowed to stand at room temperature for 24 to 36 hours. It is then cooled and the precipitated solid is collected by filtration, washed 2 times with 50 ml. of water and dried. The crude product can be purified by any suitable method, e.g., it can be recrystallized from a suitable solvent. If the neo-acid does not precipitate on cooling, it can be recovered by extraction with a suitable solvent, e.g., ethyl ether.

Example 2: Preparation of 3-Phenyl-3-Hydroxy-2,2-Dimethyl-1-Propionic Acid — A mixture of 141 g. of 2-(1-methylethyl)-4,4-dimethyl-2-oxazoline and 106 g. of benzaldehyde is heated at 99° to 105°C. for 8 hours to produce 2-(1,1-dimethyl-2-hydroxy-2-phenyl-ethyl)-4,4-dimethyl-2-oxazoline, a Group 1 oxazoline. This compound is hydrolyzed according to the general procedure. 3-phenyl-3-hydroxy-2,2-dimethyl-1-propionic acid is obtained.

Example 3: Preparation of 2,2-Bis(Hydroxymethyl) Oleic Acid — The experiment of Example 2 is repeated except that the oxazoline employed is 2-heptadecenyl-4,4-dimethyl-2-oxazoline and the product obtained by condensation with formaldehyde is 2-[1,1-bis(hydroxymethyl)-2-heptadecenyl]-4,4-dimethyl-2-oxazoline. It is hydrolyzed according to the general procedure and 2,2-bis(hydroxymethyl) oleic acid is obtained.

NONCATALYTIC PROCESSES

From Haloalkanols

In the process of R.V.J. Achard and J. Morel; U.S. Patent 3,404,166; October 1, 1968; assigned to Rhone-Poulenc SA, France trans-ω-hydroxy-2-alkenoic acids are made from ω-haloalkanols of 2 fewer carbon atoms by oxidation to the corresponding ω-haloalkanal, reaction of the latter with malonic acid or a derivative thereof, followed by decarboxylation and hydrolysis to give the desired acid.

The process comprises oxidizing an ω-haloalkanol of the formula, $Hal(CH_2)_nCH_2OH$ in which Hal represents a chlorine, bromine or iodine atom and n is an integer higher than 4 so as to produce an ω-haloalkanal of the formula, $Hal(CH_2)_nCHO$, condensing this haloaldehyde with malonic acid or an acid alkyl malonate with simultaneously an at least partial decarboxylation completed by heating, so as to produce an acid of the formula, $Hal(CH_2)_nCH=CH-COOH$, or an alkyl ester thereof when an acid alkyl malonate has been employed, hydrolyzing the product, and separating the ω-hydroxy-2-alkenoic acid produced.

The haloalkanol is preferably an ω-chloro-alkanol and when an acid alkyl malonate is used the alkyl group is preferably methyl or ethyl. In the process, ω-halogenoalkanals of formula $Hal(CH_2)_nCHO$ are prepared by oxidizing ω-halogenoalkanols of formula $Hal(CH_2)_nCH_2OH$ by known methods of oxidizing primary alcohols to aldehydes, for example, using manganese dioxide or, preferably, using an aqueous mixture of sulfuric and chromic acids. It is especially preferred to add an aqueous alkali metal dichromate solution gradually to a mixture of dilute sulfuric acid and the ω-haloalkanol at the boiling point so that the ω-haloalkanal is steam-distilled out of the reaction mixture as it is formed. The degree of dilution of the sulfuric acid is not critical and the dilutions recommended for similar oxidations may be used. The ω-haloalkanal is then condensed with malonic acid or an acid alkyl malonate, the operation being carried out in an organic diluent comprising an organic base, e.g., pyridine. It is preferred to use pyridine both as diluent and base. The reaction continues from 2 to 60 hours from 20° to 50°C.

The reaction is accompanied by at least partial decarboxylation of the dicarboxylic acid (or acid ester) formed. The decarboxylation is, if necessary, finally completed by heating the reaction mixture for 1 to 2 hours to 60° to 100°C., to give the acid of formula $Hal(CH_2)_nCH=CH-COOH$. The ω-halo-2-alkenoic acid is then hydrolyzed with a base to the trans-ω-hydroxy-2-alkenoic acid of formula $HO(CH_2)_nCH=CH-COOH$. This operation is carried out, for example, by heating under reflux for 4 to 5 hours an aqueous solution of an alkali salt of the ω-halo-2-alkenoic acid with an aqueous solution of an alkali metal hydroxide or carbonate, the quantity of alkaline agent employed being at least equal to the stoichiometric quantity.

When an acid alkyl malonate is used in place of malonic acid itself, the alkyl ω-halo-2-alkenoate obtained is similarly hydrolyzed to give the ω-hydroxy-2-alkenoic acid. It is unnecessary in the process to use particularly pure starting materials or to purify carefully the intermediate products. It is also unnecessary to isolate the ω-halogenoalkanal after oxidation before passing to the following stage. The mixture obtained, which still contains unconverted alcohol, may be condensed as it is with malonic acid.

Under these conditions, there is obtained, after the condensation, a mixture which is first separated from pyridine, or other organic base, by extraction with an organic solvent in acid medium. From the organic phase thus isolated, the desired ω-halo-2-alkenoic acid is extracted (as a salt) by treatment with an aqueous solution of an alkali metal hydroxide.

Example: The preparation of trans-8-hydroxy-2-octenoic acid is as follows. 6-chlorohexanal is prepared first. Into a 5 l. three-necked, round-bottomed flask provided with a stirrer, a dropping funnel, a distillation condenser and a thermometer are charged: water, 2,500 cc.; sulfuric acid (d. = 1.83), 400 cc.; and 6-chlorohexanol, 400 g. The reaction mixture is boiled and a solution of 400 g. of sodium dichromate ($Na_2Cr_2O_7 \cdot 2H_2O$) in 5 l. of water is run in through the funnel at a rate substantially equal to that at which the mixture distills. This addition lasts 4 hours in all. There are then added 500 cc. of water, while 500 cc. of the reaction mixture are distilled. The distillate is extracted with ether and the ethereal solution obtained is dried over anhydrous sodium sulfate and then concentrated on the water bath in vacuo. There is thus obtained a residue of 293.7 g. containing 147.7 g. of 6-chlorohexanal (determined by reaction with hydroxylamine hydrochloride) and 146 g. of 6-chlorohexanol. The percentage of conversion of 6-chlorohexanol is therefore 63.5% and the 6-chlorohexanal yield based on the 6-chlorohexanol used is 59%.

This is followed by preparing 8-chloro-2-octenoic acid. Into a 2 l. three-necked, round-bottomed flask provided with a stirrer, a thermometer, a reflux condenser and a bubble counter, are charged, in the following order: the mixture of 6-chlorohexanal and 6-chlorohexanol prepared in the above example, 289.7 g. (i.e. 145.7 g. of 6-chlorohexanal); pyridine, 300 cc.; and malonic acid, 135 g. The reaction mixture is maintained at 30°C. for 60 hours, heated for one hour at 60°C., and then for one hour at 90° to 95°C. The product is cooled to 50°C. and poured on to a mixture of 600 g. of ice and 500 cc. of hydrochloric acid(d. = 1.18).

The product is extracted with three 300 cc. portions of ether and the pyridine remains in the aqueous medium as its hydrochloride. The ethereal solution is stirred with a mixture of 400 cc. of water and 200 cc. of sodium hydroxide solution (d. = 1.33). The ethereal solution, after drying over sodium sulfate and evaporation, gives a resdue from which 144 g. of 6-chlorohexanol can be recovered. The aqueous alkaline solution is treated with activated charcoal, filtered through a Clarcel filtration adjuvant and then acidified with 250 cc. of hydrochloric acid (d. = 1.18). The crude 8-chloro-2-octenoic acid (157 g.) is extracted with ether. Yield, 82.2% calculated on the 6-chlorohexanal. On recrystallization at -10°C. from petroleum ether, there is obtained an acid whose solidification point is 17.6° to 18°C.

The preparation of the trans-8-hydroxy-2-octenoic acid then continues. Into a 1 l. round-bottomed flask provided with a reflux condenser are charged: crude 8-chloro-2-octenoic acid, 137 g.; water, 1,750 cc.; and sodium carbonate, 137 g. The mixture is heated for 4 hours under reflux. After cooling, the product is treated with activated charcoal, filtered and then acidified with 250 cc. of hydrochloric acid (d. = 1.18). By extraction with ether, there are isolated 94 g. of a product which, on recrystallization from 200 cc. of acetonitrile, gives 66 g. of trans-8-hydroxy-2-octenoic acid, MP 62°C. (yield, 54%).

Recrystallization of this acid from a mixture of cyclohexane and ethyl acetate (50/50) raises the MP to 63°C. Elemental and functional analysis, the infra-red spectrum and the nuclear magnetic resonance confirm the constitution given for this product, which on hydrogenation gives 8-hydroxy-octanoic acid, MP 58°C.

Synthesis of Hydroxy Acids

From Alpha-Nitratocarboxylic Acids

In the process of W. Müller, J. Schweighofer and F. Weinrotter; U.S. Patent 3,449,385; June 10, 1969; assigned to Osterreichische Stickstoffwerke AG, Austria saturated aliphatic α-hydroxycarboxylic acids with up to 18 carbon atoms which are unbranched in α-position are produced by reacting the corresponding α-nitratocarboxylic acids or their water-soluble salts with at least one mol of a water-soluble salt of sulfurous acid at a temperature between 20°C. and the boiling point of the reaction mixture.

The crude nitrate esters, as produced on reaction of α-olefins with dinitrogen tetroxide in the presence of oxygen, may be used directly for the reaction, without previous purification. The nitro-compounds which occasionally occur as impurities in the nitrate esters do not interfere with the course of the reaction, since they react with sulfites to give sulfonic acids which are soluble in water but insoluble in ether and which can easily be separated off during the further working up. In the process any sulfite-containing compound may be used as long as it is water-soluble. Particularly suitable compounds are the ammonium, alkali metal and alkaline earth metal sulfites and bisulfites.

Furthermore, technical ammonium sulfite lye, which may also contain a certain amount of sulfate, as produced on purifying the waste gases from sulfuric acid manufacture, may be used as a reagent. The addition of a sulfite-containing compound produces, simultaneously with the hydrolysis of the nitratocarboxylic acid to the α-hydroxycarboxylic acid, a reduction of the nitrate nitrogen, whereby the sulfite is mainly oxidized to sulfate. As a result of the reduction of the nitrate nitrogen the undesired oxidation reactions are practically completely suppressed. Pure α-hydroxycarboxylic acid is obtained in practically quantitative yield.

The molar ratio of sulfite to nitratocarboxylic acid preferably should be at least 1:1. It is advantageous to use 2.5 mols or more than 2.5 mols of sulfite per mol of nitratocarboxylic acid. In carrying out the process, it has proved advisable to introduce the α-nitratocarboxylic acid into the aqueous sulfite solution. It is however, also possible to add the reagents simultaneously to an already reacted, or still reacting, aqueous solution of a salt of the α-hydroxycarboxylic acid which it is intended to manufacture. This latter procedure is advisable when carrying out the process continuously.

In all variations of the process good mixing of the reaction solution should be ensured. The amount of water present in the reaction charge need not suffice to dissolve the water-soluble sulfite, i.e., the sulfite can be used both as a solution or with part of it in the form of a slurry. Instead of the free nitratocarboxylic acid, a water-soluble salt thereof, above all the

ammonium or alkali metal salt, is also suitable as a starting material. The
α-hydroxycarboxylic acid may be isolated from the reaction mixture by any
known method. Thus a long-chain water-insoluble acid may after acidification with mineral acid, e.g., sulfuric acid or hydrochloric acid be directly
separated from the aqueous phase. The α-hydroxycarboxylic acids so obtained are practically free from impurities and may optionally be esterified
with alcohols, or acylated with acids, without further purification. Depending on the manufacturing conditions, the α-hydroxycarboxylic acids may
contain varying amounts of the corresponding hemilactides, which arise by
intermolecular dehydration and which may be regarded as internal esters.

These are also a constituent of commercially sold α-hydroxycarboxylic acids.
The hemilactide can, by saponification with alkaline or acid materials,
easily be converted to the monomolecular α-hydroxycarboxylic acid.
Straight-chain aliphatic α-hydroxycarboxylic acids, and the esters of such
acids produced from them, are valuable industrially usable products. They
may for example be used as wetting agents and in plant protection.

Example 1: 140 g. of crude α-nitratocaprylic acid (approx. 85% strength,
made from octene-1 and N_2O_4) are introduced at 60°C. into a solution of
270 g. of sodium sulfite in 450 ml. of water over the course of 45 minutes,
with stirring. The reaction is exothermic and the temperature is adjusted to
60°C. by cooling. When addition is complete the mixture is warmed to 90°
to 95°C. and kept at this temperature for 3 hours. After cooling the reaction mixture is acidified with 40% sulfuric acid whereupon it separates into
2 phases. The organic phase is washed 4 times with 150 ml. of water and is
subsequently dried over sodium sulfate.

The mother liquor and the combined wash waters are extracted with ether in
order to increase the yield, and the extract is dried and after evaporation of
the ether is combined with the organic phase. The bulk of the impurities
from the α-nitratocaprylic acid remains in the aqueous phase as sulfonic
acids. The crude product so obtained consists of free α-hydroxycaprylic
acid with varying contents of 2-(α-hydroxycaproyloxy)-caprylic acid and
may be directly used for most purposes, e.g., for esterification. The yield
is 95% of theory.

The pure α-hydroxycaprylic acid may be obtained by recrystallization from
n-heptane, and in the course of this the mother liquors which no longer crystallize (enriched hemilactide) may, by saponification with caustic alkali or
with acid, be practically quantitatively converted to the monomeric product.

Example 2: 345 g. of α-nitratostearic acid are introduced at 70°C. into a
solution of 309 g. of sodium sulfite and 104 g. of sodium bisulfite in 1,400
milliliters of water over the course of 1 hour, with stirring. The reaction is

exothermic and the temperature is adjusted to 70°C. by cooling. When addition is complete, the mixture is warmed to 90° to 95°C. and kept at this temperature for 7 hours. After cooling the reaction mixture is acidified with 40% sulfuric acid with stirring, whereupon the solid α-hydroxystearic acid is precipitated. The acid is separated by filtering off, washed with water and dried. The α-hydroxystearic acid is obtained in a yield of 90% of theory. The products so obtained consist of free α-hydroxystearic acid with varying contents of 2-(α-hydroxystearoyloxy)-stearic acid. The pure α-hydroxystearic acid may be obtained by saponification of the anhydro-hydroxystearic acid with caustic alkali.

Use of Alkanol Reaction Medium

Hydroxy unsaturated acids having allylic or homoallylic systems with a double bond between the hydroxyl and carboxyl group, and their salts, esters, and amides yield a product containing an enhanced proportion of the corresponding omega-hydroxyalkanoic acid according to the process of *M.J. Diamond; U.S. Patent 3,466,310; September 9, 1969; assigned to the U.S. Secretary of Agriculture.* In accordance with the process, a compound selected from the group consisting of acids, salts, esters, and amides, which contains the radical

$$CH_3-(CH_2)_x-CHOH-(CH_2)_y-CH=CH-(CH_2)_z-\overset{O}{\underset{\|}{C}}-$$

(wherein y is an integer from 0 to 1, and x and z are each an integer from 0 to 16 with the limitation that the sum of x and z does not exceed 16) is reacted with a strong alkali of a temperature of about 178° to 210°C. in the presence of a medium consisting chiefly of a monohydroxy primary or secondary alkanol which has a boiling point (at atmospheric pressure) of at least 178°C., typically 1-octanol or 2-octanol. The key item is the use of the medium in that it directs the course of the cleavage to yield a reaction product containing a higher ratio of hydroxy acid $HO-(CH_2)_{z+2}-COOH$ to dibasic acid $HOOC-(CH_2)_{z+1}-COOH$.

The advantageous result obtained is graphically illustrated by the following equations, wherein x, y, and z have the values stated above:

$$CH_3-(CH_2)_x-CHOH-(CH_2)_y-CH=CH-(CH_2)_z-COOH$$

Reaction 1 Promoted / Reaction 2 Suppressed

$HO-(CH_2)_{z+2}-COOH$ $\quad\quad$ $HOOC-(CH_2)_{z+1}-COOH$
$+$ $\quad\quad\quad\quad\quad\quad\quad\quad\quad\quad\quad$ $+$
$CH_3-(CH_2)_x-\overset{O}{\underset{\|}{C}}-(CH_2)_yH$ $\quad\quad$ $CH_3-(CH_2)_x-CHOH-(CH_2)_yH$

For use in the process, 2-octanol is generally preferred as it is very effective and relatively inexpensive. However, many other primary or secondary monohydroxy alkanols may be used. Since the reaction is conducted at about 178° to 210°C., the selected alkanol should have a boiling point (at atmospheric pressure) of at least 178°C. Especially good results are obtained with alkanols which are unhindered, that is, those which are free from branching on the carbon atoms alpha or beta to the carbon atom which bears the hydroxyl group.

For example, such alkanols as 1-octanol or 2-octanol (free from any branching) provide better resuls than diisobutyl carbinol which contains branching on both carbons beta to the carbon atom which bears the hydroxyl group. Illustrative examples of alkanols, in addition to those cited above, which may be used are: 5-ethyl-nonanol-2; 7-ethyl-2-methylundecanol-4; nonanol-2; decanol-4; nonanol-1; undecanol-1; and cyclooctanol. Also useful are commercial mixtures of primary and secondary alcohols such as the products sold on the market as isooctanol and isodecanol.

Although it is generally preferred to use the alkanol as the sole added medium in the reaction, it is within the broad ambit of the process to use a reaction medium wherein the alkanol is the chief or major ingredient, the remainder being a conventional inert solvent such as a high-boiling hydrocarbon, typically decalin or white mineral oil.

The reaction is carried out as follows. There is provided a reaction kettle of material resistant to attack by hot caustic, equipped with heating means, stirrer, reflux condenser, etc. The kettle is first charged with the alkanol, alkali, and water. The alkanol is used in excess to function not only as a reaction director but also as a diluent to keep the reaction mixture fluid enough so it can be stirred effectively, thus to keep the various reactants in contact with one another.

Assuming that the reaction will involve the use of one mol of unsaturated hydroxy acid or its equivalent (this same basis will be applicable to the other proportions stated below), the alkanol is generally supplied in an amount to provide at least 2 mols thereof, preferably at least 4 mols. A larger proportion of alkanol may be used but will provide little if any added advantage. The alkali, e.g., sodium hydroxide, potassium hydroxide, or mixtures thereof, is provided in amount to furnish at least 2 mols thereof.

Preferably an excess is used, i.e., about 4 to 18 mols. Water is provided in relatively small amount to just dissolve the alkali or at least convert it from a solid to a fluid condition so that the alkali will properly contact the other substances in the reaction system. After charging the kettle with the alkanol, caustic, and water, the contents of the kettle are brought to the

Synthesis of Hydroxy Acids

reaction temperature, about 178° to 210°C., and maintained thereat through the course of the reaction, with continuous application of stirring. The starting material, the unsaturated hydroxy acid or equivalent, is fed into the kettle slowly over a period of at least several hours. Usually a reaction period of about 2 to 12 hours is used. Longer times may be employed but offer little added benefit. After completion of the reaction, the resulting mixture may be treated to isolate the omega-hydroxy alkanoic acid and other products by methods well known in the art.

Example: A series of runs were carried out using the following technique in each case. A 100 ml., thick-walled, Pyrex glass reaction vessel was fitted with a stirrer, dropping funnel, and reflux condenser. The reaction vessel was charged with 24 ml. of a selected organic diluent (as specified below), 1.8 ml. of water, and 6.8 g. of sodium hydroxide. The dropping funnel was charged with 6.5 g. of methyl ricinoleate. The reactor was immersed in a silicone oil bath heated to 185° to 195°C., and the ricinoleate was then introduced dropwise. After all the ricinoleate had been added the mixture was stirred for 12.5 to 13 hours longer while holding the oil bath at 185° to 195°C.

At the end of this period, a 3 g. portion of the reaction product was dissolved in 20 ml. hot water, acidified to pH 1 with 50% aqueous sulfuric acid and extracted with ether. The ether solution was dried with sodium sulfate, and the ether was removed on a rotary evaporator to yield an oily residue which was converted to mixed methyl esters in refluxing excess methanol with 0.5% concentrated sulfuric acid. The resultant ester mixture was analyzed to determine the proportions of 10-hydroxydecanoic acid, sebacic acid, and uncleaved ricinoleic acid in the reaction product. The diluents used and the results obtained are tabulated below.

Run[1]	Diluent	Type of diluent	Analysis[2]			Ratio of 10-hydroxy-decanoic acid to sebacic acid
			10-hydroxy-decanoic acid, percent	Sebacic acid, percent	Ricinoleic acid, percent	
a	1-octanol	Prim. alkanol	82.6	16.5	0.5	5.0
b	Isooctanol	Com'l mixture of prim. and sec. alkanols.	73.0	15.4	0	4.7
c	Isodecanol	do	62.0	28.6	4.8	2.2
d	2-octanol	Sec. alkanol	80.0	11.0	0	7.3
e	1:1 mixture of 2-octanol and decalin.	Mixture of sec. alkanol and hydrocarbon.	53.0	33.0	14.0	1.6
f	Cyclooctanol	Sec. alkanol	63.0	22.8	3.2	2.8
g	Diisobutyl alcohol	do	53.0	34.0	6.3	1.6
h	Phenethyl alcohol	Aromatic alcohol	14.0	31.0	51.0	0.45
i	2-methyl-2-nonanol	Tert. alkanol	18.7	75.0	6.3	0.25
j	Decalin	Hydrocarbon	31.0	55.0	14.0	0.56
k	α-methylbenzyl alcohol	Aromatic alcohol	15.0	20.0	20.0	0.75

[1] Runs h through k are not illustrative of the invention, but are included for purpose of comparison.
[2] The difference between 100 percent and the total percentages reported represents a mixture of unidentified fragments.

Lesquerolic Acid from Seed Oil

The principal constituent fatty acid of the triglycerides comprising the seed oils of the genus Lesquerella (family Cruciferae), including the species lasiocarpa and lindheimertii, is a C_{20}-hydroxy acid analog of ricinoleic acid. Specifically, this fatty acid is 14-hydroxy-cis-11-eicosenoic acid designated lesquerolic acid, having the structure

$$CH_3(CH_2)_5-\underset{\underset{OH}{|}}{CH}-CH_2CH=CH(CH_2)_9COOH$$

Lesquerolic acid is prepared in a process of C.R. Smith, Jr., M.O. Bagby and I.A. Wolff; U.S. Patent 3,057,893; October 9, 1962; assigned to the U.S. Secretary of Agriculture according to the following procedure. Coarsely ground seeds of Lesquerella lasiocarpa (431.9 g.) were Soxhlet-extracted overnight with petroleum ether. Then most of the solvent was evaporated under nitrogen on a steam bath and the balance evaporated in vacuo, yielding 113.2 g. of an oily material which was then transesterified by refluxing for 2 hours under nitrogen in 3,200 ml. of methanol containing 1% sulfuric acid.

The mixed methyl esters were isolated from the solution by diluting with 5 l. of water, saturating with sodium chloride, successively extracting with ether, extracting the pooled ether extracts with 5% potassium carbonate, successively washing the pooled ether extract with water, separating the ether layer and drying the same over sodium sulfate, and removing the ether under partial vacuum to give 111.5 g. of mixed methyl esters.

Partial distillation of 110.4 g. of the mixed methyl esters in a spinning band column left 54.5 g. of a concentrate in the still pot that by gas chromatography was found to consist of 4% methyl hydroxyoctadecenoate, 2% of the methyl ester of a C_{20} unsaturated acid, 1.1% of the methyl ester of a C_{20} saturated acid, and 92.9% of methyl lesquerolate. The above concentrate (54.47 g.) was then refluxed under nitrogen for 2 hours with 655 ml. of N ethanolic potassium hydroxide, concentrated under partial vacuum to about 200 ml., diluted with 1,200 ml. of water, successively extracted with 200 ml. portions of ether, and the combined ethereal extracts then successively washed with 100 ml. portions of water.

The combined aqueous alkaline mixture and wash water were acidified to methyl orange with hydrochloric acid and extracted with successive portions of ether. The pooled ethereal extract was washed with water, and then made slightly alkaline to indicator paper with ethanolic sodium hydroxide to form the sodium soaps. Upon removal of the solvent under reduced pressure, 52.9 g. of the mixed sodium soaps were obtained. From another preparation of the mixed methyl esters a 3.40 g. portion was subjected to a 30-transfer countercurrent distribution with acetonitrile-hexane. Methyl lesquerolate recovered from tubes 6 through 14 was found by gas chromatography to be 90 to 97% pure. Methyl lesquerolate shows IR maxima at 2.740μ; 2.770μ; (doublet); and at 5.720μ (no maximum at 10 to 11μ).

A 1.11 g. portion of the highly purified methyl lesquerolate as previously described was refluxed for 1 hour with 0.8 N ethanolic potassium hydroxide to form the corresponding potassium soap. Water was added and the unsaponifiables were removed by extracting with ether. The aqueous solution remaining was acidified strongly with hydrochloric acid to free the lesquerolic acid which was then extracted with successive portions of ether. After pooling and drying the ether extracts over sodium sulfate, the ether was evaporated to give 0.90 g. of pure lesquerolic acid, an oil material having a rotation $[\alpha]D^{22}$ of $+6\pm1°$.

Omega-Hydroxypelargonic Acid Using Polymeric Aluminum Alkyls

W.K. Henle; U.S. Patent 3,342,841; September 19, 1967; assigned to Shell Oil Company has developed a process for the production of certain straight chain C9-alkanoic acids which possess an additional substituent in the omega position relative to the carboxy group. This is accomplished by carboxylation of certain polymeric aluminum alkyls followed by optional oxidation and subsequently hydrolysis to produce the desired acidic products. The product mixture contains varying proportions of sebacic acid and/or ω-hydroxypelargonic acid, depending upon the particular reaction procedure employed.

The initial reaction step comprises the carboxylation of a polymeric aluminum alkyl. Although other polymeric aluminum alkyls are similarly operable, to obtain ω-substituted C9-carboxylic acids, it is necessary to employ a polymeric aluminum alkyl wherein all alkyl moieties are α,ω-divalent straight chain C8-moieties. Although, as in the case of any highly crosslinked polymeric material, the polymeric aluminum alkyl is not completely described by a single structure, it is considered that the aluminum reactant may be represented by the formula

$$\left[\begin{array}{c} -C_8H_{16}-Al-C_8H_{16}-Al- \\ | \quad\quad\quad | \\ C_8H_{16} \quad\quad C_8H_{16} \\ | \quad\quad\quad | \\ -C_8H_{16}-Al-C_8H_{16}-Al- \end{array} \right]_n$$

wherein n is a very large number. Although it is apparent that this polymeric material is not completely described by a simple chemical name, it will be referred to as dialumino trioctane, thereby indicating the composition ratio of 2 aluminum atoms for each 3 octane moieties. The dialumino trioctane is prepared by reacting 1,7-octadiene with a trialkyl aluminum or a dialkyl aluminum hydride, wherein the alkyls are lower alkyl, e.g., having up to 4 carbon atoms, at an elevated temperature. The reaction may be conducted in the presence of solvent, but preferably is conducted by merely mixing the reactants and heating the mixture until reaction is complete.

During reaction, the former lower alkyl substituents on the reactant trialkyl aluminum or dialkyl aluminum hydride are apparently replaced by the octadiene and the former lower alkyl substituents are observed as the corresponding olefin. For example, reaction of 1,7-octadiene with triisobutyl aluminum or diisobutyl aluminum hydride results in the production of dialumino trioctane and isobutylene. The polymeric dialumino trioctane is a hard, brittle glassy solid at room temperature which becomes viscous when heated above about 60°C.

Carboxylation is effected by contacting the polymeric aluminum compound with carbon dioxide which is in the liquid or gaseous state. To effect the initial carboxylation, the dialumino trioctane is contacted with at least a molar excess, based on the aluminum, of carbon dioxide at temperatures below about 140°C. The temperature range from about 0°C. to about 100°C. is preferred for the initial carboxylation and frequently it is convenient to employ ambient temperature. The dependency on carbon dioxide pressure will largely be determined by the physical state of the carbon dioxide and the state of particle size of the dialumino trioctane.

In general, reaction pressures from 0.5 atmosphere to about 75 atmospheres are suitable. Particularly convenient are pressures generated by the use of liquid carbon dioxide in a sealed reaction vessel. Such pressures are from about 40 atmospheres to about 60 atmospheres. In the carboxylation process, it is preferred that anhydrous conditions be employed. Subsequent to reaction with one mol of carbon dioxide per mol of aluminum present in the polymeric material, determined, for example, by following the reactor pressure decrease, the reaction may be terminated and the mono-carboxylated product recovered as a solid at ambient temperature.

If the carboxylation of a second bond is desired, the isolated monocarboxylated compound may be again contacted with a molar excess of carbon dioxide, although it is most convenient to conduct the second carboxylation without prior separation of the monocarboxylated aluminum-containing polymer. Somewhat more vigorous reaction conditions are required to effect the second carboxylation, particularly with regard to the reaction temperature. Reaction temperatures above about 150°C. are required to obtain secondary carboxylation at a desirable rate although the temperature should be no higher than about 220°C. Preferred are reaction temperatures from about 170°C. to about 210°C. The secondary carboxylation is performed at pressures that are atmospheric or above and pressures from about 1 atmosphere to about 80 atmospheres are suitable; pressures from about 35 atmospheres to about 60 atmospheres are preferred. As the monocarboxylated polymeric material is a solid at reaction temperature, continued attrition during the secondary carboxylation is desirable to obtain an optimum reaction rate.

Subsequent to the reaction, dicarboxylated product is recovered as a solid from the reactor. As an optional second step, the carboxylated aluminum-containing polymer, either monocarboxylated or dicarboxylated, is reacted with molecular oxygen to oxidize the remaining carbon-aluminum bonds in the polymeric material.

Whether or not the carboxylated product has been oxidized, the aluminum-containing polymeric product is converted to the desired carboxylic acid mixture by conventional hydrolysis methods. Hydrolysis is typically effected by contacting the polymeric product with an aqueous solution of a strong acid.

Subsequent to hydrolysis, the product mixture is separated and the carboxylic acid product is recovered by conventional methods, e.g., selective extraction, fractional distillation, crystallization or chromatographic methods.

Example 1: To a steel reactor equipped with a stirrer and a vent to release gaseous products was charged 0.41 mol of diisobutyl aluminum hydride and 0.6 mol of 1,7-octadiene. The mixture was maintained at atmospheric pressure in the absence of moisture and oxygen, and was stirred at 130°C. for 10 hours, during which time 0.8 mol of isobutylene was liberated.

The product, dialumino trioctane is a clear, colorless resinous material which is viscous above about 60°C. but becomes hard, brittle and glassy at room temperature and is easily powdered. When the production of dialumino trioctane was repeated using 0.41 mol of triisobutyl aluminum in place of the diisobutyl aluminum hydride, 1.2 mols of isobutylene were liberated during reaction and a similar polymeric material was obtained.

Example 2: In an autoclave, 39 g. of dialumino trioctane prepared according to the procedure of Example 1, was reacted under continuous attrition with carbon dioxide at room temperature at a carbon dioxide pressure of approximately 600 lbs. After 1 hour the temperature was raised to 210°C.

and the attrition was continued until two mols of carbon dioxide for each mol of aluminum present had been consumed as measured by the pressure drop within the reactor. The reactor was then cooled and opened and the carboxylation product mixture was hydrolyzed by reaction with aqueous 3N hydrochloric acid at 100°C. for 0.5 hour.

The hydrolysis product mixture was extracted with ether and the combined extract was dried over anhydrous sodium sulfate. Removal of the ether solvent afforded a mixture which was analyzed by gas-liquid chromatography and found to contain 45 mol percent of sebacic acid, an equivalent amount of pelargonic acid and 10 mol percent n-octane.

SYNTHESIS OF SALTS AND SOAPS

REACTIONS WITH ACIDS

Calcium and Magnesium Soaps Using Liquefied Acids

The usual methods of making calcium and/or magnesium soaps of C_{12} to C_{22} fatty acids fall into two groups; processes in which the soaps are formed by precipitation out of aqueous solution (these soaps of course being water-insoluble); and those processes in which the ingredients are brought together under such conditions that a molten calcium or magnesium soap is formed, which is later allowed to cool.

Both types of processes have disadvantages, the first involving operating with relatively large quantities of water and entailing the disadvantages of filtration, thickening, drying and the like. The fusion processes require relatively elaborate equipment and a considerable loss of heat energy, since the temperature required for the fusion of calcium and magnesium soaps of fatty acids is quite high, ranging generally from about 220° to 550°F.

J.W. Freeland; U.S. Patent 3,376,327; April 2, 1968 provides a process for the production of calcium and magnesium (and mixtures thereof) soaps of fatty acids described below, in a solid composition form by a simple, quick, economical and effective process which avoids the difficulties entailed in the known precipitation and fusion methods.

A fatty acid is selected having from 12 to 22 carbon atoms and a titer of not more than 150°F. (and the fatty acid may of course comprise a mixture of several, such as a mixture of partially hydrogenated sardine oil fatty acids and of tall oil fatty acids); and heated to a temperature within the relatively low range of 90° to 150°F. with the proviso, however, that the temperature selected should be at least sufficient to liquefy the fatty acid. The heated fatty acid is contained in a suitable container which is provided with a means of agitation, which may be an ordinary propeller mixer. An alkaline earth compound is selected from the class consisting of calcium oxide, calcium hydroxide, magnesium oxide and mixtures thereof, the alkaline earth compound being comminuted to at least -100 mesh.

The relative amount of the alkaline earth compound used is such as to be from 1.25 to 5 equivalent weights of the fatty acid. The alkaline earth compound is added as quickly as conveniently possible to the fatty acid, and with agitation. It will be found that within a short time, generally from 1/2 to 1 minute, the temperature of the admixture so-formed suddenly begins to rise. This is first clearly perceptible when the increase in temperature has reached about 20°F. increase.

The admixture is immediately poured onto a horizontal surface, taking care to do this before the temperature has increased so much that the admixture has passed from a liquid to a solid state. The admixture which now has been poured onto the horizontal surface, which may be to a depth conveniently to about 1/2", continues to increase in temperature and more or less suddenly solidifies.

Thereafter, the temperature gradually decreases again, allowed to remain until it has come back to room temperature. The slab may be broken up into pieces for storage or shipment and eventually, when desired, it may be passed through a suitable mill and ground to the desired fineness. For many types of usage, it may be ground to pass a 100 mesh screen, or even a 200 mesh screen.

Example: 60 pounds of tall oil fatty acids (which comprise about 50% oleic, 40% linoleic and 4% linolenic acids, with a titer of about 60°F.) are placed in a 12 gallon open top fiber drum and heated by circulation with a pump and an electric heating unit to 90°F. 12 pounds of commercial -200 mesh magnesium oxide are added while the fatty acids are agitated with a propeller mixer, the addition being made within about 20 seconds.

Agitation is continued and after about 1 minute the temperature suddenly commences to rise. The propeller is quickly withdrawn and the fluid mass poured out onto a steel pan, the temperature at this point having reached about 130°F. After pouring, the temperature continues to rise to about 180°F. in a period of an additional minute or two, whereupon evolution of heat ceases, the layer of composition is now solid, about 1/2" thick, and it then slowly cools to room temperature. The slab is broken up easily with a hammer into light yellow pieces, and subsequently passed through a hammermill to give a powdered product of about −100 mesh.

Metal Soaps by Catalytic Grinding Process

In the process of R.E. Lally and J. Cunder; U.S. Patent 3,476,786; November 4, 1969; assigned to Diamond Shamrock Corporation finely divided water-insoluble metallic salts of higher fatty acids are produced by grinding solid fatty acids with particular solid metals, metal oxides, metal hydroxides, metal carbonates or mixtures thereof in the presence of a catalyst and in the absence of water.

The fatty acid used can be either saturated or unsaturated acid having a carbon chain of from 10 to 22 carbon atoms as well as a mixture of two or more of the above acids. Furthermore, the acids may be substituted or unsubstituted. Typical functional groups which may be present in the acid include hydroxy, chlorine, bromine, etc.

The metal soaps to which this process applies are those of polyvalent metals, particularly the divalent or trivalent metals such as calcium, magnesium, lead, barium, strontium, zinc, iron, cadmium, aluminum, nickel, copper, tin and mixtures of the above. The solid metallic component which is ground with the fatty acid to form metal soaps can be either the metal itself or metallic oxides, metallic hydroxides or metal carbonates or may consist of mixtures of the above.

One or more anhydrous catalysts are incorporated into the mixture of the metallic component and the fatty acid to produce the powdered metal soap in accordance with this process. Typical catalysts which are utilized include any anhydrous water-soluble inorganic basic salt, any anhydrous water-soluble inorganic acid salt, any water-soluble organic amine base and mixtures thereof. The amount of catalyst utilized can be varied, however, it is generally preferred to utilize from about 0.1 to 5.0% by weight of the catalyst based on the weight of the fatty acid used.

Generally the method can be carried out by adding a fatty acid in a solid anhydrous form to a solid, anhydrous metallic component in the presence of particular catalysts and in the absence of water to form a mixture of these two solid substances.

Any means of abrasion or grinding of this mixture containing the aforementioned solid particles may be employed to produce the metal soap of a fatty acid in a fine, powdery, anhydrous state. Typical methods of grinding to subdivide continually the particles which may be utilized in accordance with this process include high speed agitation, ball milling, air milling, jet milling, hammer milling, stone milling, tumbling in barrels, etc.

Any method of continual subdivision of these particles may be utilized. Continuous subdivision of the particles by means of grinding should take place for a period of at least 10 minutes. Generally, it is preferred to carry out the continuous subdivision of these particles for a period of from about 15 minutes to 30 hours or longer. When these grinding procedures are used for periods of less than about 10 minutes a complete interreaction between the metallic component and the solid fatty acid particles is not obtained.

Grinding times for periods of above 30 hours may be utilized, however, in most cases no additional benefits result from using grinding times above 10 hours. Therefore, it is seldom, if ever, necessary to utilize such prolonged periods of grinding. Elevated reaction temperatures are not necessary although heat may be applied. However, if heat is applied, care should be taken so that the temperature of the mixture never exceeds the melting point of the resultant metal soap.

Example 1: 800 parts by weight dry, powdered stearic acid, 180 parts by weight of anhydrous powdered calcium hydroxide and 16 parts by weight of anhydrous ammonium carbonate as a catalyst were mixed in a small drum. This mixture was then ground by rolling on a roller mill for 1 1/2 hours. After this period the material was ground by one pass through an air mill. The product thus obtained was an unctuous free-flowing powder having a free fatty acid content of 19% indicating that stearic acid and calcium hydrate had substantially reacted.

Example 2: 200 parts by weight of flaked stearic acid, 252 parts by weight of powdered anhydrous lead oxide were mixed in a small tank. This mixture was ground for 24 hours in a 1 gallon porcelain ball mill which was one-half filled with 1" diameter porcelain balls. The reaction product was still yellow in color indicating that reaction was incomplete after 24 hours of grinding.

Example 3: 100 parts by weight of flaked anhydrous stearic acid, 126 parts by weight of powdered anhydrous lead oxide and 10 parts by weight of powdered anhydrous ammonium carbonate as a catalyst were mixed in a small tank. This mixture was ground for 24 hours in a 1 gallon porcelain ball mill which was one-half filled with 1" diameter porcelain balls. The final product was a fine white powder having a free fatty acid content of about 3%. The reaction product was white in color indicating that reaction was substantially complete after 24 hours of grinding.

Steam Distillation Process for DMOA

The process of J. Rinse; U.S. Patent 3,546,262; December 8, 1970 involves the preparation of divalent metal oxide acylates (DMOA) which consist simply of 2 metal atoms connected by an oxygen atom and with an acyloxy (carboxylic acid of dialkylphosphoric acid) group on each metal atom. However, two or more of these simple molecules form strongly bound associates (by secondary forces) which result in a noncrystalline, resinous structure.

Divalent metal diacylates, e.g., acetates and the method of preparing them are known. Corresponding diacylates are prepared in the same manner as the known diacylates from virtually any divalent metal. DMOA is prepared from a metal (carboxylic acid) diacylate (MX_2) by removing one acyloxy group (X) by steam, followed by vacuum heating

(1) $\qquad MX_2 + H_2O \longrightarrow HOMX + HX$

(2) $\qquad 2HOMX \longrightarrow XMOMX + H_2O$

This removal of one acyloxy group is facilitated if the group has a small number of carbon atoms, e.g., 2 to 5. The resulting acids (HX) are volatile and distill off with steam. However, if acids of medium volatility, such as ethylhexoic and naphthenic acids are used simultaneously, small quantities of such acids may also be removed. Therefore, a slight excess, e.g., 10% by weight, of such acids is used either in the beginning of the reaction or after the steam process to replace remaining, e.g., acetate groups. The higher fatty acids, such as those from tall oil and stearic acid, will not be removed under the conditions of the reaction.

Solutions of DMOA in organic solvents, applied in a thin layer on a solid substrate, e.g., glass, dry to tack-free, glossy, extremely adherent coatings. Any moisture on the surface of the substrate to which the solutions are applied apparently reacts with the resin (DMOA) and facilitates the formation of the resulting coating. DMOA also reacts with organic acids, such as those present in bodied linseed oils and in alkyd resins, binding the metal to the organic polymer.

Although DMOA differs from its corresponding regular metal soap with respect to solubility with low viscosity, reaction with moisture and acids, and adhesion, the functionality of the metal atom, e.g., as a drying or a stabilizing agent (vinyls) remains fully available and is even strengthened because of the higher metal content per unit weight.

In those cases where viscosity increase by metal soaps is undesirable, the corresponding compounds are preferably employed in lieu thereof. Although specific details may vary, each DMOA is prepared according to the same general processes irrespective of the divalent metal employed.

The melting point of the DMOA varies with the divalent metal when the same carboxylic acid acylate or alkyl phosphate ligand is maintained; low melting point resins are obtained with such metals as zinc, lead and copper; intermediate melting point resins, with such metals as cobalt and manganese; and melting points in excess of 200°C. with such metals as alkaline earth metals, e.g., calcium and magnesium.

The low melting point range may be considered from about 20° to 100°C.; the intermediate melting point range, from 100° to 160°C.; and the high melting point range, above 160°C. Although the preceding reflects a general relationship, the ligand may also be a determining factor in the melting point range. Abietic acid ligands, e.g., cause much higher melting points than those of ethylhexoic acid.

The solubility of DMOA in organic solvents is very good, particularly in aromatic hydrocarbons, such as toluene and xylene; in aliphatic hydrocarbons, such as mineral spirits; in lower alkanols; and in ketones. With these and similar solvents solutions of DMOA are frequently obtained with from 60 to 90% by weight of solids based on the weight of the total solution.

Both divalent metal atoms in DMOA need not be of the same divalent metal. The same procedure as is represented by equations (1) and (2) is employed to combine two different divalent metals in a single molecule of DMOA, e.g., XZnOCdX and XCuOHgX, each X being either a carboxylic or dialkylphosphoric acyloxy ligand bonded directly to a metal atom. The particular ligand influences the solubility of the DMOA whether both divalent metal atoms are the same or different.

The preferred carboxylic acyloxy ligands are those having at least 7 carbon atoms. Although there is no critical upper limit on the number of carbon atoms, from 20 to 22 carbon atoms is a practical upper limit. The acyl of the acyloxy is preferably a hydrocarbon, monobasic aliphatic, cycloaliphatic or combined cycloaliphatic aliphatic carboxylic acid acyl from a monobasic acid with at least 1 cycloaliphatic ring and from 6 to 29 carbon atoms, lauric acid, palmitic acid, stearic acid, oleic acid, linoleic acid, linolenic acid, abietic acid or behenic acid; it can also be from an aromatic acid.

As is known, some metal oxides, such as those of lead, mercury and copper, react with unsaturated fatty acids; when these particular metals are employed, it is therefore preferred to use only saturated (alkanoic) acyloxy ligands. Each alkyl group of the dialkylphosphoric acid acyloxy ligands has at least 5 carbon atoms. Again, there is not a critical upper limit, but there is a practical upper limit of about 18 carbon atoms in each such alkyl group. The dialkylphosphoric acid is an orthophosphoric acid.

Synthesis of Salts and Soaps

In the same manner that the divalent metals may differ, the ligands attached thereto may also differ in the same DMOA molecule. One ligand may be a carboxylic acid acyloxy ligand and the other, a dialkylphosphoric acid acyloxy ligand.

To prepare DMOA, a reaction is initiated between either a mixture of divalent metal diacylate (the acyl of which has from 2 to 6 carbon atoms) and an aliphatic carboxylic acid of low volatility (having a carbon-to-carbon chain of at least 7 carbon atoms, e.g., ethylhexanoic acid) or a mixture of (a) divalent metal, divalent metal oxide, divalent metal hydroxide or divalent metal carbonate and (b) an equivalent mixture of aliphatic carboxylic acid of high volatility (having a carbon-to-carbon chain of from 2 to 6 carbon atoms) and either aliphatic carboxylic acid of low volatility or dialkylphosphoric acid.

Exemplary divalent metal diacylates are: zinc diacetate, cobalt diacetate and calcium diacetate. Suitable divalent metals are: zinc, lead and copper. Illustrative divalent metal oxides are: mercuric oxide and lead oxide. Typical divalent metal hydroxides are: copper hydroxide and calcium hydroxide. The divalent metal carbonates include, e.g., zinc carbonate and magnesium carbonate.

Usually some solvent, such as a hydrocarbon solvent, e.g., xylene or mineral spirits (having a boiling point either from 150° to 170°C. or from 220° to 240°C.), is employed to maintain the batch as a liquid. After the liquid batch becomes clear, steam is blown into it at constant temperature, or water is dropped in slowly, keeping the temperature at a predetermined level.

The viscosity of the batch during steaming decreases rather rapidly and, with most metals, becomes very low, e.g., from about 100 to 1 poise, at a temperature of 200°C. or lower. Metals, such as calcium, magnesium and, to a lesser extent, cobalt and manganese, require heating above 200°C., sometimes even above 250°C., before the batch thins down. Usually, after 15 to 20 minutes the distillation of acids ends, steaming is terminated and vacuum of up to 5 cm. H_2O is applied. Most DMOA releases water and solvent slowly.

The condensation of the basic metal acylates to their anhydrides proceeds slowly, but always practically completely. Complete removal of solvents is not always possible. Low viscosity during vacuum, without any more condensate, indicates the end of the reaction. The addition of a small quantity of toluene or other volatile solvent, e.g., hexane, assists in the removal of water and high boiling solvents. The preferred highly volatile acids are acetic and propionic acid; butyric and valeric acids may also be used. However, with some metals small quantities of the latter acids may remain after the steam distillation. For economic reasons acetic acid is used most frequently. The specific metal also determines the rate of removal of the acid, which is more difficult for calcium and barium than for zinc, copper or mercury. The reaction temperature varies from 105° to 260°C., being lowest for copper and mercury.

The steaming process requires from 10 to 60 minutes. A convenient variation is to drop water slowly into the reacting batch under good agitation, keeping the temperature at a level determined experimentally for each metal. The end point of the reaction is reached when no more acid appears in the distillation or, in some cases, by the appearance of turbidity in the batch.

The structure XMOMX has been confirmed by infrared spectographic analysis, indicating the absence of hydroxy groups and the presence of predominantly one type of acyloxy groups. The use of more than one equivalent of nonvolatile acid per metal atom will decrease the yield of metal oxide acylate and increase the metal diacylate yield. In general an excess of one-half equivalent of nonvolatile acid per metal atom does not considerably change the nature of the products. As the excess of acid is increased beyond that amount, the properties gradually approach those of the regular metal diacylates.

Example: 11.7 g. of magnesium hydroxide are added to a solution of 12 grams of acetic acid and 56 g. of tall oil fatty acids in 50 g. Isopar M (a hydrocarbon solvent with BP 220° to 240°C.); 20 g. of water are added to the resultant at 220°C. and the temperature is then raised to 250°C., adding 30 g. more of Isopar thereto when the viscosity increases.

Thereafter, 35 g. of water are slowly dropped in, alternating with 25 g. of butanol. After applying a vacuum, 55 g. of a hard light brown resin (MP 190°C.), which is soluble in a mixture of xylene and butanol, is obtained. (Apparently 7 g. of tall oil fatty acid is also removed by the high temperature.) The resin is useful as a varnish component.

Replacing the magnesium hydroxide [$Mg(OH)_2$] with an equivalent of stannous hydroxide [$Sn(OH)_2$] results in the preparation, in similar manner, of the corresponding tin oligomers. Replacing the tall oil fatty acids with an equivalent of n-heptanoic acid results in the preparation, in similar manner, of the magnesium oligomer with the corresponding ligand.

Divalent Metal-Zirconium Compounds by Water Removal Process

The process of S.E. Harson; U.S. Patent 3,419,587; December 31, 1968;

Synthesis of Salts and Soaps

assigned to Hardman & Holden Limited, England provide compounds and complexes of divalent metals, zirconium and carboxylic acids with or without phenols or oxygenated organics, formulated to give good solubility in organic media.

Metal-organic compounds containing zirconium and one or more divalent metals are prepared by first reacting zirconyl carbonate with a monocarboxylic acid and then reacting with one or more divalent metals in powder form or in the form of oxides, hydroxides or carbonates and distilling to remove the water which is liberated. An alkyl phosphoric or phosphorous acid or a sulfonic acid may be added in addition to the carboxylic acid. The compounds and complexes and compositions of matter can be represented by the following general formula:

(1) $\qquad DZr(OH)_n X_m$

where D = divalent metal; X = carboxylic acid or mixture of carboxylic acids with or without phenolic compounds; m = 2 to 4 and n = may be variable but probably not greater than 3.

(2) $\qquad D_2 Zr(OH)_n X_m$

with definitions as above and m is 4 to 6

(3) $\qquad D^1 D^2 Zr(OH)_n X_m$

with m as 4 to 6 and D^1 and D^2 represent different divalent metals

(4) $\qquad$ Mixtures of (1) to (3)

(5) $\qquad D_n Zr X_m$

in which m is a quantity not exceeding 2 and n is a quantity less than 1.0. In addition it is often found to be advantageous to include a proportion of polar oxygenated organic compound capable of coordinating with zirconium to facilitate processing and to improve stability and compatibility. A convenient commercially available compound is isobutyl alcohol which can be used as an azeotroping solvent in the removal of water but a variety of other compounds can be substituted.

The divalent metals or mixtures include magnesium, calcium, strontium, barium, zinc, cobalt, cadmium, mercury, copper, iron, lead, manganese and nickel. In addition there may be present a small amount of sodium, potassium or ammonium base. A convenient method of manufacture can be based on commercially available zirconyl carbonate but other suitable reactive forms of freshly precipitated or basic inorganic zirconium compounds may be used. In practice good reaction rates are obtained with water wet cake or damp crumb (paste) which may also contain residues of sodium or ammonium radicals. No particular processing difficulty has been experienced with basic residues up to about 0.2 mol (as sodium) per zirconium, though in some cases slight adjustment of formulation may be made to take account of this factor.

With regard to carboxylic acids high metal contents can be rendered organically soluble with as little as one C_8 to C_{11} carboxylic acid per DZr combination and lower carbon ratios are not excluded provided adjustment is made in the nature of the solvent when necessary. In general, increase in the carboxylic carbon to DZr ratio gives improved solubility in nonpolar diluents though this is of course also affected by the increase in the value of m towards 4 or 6 in the general formula (1) to (4) above.

With carboxylic acids smaller than propionic or more polar, processing generally is facilitated by adjustment of the nonpolar to polar constituents to the processing diluents or, if necessary, by ageing of intermediates. Carboxylic acids of the solubilizing type referred to (C_8 to C_{30}) include natural fatty acids, synthetic straight or branched chain acids including Versatic acid 911 and I.C.I. 810 ($C_8C_9C_{10}$ branched chain acids), petroleum derived carboxylic acids such as naphthenic acid, other acids, aromatic or substituted aromatics or halogenated carboxylic acids or unsaturated acids.

However, in a preparation of the type $PbCoZrX_{4 \text{ to } 5}$, for example, the same solubilizing C_8 to C_{11} synthetic acids would not necessarily be chosen for lead and cobalt respectively. With regard to phenols, alkyl substitution up to C_8 or more may be used and a proportion of halogenated phenol may also be incorporated for specific applications. Dicarboxylic acids may also be incorporated if desired, with appropriate choice of reaction procedure and composition.

It is difficult to generalize with regard to the divalent metals since differences in behavior can be detected between close neighbors such as zinc and cadmium and calcium and barium. With regard to both calcium and barium, however, it can readily be demonstrated that the zirconium complexes have the practical advantage of easy processing and lack of heat sensitivity. This is however, also enhanced by selection of appropriate m ratio in the Formula (1) to (4).

Processing may be aided by the inclusion of a proportion of diluent or solvent and removal of water can conveniently be carried out in Dean & Stark type equipment. The products may be partially or fully dehydrated. The process may be continued if necessary with removal of volatile diluent and substitution of volatile or nonvolatile diluents or coordinating agents. The divalent metals can be used conveniently in the form of the metal powder, metal oxide, hydroxide or carbonate. In the use of metal powders care may be necessary to give controlled rate of hydrogen evolution. In the following examples Pr indicates propionate; T, tallate and M, methacrylate.

Example 1: Cadmium Zirconium Propionate Tallate $CdZrPr_{1.5}T_{1.7}$ — 289.5 g. (1 mol) of zirconyl carbonate paste, 86 g. of isobutyl alcohol and 86 g. of white spirit were weighed into a three-necked reaction flask and an addition made while stirring at room temperature of 111 g. (1.5 mol) of propionic acid followed by 203 g. (0.7 mol) of tall oil fatty acids. This procedure minimizes frothing due to CO_2 release. The mixture was heated and became transparent at 60°C. when a further 290 g. (1 mol) of tall oil fatty acid was added, followed by 128.4 g. (1 mol) of cadmium oxide. Some initial granular aggregates of cadmium oxide dissolved on heating at 100°C. for about 40 minutes under reflux.

The product was dried by Dean & Stark procedure with the recovery of 171 cubic centimeters of aqueous distillate at a vessel temperature of 132°C. White spirit 141 g. was added to give a viscous clear light brown solution containing 10% cadmium and 8.1% zirconium. A repeat product substituting methacrylic acid for propionic acid gave a clear tough plastic solid final product containing 10% cadmium and 8.1% zirconium.

Example 2: Zinc Zirconium Methacrylate Tallate $ZnZrM_{1.0}T_{2.0}$ — 287 g. (1 mol) of zirconyl carbonate paste, 90 g. of isobutyl alcohol and 90 g. of white spirit were weighed into a three-necked reaction flask and an addition made, while stirring, of a mixture of 86.1 g. of methacrylic acid and 290 g. of tall oil fatty acids, resulting in an opaque yellow emulsion. Heating to 72°C. yielded a considerably clearer emulsion and an addition was then made of 290 g. of tall oil fatty acid followed by 81.4 g. of zinc oxide.

After 5 minutes at 75°C. some white zinc oxide was visible and the product was heated to 85°C. for a further half hour and allowed to stand overnight. The product was then in the form of a white waxy solid which was remelted and heated to 96°C. under reflux for 1 hour. Drying by Dean & Stark procedure yielded 192 cc of aqueous distillate in 6 hours at a final product temperature of 190°C. The final product was in the form of a moderately viscous light brown liquid on cooling to room temperature. On standing it changed to a soft semisolid low-melting semiopaque form.

Basic Cadmium Salts as Vinyl Resin Stabilizers

Vinyl resin compositions are known to be sensitive to the action of light and heat, and the acid degradation products produced by such action react to effect deterioration of the resin composition. This deterioration, primarily evidenced by color changes in the resin compositions, which are in themselves undesirable, also seriously affects other physical characteristics of the resins such as flexibility and tensile strength. Since the resin compositions are necessarily exposed to heat during compounding and processing, and to light during ordinary use, it is desirable to incorporate agents which tend to stabilize the physical properties of the resin composition.

Cadmium salts of aliphatic carboxylic acids have heretofore been employed as stabilizers for vinyl resin compositions. The cadmium salt stabilizers are particularly valuable because they impart clarity to the resin compositions as well as stabilization properties. Their employment has therefore been indicated where clarity is desired in the finished product.

The widespread use of vinyl resins for electrical insulation purposes has given rise to another requirement for stabilizers. Such a stabilizer should not, of itself, impair the electrical resistivity of the resin composition. Moreover, it should be of such a nature that it overcomes the effects on resistivity of electrolytes (e.g., HCl) generated in the course of degradation of the resin, and does not react, in the process, to produce compounds which have untoward effects on electrical resistivity.

J.G. Hendricks and L.M. Kebrich; U.S. Patent 3,225,075; Dec. 21, 1965; assigned to National Lead Company provides for the production of basic cadmium salts of aliphatic carboxylic acids and vinyl resin compositions stabilized by basic cadmium salts of aliphatic carboxylic acids.

The process contemplates a method of producing a basic cadmium compound which comprises mixing a cadmium compound selected from the group consisting of cadmium oxide and cadmium hydroxide and an aliphatic carboxylic acid in an aqueous medium or in addition containing a water-soluble organic compound selected from the group consisting of alcohols and ethers, and mixing the same until the cadmium compound and aliphatic carboxylic acid are chemically combined. This process also contemplates a vinyl halide composition containing, as stabilizer, a basic cadmium compound corresponding to the formula

$$CdO \cdot Cd(C_nH_{2n \pm 1}COO)_2$$

where n is an integer from 3 to 21, the cadmium compound being substantially free of electrolyte. It has been found that the basic cadmium aliphatic carboxylates when prepared as herein described, result in extraordinary electrical resistivity heretofore unattainable with organic cadmium salts.

Since a basic cadmium aliphatic carboxylate, by itself contributes a degree of heat and light stabilization, it may be used alone or if it is desired, in conjunction with other metal salt or organic stabilizers, such as alkaline earth metal salts and phenolic compounds, epoxides, polyols, etc. Monobasic cadmium caprate having the formula $CdO \cdot Cd(C_9H_{19}COO)_2$ is the preferred stabilizer because it contributes a highly beneficial combination of properties to the vinyl resin products, namely high electrical resistivity, clarity, heat and light stability.

Other stabilizers found to be effective in regards to their high electrical resistivity characteristics are: monobasic cadmium valerate, monobasic cadmium behenate, monobasic cadmium crotonate and monobasic cadmium oleate. Other acids capable of reacting to form basic cadmium salts are butyric, caproic, caprylic, lauric, myristic, stearic and palmitic. In general, the acids that are useful in this process are those containing from 4 to 22 carbon atoms in a saturated or unsaturated carbon chain.

It is preferred to add the basic cadmium aliphatic carboxylate to the resin batch on the initial mixing of the ingredients, but it may also be introduced at any stage of manufacture. The basic cadmium aliphatic carboxylate disperses readily in vinyl resin or vinyl resin compositions containing other compounding agents so that uniformity is easily obtained. As other compounding agents we mention plasticizers, such as dioctyl phthalate; electrical grade clays; fillers and coloring agents.

The vinyl resin compositions may, after a blending operation, be processed at wide ranges of temperature, dependent upon, for instance, the molecular weight of the resin, the actual process involved, the formulation of the resin composition, etc.

The compositions used in the examples were weighed, mixed, processed on a two-roll mill at a temperature of 315°F. and sheeted in a 4-minute cycle. Samples of these sheets were then tested for heat stability and volume resistivity. The effectiveness of this process is independent of the method or process employed in producing objects or items, those operations including milling, calendering, molding, extruding, etc.

Basic cadmium compounds to provide the desired beneficial effects should be present in the amount of from 0.01 to 5% by weight based on the resin. Amounts lower than 0.01% have limited stabilizing action whereas amounts in excess of 5% do not serve any additional stabilizing purpose. The desired results can normally be attained by using amounts of a basic cadmium compound totaling between 0.05 and 3.0% based on the weight of the vinyl resin. In place of cadmium oxide, cadmium hydroxide may be substituted. The mol ratio of acid to base is not limited to 2:2 and generally satisfactory stabilization can be attained using combinations of normal and basic cadmium carboxylates in which this ratio may be, for example, 2:1.5. The process is best conducted in a heated pebble mill, at a temperature of between 30° and 100°C., in an aqueous medium and may contain a small amount of a water-soluble alcohol, glycol ether or the like, e.g., secondary butanol, isobutanol or ethylene glycol monobutyl ether. The water-soluble organic compound seems to catalyze the neutralization and form workable dispersions of the water-repellent product.

Example 1: Monobasic Cadmium Caprylate — 51.4 g. (0.40 mol) of cadmium oxide and 57.7 g. (0.40 mol) of caprylic acid were reacted in a solution of 300 ml. of water and 25 ml. of isobutanol. The reaction was conducted at $35° \pm 5°C.$ for 24 hours in a porcelain pebble mill. The white product, which after filtration and drying weighed 103.9 g., was found to be a single phase solid having an average refractive index of 1.56 and a density of 1.70.

Example 2: Two vinyl halide resin compositions were weighed, mixed, heated on a two-roll mill at a temperature of 315°F. and milled for 3 minutes until substantially uniform. The compositions were then sheeted into 20 mil sheets. Composition 1, containing monobasic cadmium caprate prepared as in Example 1 and Composition 2, containing monobasic cadmium caprate prepared by a metathesis reaction that was repeatedly washed to remove, as much as possible, the sodium sulfate remaining in the product, were evaluated for volume resistivity according to the following procedure.

The composition having a thickness of 20 mils was coated with colloidal graphite to insure intimate contact between the specimen and the electrode. The specimen after coating is carefully preconditioned to a temperature of 70°C. for 30 minutes after which time the specimen is placed between 2 standard electrodes. An applied voltage of 500 v. DC, is applied, and after an electrification period of 1 minute the electrical resistivity is measured using a megohmmeter. Typical analysis shows the basic cadmium salt contained 0.005% sodium when prepared in a pebble mill and greater than 0.045% sodium when prepared by methathesis with repeated washings. The table shows the plastic formulations and the results of volume resistivity measured at 70°C.

Component	Composition 1, parts by weight	Composition 2, parts by weight
Geon 101 (polyvinylchloride resin)	100	100
DOP (dioctyl phthalate)	50	50
Electrical grade clay	5	5
Barium caprate	1.0	1.0
Bisphenol A	.02	.02
Monobasic cadmium caprate (pebble mill)	1.0	
Monobasic cadmium caprate (metathesis)		1.0
Volume resistivity, 70°C., 10^{12} ohm-cm	15.0	3.0

Composition 1 was by far superior to Composition 2 with a volume resistivity of 15×10^{12} ohm-cm. as compared to 3.0×10^{12} ohm-cm. Composition 1 was compared also to a commercial electrical lead stabilizer. The results showed Composition 1 to be at least equal in volume resistivity and superior in heat stability.

Water Removal Process for Molybdenum Salts

The process of *M. Becker; U.S. Patent 3,578,690; May 11, 1971; assigned to Halcon International, Inc.* comprises the direct reaction of a molybdenum compound with a carboxylic acid at elevated temperatures, while removing the water from the reaction mixture, to form a molybdenum carboxylate. It is a critical feature of this process that free water is removed during the reaction; this includes water that may be initially present and the water that is formed during the reaction.

The molybdenum compounds contemplated by this process are molybdenum halides such as molybdenum hexafluoride and molybdenum pentachloride, the various oxides of molybdenum such as molybdenum dioxide, trioxide and sesquioxide and the like; alkali and alkali earth molybdates such as cesium molybdate, sodium molybdate, potassium molybdate, calcium molybdate and the like; and ammonium molybdate or molybdic acid 85%, (the latter two are the same compound, however, the specification of molybdic acid 85% usually shows a slightly lower MoO_3 content). In the preferred aspect ammonium molybdate (molybdic acid 85%) and molybdenum trioxide are employed and especially ammonium molybdate.

The carboxylic acids contemplated by this process are monocarboxylic acids, such as monoaliphatic acids, monoalicyclic acids and monoaromatic acids. The aliphatic acids may be lower aliphatic acids of 2 to 6 carbon atoms, intermediate aliphatic acids of from 7 to 11 carbon atoms, and higher aliphatic acids of from 12 to 30 carbons. The starting molybdenum compound and carboxylic acid may be reacted in the presence of an inert solvent and in fact unless the carboxylic acid is a liquid at the temperature of reaction, a suitably inert solvent is employed.

As indicated previously, the removal of water is a critical feature. If the reaction is carried out without the removal of water, essentially no molybdenum compound is formed. However, although water removal is necessary, the manner in which it is removed is unimportant and therefore, one may employ any known techniques for water removal. For example, the water may be removed by the use of dehydrating agents such as calcium chloride or more preferably one may employ an azeotropic agent. Any azeotrope may be used which would be inert to the reaction itself. The preferred azeotropes are benzene or aralkyl compounds such as lower alkyl benzenes containing from 1 to 3 alkyl groups and each alkyl group containing from 1 to 4 carbon atoms (ethylbenzene, xylene, cumene and the like) or any other straight or branched chain hydrocarbon such as an alkane of from 5 to 12 carbon atoms (hexane, octane, decane and the like). In the preferred method a lower alkyl benzene is employed such as ethylbenzene. If it is so desired, the azeotrope may also be used as a solvent in the system or the azeotropes may be used in addition to a solvent. The amount of azeotrope necessary depends upon the amount of water to be removed and will vary from one system to another.

The reaction is suitably carried out at a temperature of from 100° to 300°C. In its preferred aspects, the reaction is carried out at a temperature of 150° to 250°C. and especially 190° to 225°C. It is to be understood that among other factors the temperature of the reaction will depend upon the carboxylic acid employed, in that the temperature should be at or below the boiling point of the carboxylic acid at the pressure employed.

Accordingly, the time of reaction is not critical and the reaction is carried out for a sufficient length of time to allow for substantial reaction to take place. Suitably, the reaction is carried out from 2 to 48 hours or more. The concentration of reactants is not critical and accordingly may suitably be adjusted with regard to the specific reactants and conditions.

Example: (a) A mixture consisting of 60 g. octanoic acid, 17.7 g. molybdic acid, 85%, and 30 g. ethylbenzene is charged to a 250 cc flask equipped with a thermometer, reflux condenser and a Dean-Stark tube. This flask is then placed in a constant temperature oil bath which is kept at 200°C. The flask content is refluxed atmospherically for 48 hours, followed by filtration to remove any undissolved solids; yield 15.2 weight percent molybdenum. Similarly, when the above reaction is carried out at 100°, 150°, 250° or 300°C. until water is no longer evolved, similar results are obtained.

(b) Similarly, when an equivalent amount of molybdenum trioxide is used in place of molybdic acid in (a) above, there is obtained molybdenum octanoate; yield 3.4 weight percent molybdenum. Similarly, when an equivalent amount of molybdenum hexafluoride, molybdenum pentachloride, molybdenum dioxide, molybdenum sesquioxide, potassium molybdate or calcium molybdate is used in place of molybdenum trioxide, similar results are obtained.

Molybdenum and Vanadium Salts Using Oxalate

J. Kollar; U.S. Patent 3,362,972; January 9, 1968; assigned to Halcon International Inc. provides a process for preparing a salt of a metal of the

Synthesis of Salts and Soaps

group consisting of Mo and V which is soluble in a hydrocarbon medium, which process comprises heating an oxalate compound of a metal of the group consisting of Mo at a valence of +6 and of V at a valence of +5 with a hydrocarbon carboxylic acid of 4 to 50 carbon atoms having about at least 4 carbon atoms per carboxylic group, whereby the hydrocarbon-soluble salt is formed.

Example 1: Molybdenum hexanoate is prepared by heating MoO_3 (144 g.), water (400 g.), oxalic acid dihydrate (126 g.) and hexanoic acid (90 to 95% purity) (1,940 g.), at a temperature of 100°C. with vigorous agitation for about 1 hour. All the MoO_3 goes into solution. Then water is stripped or flashed off by heating and the temperature is gradually raised to 150° to 200°C., and heating is continued at this temperature for 4 to 6 hours, with vigorous stirring. The desired hexanoate composition is formed directly with about 5% (wt.) content of the metal component (Mo) and is substantially free of undesirable materials.

While there is no intent to be limited by theory, it is believed that during the reaction, the valence of the molybdenum may change from +6 to a lower value and that oxalate ion may be decomposed to carbon dioxide and water in a redox reaction. Vapors are evolved and they contain water and carbon dioxide (determined by qualitative analysis).

This is a most surprising result, especially since in the absence of oxalic acid, the hexanoate is not formed, i.e., no hydrocarbon-soluble material is formed. Additionally, substitution of formic acid for the oxalic acid on a mol for mol basis does not give the hexanoate, i.e., no hydrocarbon-soluble material is formed. Also if the molybdenum is initially in a lower valence form, e.g., a valence of four, the hexanoate is not formed; i.e., no hydrocarbon-soluble material is formed.

The hexanoic acid need not be of high purity but can be a distilled cut containing a small portion of 7 carbon and/or 8 carbon atom acids as well as 5 carbon and/or 4 carbon atoms acids. The resulting molybdenum hexanoate composition is particularly suitable and effective for use as a catalyst in the oxidation of propylene oxide by means of a peroxide type oxidizing agent. The hexanoate is soluble in hydrocarbons.

Example 2: The procedure of Example 1 is repeated using 182 g. V_2O_5, 252 g. oxalic acid dihydrate, 500 g. water and 1,900 g. of hexanoic acid (90 to 95% purity). After 2 hours at 100°C. the H_2O is flash distilled and the temperature is raised. Heating at 180° to 200°C. is for 2 to 6 hours. The product contains about 5% V as hexanoate in solution. Similar results to those of Example 1 are obtained by using hexanoic acid with molybdenum oxalate (in the same proportion of hexanoic acid and Mo) and heating at

150° to 200°C. for 4 to 6 hours. Also the Example 1 procedure may be modified by adding the hexanoic acid after removal of water, and similar results are obtained. Comparable results to the foregoing may be obtained with various modifications thereof, including the following. In place of the molybdenum trioxide or vanadium pentoxide, other highest valence compounds of these metals or mixtures of such compounds may be used, e.g., the corresponding peroxy acids, acids and the like, corresponding hexanoate formed.

Mixtures of such metal compounds may be used; instead of hexanoic acid, an alkyl, alkenyl, aralkyl and the like carboxylic acids of up to 50 carbon atoms or mixtures thereof, may be used. The acids may contain 1, 2 or more carboxylic groups, however, it is preferred that there be present at least 4 hydrocarbon carbon atoms per carboxylic carbon in order to provide the desired solubility in a hydrocarbon or the like organic medium.

Monocarboxylic acids are preferred. These may be pure fatty acids of the formula RCOOH, where R is an alkyl group of 4 to 30 carbon atoms, distilled cuts of fatty acids or mixtures, naphthenic acids, acids derived from natural oils and waxes, tall oil acids, abietic acid, tung oil acids, linoleic acid, oleic acid and the like.

Generally, one mol of oxalic acid is used per mol of the heavy metal oxide (e.g., MoO_3) or compound used; however, somewhat lesser or greater proportions are operative, e.g., 0.8 to 1.3 mols of this acid per mol of the heavy metal compound. All of the metal compound reactant used should go into solution in water. The proportion of carboxylic acid groups (e.g., of acids of 5 to 50 carbon atoms) may be 1 to 100 mols per mol of the heavy metal compound (MoO_3, or the corresponding oxalate) desirably 1.5 to 50 mols and preferably 2 to 20 mols.

The proportion of water used is 0.5 to 50 parts by weight per part of oxalic acid, desirably 0.75 to 30 parts and preferably 1 to 15 parts. The amount of water is kept low, but sufficient water is used to fluidize the reaction mixture. The heating of the aqueous mixture is at 100°C. for 1 to 2.5 hours; then water is removed, e.g., by evaporation; higher temperature may be used with elevated pressure, e.g., 150°C. The heating of the water-free mixture is at about 140° to 240°C. for 2 to 6 hours; at such temperature, oxalate decomposes.

Silver Salts from Silver Complexes

T.T. Bryan; U.S. Patent 3,458,544; July 29, 1969; assigned to Minnesota Mining and Manufacturing Company provides a process for preparing silver salts of organic carboxylic acids, such as silver behenate, in which an organic carboxylic acid dissolved in a water-immiscible phase is admixed with an alkali-soluble silver complex in an aqueous phase (pH at least 7.5) and recovering precipitated silver salt as a finely divided, highly pure, free-flowing product. The process is carried out by preparing an oil-in-water dispersion or emulsion having in the oil phase an organic acid, the silver salt of which is water-insoluble, preferably a fatty acid, and in the aqueous phase an alkali-soluble silver complex having a dissociation constant (to silver ion) greater than the silver salt of the organic acid, and agitating the dispersion, e.g., by homogenization, the pH of the aqueous phase being maintained above about 7.5.

The water-insoluble silver salt forms as a precipitate at the interface of the two immiscible phases and is recovered, usually by settling, filtration, washing with distilled water until the filtrate is free of undesired anions (including those introduced into the aqueous phase along with the silver) and drying. In general the average particle size of the oil phase in the dispersion is preferably maintained in the range of 1 to 10 microns.

The alkali-soluble silver complex in the aqueous phase is preferably silver ammonium complex, although other silver complexes (silver amine complexes, such as the silver complexes of methylamine or ethylamine) can be used if they are alkali-soluble (i.e., do not form insoluble silver compounds in alkaline media) and if their dissociation constant is higher than that of the desired water-insoluble silver salt product.

The percent conversion to the desired silver salt increases with the increase in pH, and essentially complete conversion is obtained at a pH of 7.5 or above. The presence of an acid acceptor, such as ammonia, as part of the silver complex in the aqueous phase serves to neutralize the hydrogen ions as they are formed and hence direct the equilibrium toward the formation of the desired silver salt and to maintain the pH value above 7.5. When the silver complex does not produce an acid acceptor upon dissociation, a separate water-soluble acid acceptor may be added to the aqueous phase to maintain the desired alkalinity.

The final product is a free-flowing powder having an average particle size between 5 and 50 microns and, accordingly, a high surface area per unit weight. Because of the fine particle size and high purity (usually at least 98% purity) of the insoluble silver salt product, it can be readily dispersed in a resin system without extended ball milling or grinding to produce a highly transparent coating when deposited onto a film base.

The process also permits the commercial synthesis of silver soaps in a continuous process, and the aqueous solution of silver complex and an oil-in-water emulsion of an organic acid (preferably behenic acid) can be reacted during mixing as they are fed simultaneously through a centrifugal pump, the product thereafter filtered, washed and dried. By varying the flow rate of the two solutions and/or their relative concentration, silver soap of varying degrees of purity can be obtained. However, in general, with either a continuous or a batchwise process it is desirable to use approximately equivalent stoichiometric amounts of the reactants, i.e., water-soluble silver complex and oil-soluble organic carboxylic acid.

The speed of the reaction can be effected within limits by regulating the temperature of the two-phase system in which the interfacial reaction takes place. Preferably temperatures of from about 20° to 70°C. are used, temperatures below 20°C. being suitable only if the lower rate of reaction can be tolerated and temperatures above 70°C. being useful only if the solvents employed are not lost by boiling. In some cases, elevated pressures may be useful.

Example: A 0.01 molar solution of behenic acid in benzene is heated to 60°C. This solution is homogenized in an equal volume of water at 60°C. until the emulsion has an average particle size of 1 to 10 microns. To the resulting oil-in-water emulsion an equivalent stoichiometric amount of 0.1 normal aqueous silver ammonium nitrate solution having a pH of about 9 is added with stirring. The precipitate formed is allowed to settle, filtered using suction, washed with distilled water until the filtrate is free of nitrate ions, and then dried. Silver behenate product, analyzing 24.17% silver, is recovered in a yield of 98%.

REACTIONS WITH ALCOHOLS

Alkali Salts by Oxidation in Presence of Cu(II) and Noble Metal

H. Hartel and G. Bier; U.S. Patent 3,449,413; June 10, 1969; assigned to Dynamit Nobel AG, Germany describe a process for the preparation of alkali salts of carboxylic acids. The salts are prepared by the oxidation of primary alcohols comprising reacting such alcohol in an alkaline aqueous medium with a mixture of a copper(II) oxide or hydroxide and a noble metal or its oxide or hydroxide.

The copper(II) hydroxide may be produced by the precipitation of a chlorine-free water-soluble copper(II) compound. The complete or partial regeneration of the oxidant used up in the reaction can be carried out during the oxidation of the alcohols in the same reaction vessel or separately in an alkaline aqueous medium by treatment with oxygen or gases containing oxygen at temperatures up to about 100°C. The composition of the oxidant can vary widely.

It is advantageous to use the copper(II) oxide or copper(II) hydroxide in the presence of about 1 to 10 mol percent of the noble metal and/or its oxide or hydroxide, but other proportions can also be satisfactorily employed. It is advantageous to select the concentration of the remaining components so that, following completion of the alcohol oxidation, the concentration of alkali salts of the carboxylic acids formed and present in the solutions will be as high as possible.

Suitable primary alcohols to be reacted according to this process are the known saturated and unsaturated aliphatic alcohols. Highly volatile alcohols can also be reacted in this manner under elevated pressure, but such a procedure is unnecessary even in the case of the simplest unsaturated primary alcohol. The reaction may be carried out with the water-soluble alcohols being used per se or in the form of their dilute aqueous solutions. The water-insoluble alcohols or those of only limited solubility are made suitable for use in the oxidation reaction by means of an inert solvent, that means, inert against the alkaline and the oxidative agents, such as, dioxane, benzene, cyclohexanone.

A particular advantage of the procedure is that the reaction is easily completed at temperatures from about room to 100°C., and further, due to the presence of the copper compounds which simultaneously possess inhibiting properties, no polymerization of the reactants takes place. The noble metals and/or their oxides or hydroxides which can be used in accordance with the process include silver, gold, mercury, platinum, ruthenium, rhodium, palladium, osmium, or iridium.

Selective Process for Straight Chain Soaps

In the process of W.R. Eller; U.S. Patent 3,560,537; February 2, 1971; assigned to Ethyl Corporation alcohols having from about 6 to 30 carbon atoms per molecule are selectively reacted with alkali metal hydroxide when in the presence of less reactive branched primary alcohols to produce carboxylic acid soaps of predominantly straight chain carbon skeletal configuration and also to produce hydrogen.

The selectivity of reaction of straight chain alcohols and freedom from methylene group attack is enhanced by using proper elevated temperatures in combination with a deficiency of alkali metal hydroxide based on stoichiometric proportions for the total alcohol content of the reaction system and in the absence of oxidants for methylene groups at the temperatures involved. The soaps are usable as such or as synthesis intermediates for derivatives such as corresponding acids. The selective caustic fusion operation is a manipulation in which the temperature of reaction, the proportions of reactants and the composition of copresent materials are controlled to secure the desired result, avoiding the need for catalysts added to the system and the use of oxidizing agents that are prone to the production of methylene group attacks. Freedom from methylene group attack is enhanced by the presence in the system of by-product hydrogen which provides valuable economic advantage as well. The mixture of alcohol and alkali metal hydroxide fed to the system may be heated to temperature directly or may be subjected to a pretreatment prior to reacting the mixture at the elevated temperatures. A preferred feed is a mixture of primary alcohols of the following composition.

Alcohol	Weight Percent
Dodecanol	65
Tetradecanol	25
Hexadecanol	6
Mixed isomers (branched)	4

For selectivity and high conversion, it appears highly advantageous and desirable to perform the fusion reaction at a temperature from 240° to 340°C., preferably 330°C. The higher region, say about 330°C., is preferred from a rate viewpoint; however, temperatures above about 340°C. usually result in excessive destruction of the alcohol molecules where yields of 95% and higher are desired.

It is surprising that the selectivity of reaction of normal alcohols relative to branched alcohols with NaOH appears to be significantly better at 330°C. than at 300°C., a fact that leads to the belief that the melting point of the caustic may be a significant factor in this connection. At temperatures below 300°C., viscosity increases magnify the difficulty of securing good contact between materials as well as the foaming problem which is inherent in this operation because of the release of hydrogen. A preference for 330°C. is shown where maximum selectivity is desired.

As a practical matter, it is generally preferred to use an amount of caustic which corresponds about to the normal alcohol content of the feed material on a molar basis. In this way the normal alcohols react at a much higher rate than the branched alcohols so for all practical purposes the caustic is virtually consumed on straight chain alcohol and is unavailable for subsequent reaction of the branched alcohols.

Various caustic materials used in prior art caustic fusion are in general suitable. Preferred caustic materials because of reactivity and cost considerations are the hydroxides of metals of Groups IA and IIA having atomic numbers of 3 to 56, both inclusive. Particularly desirable are the hydroxides of the Group IA metals because the soaps produced therefrom are water-soluble; however, others can have benefit through modification of the properties of the Group IA materials. Of these caustic materials, sodium hydroxide and potassium hydroxide are preferred on a cost-effectiveness basis whereas sodium hydroxide is the most preferred in this regard.

Desirable results are obtainable with a ratio of straight chain alcohol to caustic ranging from about 1:1 (molar) to about 1.25:1 (25% excess alcohol), the former ratio preferred for optimum conversion of alcohol, the latter preferable for selectivity, with a preferred range being from 1:1 to 1.10:1. Generally, the higher ratios of alcohol to caustic will be preferred at lower temperatures and the lower ratios at the higher temperatures.

Under conditions such as the foregoing, the only soaps obtained from the caustic fusion reaction are soaps of straight chain structure. The branched alcohols remain in the unsaponifiables and are readily separable either by solvent extraction or with stripping as with nitrogen or steam at 60° to 310°C., preferably with steam at the higher temperatures.

Example 1: A mixture of 0.18 mol of 2-methyl dodecanol and 0.18 mol of n-tetradecanol was heated at 300°C. in a well stirred, 250 ml. Magne-Drive autoclave with 0.15 mol of powdered reagent grade anhydrous sodium hydroxide. Evolved hydrogen was allowed to escape through a pressure control valve which maintained a constant pressure of 175 to 200 psig. When hydrogen evolution ceased, the reactor was cooled and the contents (essentially a mixture of unreacted straight chain and branched alcohols plus sodium soaps of straight chain and branched carboxylic acids) were cooled and weighed.

An aliquot of the product mixture was charged into a 250 ml. blender with 150 to 175 ml. of pentane and a weighed portion of n-decane. After thorough blending a small sample of the pentane extract was injected directly into a gas chromatograph. The weights of unreacted straight chain and branched alcohols in the product mixture were then calculated, using the n-decane peak as an internal standard and calibration factors measured previously for the pure straight chain and branched alcohols. The blender contents (pentane extract plus mixture of straight chain and branched soaps) were filtered and the solid filter cake (soap mixture) was dried and dissolved in 100 to 125 ml. of water.

The filtrate (pentane extract) was washed with water and the aqueous washings were added to the dissolved filter cake. The resulting aqueous soap solution was acidified, and the resulting mixture of straight chain and branched carboxylic acids was washed with water, dried, weighed, esterified with diazomethane, and analyzed as the methyl esters by gas chromatography, again using calibration factors previously measured for the pure compounds. These techniques permitted calculation of independent material balances for straight chain and for branched products. In a number of experiments of this type, these material balances were consistently above 92% and averaged about 95%. On the assumption (established by independent kinetic studies) that the caustic dehydrogenation is first order in alcohol concentration, a relative rate constant was defined as the ratio of the dehydrogenation rate for the straight chain alcohol to the dehydrogenation rate for the branched alcohol and calculated from the expression:

$$r = \text{Relative Rate} = \frac{\log (a/a_0)}{\log (a'/a'_0)}$$

where a_0 and a are the initial and final concentrations of straight chain alcohol respectively, and a'_0 and a' are the initial and final concentrations of branched alcohol respectively. For this experiment, these calculations gave $r = 5.69$.

Example 2: Example 1 was repeated, except that the temperature for the dehydrogenation reaction was 330°C. instead of 300°C. For this experiment, r was found to be 7.35.

Example 3: Examples 1 and 2 were repeated, using a different alcohol mixture consisting of equal parts of 2-ethyl dodecanol and n-dodecanol and same reactant stoichiometry. The relative rate at 300°C. was $r = 6.94$ and at 330°C. was 17.11.

Monounsaturated Soaps by Selective Hydrogenation

The process of A.E. Fishman; U.S. Patent 3,503,896; March 31, 1970; assigned to Ethyl Corporation produces, synthetically, soaps of monounsaturated acids. The process comprises reacting aliphatic alcohols having from 12 to about 22 carbon atoms in the molecule with one or more alkali or alkaline earth metal hydroxides at a temperature in the range of from 280° to about 350°C. and at a pressure of up to about 25 atmospheres whereby the alcohols are converted to soaps and hydrogen is liberated. The reaction is conducted in the presence of soaps of polyunsaturated acids whereby at least part of the liberated hydrogen selectively and partially saturates the soaps of monounsaturated acids with soaps of saturated acids.

It is possible to replace a significant portion of the commercially used naturally derived carboxylic acids with synthetically produced acids which are direct and even superior substitutes for the coconut oil derived natural acids. Not only were the coconut range natural acids employed in the formulation of soap, but also practice has dictated the joint use of another naturally derived series of acids, namely, the tallow acids.

One of the objects of the process is to provide a method whereby soap compositions can be made wherein the entire acid content of soaps can be provided by acids synthetically derived from low cost materials. A portion of the raw materials is available in significant quantities from waste materials and although the source of such is in a sense natural or agricultural, it does not depend upon year by year weather or growing conditions and hence represents a predictable supply and demand picture.

The preferred process whereby the high quality synthetic coconut range acids are derived is by the reaction of certain high quality normal alcohols with caustic at elevated temperature. In the preferred alcohol-caustic reaction, the alcohols are converted to the corresponding soaps or salts of the caustic employed in extremely high yield and without the formation of significant quantities of difficulty removable by-product materials. The only significant by-products are unreacted or excess alcohols which are readily removed from the soaps by steam stripping. For the most part, isomeric alcohols react slowly or not at all under the conditions preferred for the caustic fusion reaction.

A low cost acid material having significant quantity of molecules in the 18 carbon atom per molecule range and possessing unacceptable plural unsaturation is combined with the high quality alcohols fed to the caustic fusion reaction with the surprising result that without any need for vigorous catalytic activity beyond that inherently present, the plurally unsaturated molecules are selectively partially saturated so as to yield monounsaturated molecules providing an excellent and even superior substitute for the tallow fatty acid content used in soap manufacture.

The result of this is that superior synthetic tallow range acids are produced for soap manufacture through simple processing and in substantial quantity at low cost and furthermore that the synthetic acids, like the synthetic coconut range acids, are also superior to the naturally derived acids used for this purpose particularly with regard to the important properties of color, odor, stability and freedom from sterols, proteins and naturally occurring impurities so important to soap manufacturers. The tall oil fatty acids can be saponified prior to admission to the caustic fusion reaction or can be saponified concurrently with the reaction since transient or intermediate formation of esters do not cause problems under the fusion reaction conditions.

It is considered particularly significant that the process achieves hydrogenation of a selective nature to the level desired using hydrogen which is inherently generated in the processing due to the reaction of the alcohols and that the desired result is obtained without the necessity for the addition of any catalyst or supplemental hydrogen that must be recovered for economy purposes or removed from the product to provide required purity of product. One of the preferred natural materials used is a mixture of tall oil fatty acids (or their alkali soaps or salts). Another typical material is fish oil which is also rich in materials of the foregoing type and which contains plurally unsaturated molecules as well as the others that are desired.

Example 1: A synthetic 80/20 tallow fatty acid/coconut acid soda soap composition was made using the following constituents. (Toilet bar soap of commerce)

	Parts by Weight
Normal alcohols:	
C_{12} alcohol (lauryl)	130
C_{14} alcohol (myristyl)	50
C_{16} alcohol (palmityl)	220
C_{18} alcohol (stearyl)	200
Tall oil fatty acids:	
Oleic acid	200
Linoleic acid	200
Sodium hydroxide (100% active basis)	160

The mixture of alcohols and tall oil fatty acid was reacted with the caustic at 340°C. and 400 psi until hydrogen liberation ceased. This took approximately 15 to 30 minutes. The molten soap was cooled in a nitrogen atmosphere to ambient temperature. The anhydrous soap so produced was white, of very bland odor and exhibited good foaming and cleaning properties in hand washing tests conducted with 60° to 100°F. wash water.

The titer of fatty acids sprung from the soap was 39°C. and the iodine value was 30 centigrams of I_2 per gram of acid. Both specifications are typical of an 80/20 tallow fatty acid/coconut oil fatty acid soap stock. In the caustic fusion process the iodine value had been reduced from 52 to 30 centigrams I_2 per gram of acid. All data were consistent with the reduction of diunsaturates of the tall oil fatty acids to monounsaturates. The soap had excellent keeping qualities. No antioxidant was added. Color over a 3 month storage period remained white and odor bland or mild.

Example 2: A low titer soap was produced from the following principal components.

	Parts by Weight
C_{12} normal alcohol	500
Tall oil fatty acids:	
Oleic	250
Linoleic	250
Sodium hydroxide (100% active basis)	173

The components were caustic fused as in Example 1. The resulting soap had excellent solubility and detergency in low temperature washing 100°F. These low temperature washing properties are desirable in washing of woolens and delicate synthetic fibers. These fibers may be damaged by washing at higher temperatures. The soap is also useful for preparing automobile washing compounds, liquid hand soap, and scrub soaps for floor cleaning.

Caustic Fusion Improvement by Pretreatment

The process of R.J. Fanning; U.S. Patent 3,558,678; January 26, 1971; assigned to Ethyl Corporation, a caustic fusion process for producing carboxylic acid soaps from alcohols, is improved by employing a preliminary heat treatment of the reactants prior to the actual fusion reaction. The heat treatment or pretreatment is characterized by the performance thereof at a temperature or over a temperature range up to but usually somewhat below that at which a significant evolution of gas or vapor material from reactants, diluents or products is experienced at a pressure up to about 300 to 400 psig.

A principal result of performing the heat treatment is that when the main caustic fusion reaction to produce soaps is subsequently performed, forcefully liberating the normal copious quantities of by-product hydrogen at higher pressures than the 300 to 400 psig, unreacted alcohols are not stripped out, reaction is faster, and higher yields of product soaps are obtained.

Although this treatment is useful with individuals or combinations of alcohols of a wide range of molecular weights such as alcohols having from about 2 to 30 carbon atoms per molecule, this process is particularly advantageous with the more volatile lower alcohols, particularly those having from 6 to 8 carbon atoms per molecule whose soaps and acids are highly desired for ester production.

The process is concerned particularly with the caustic fusion reaction of short chain or lower molecular weight alcohols under conditions of temperature and pressure such that a significant amount of the alcohols would ordinarily be vaporized from the reaction mass under the reaction conditions but for the involvement of the improvement of the process.

At first glance it would appear that such vaporization poses no particular problem since the vaporized alcohol seemingly could be collected and recycled; however, practical experience has shown that alcohols so vaporized experience a significant degree of dehydration or other alteration so that when the resulting materials are condensed and recycled to the reaction mass a significant proportion of the return material is not usable alcohol for the reaction but rather appears to be a partially dehydrated material including components such as olefins which are of no value for reaction with caustic to produce soaps. The improvement is applied to a process for producing carboxylic acid soaps by performing an overall reaction of alcohols RCH_2OH with caustic $M(OH)_n$ at a reacting temperature from about 540° to 630°F. in about a 1:1 molar ratio of alcohol to (—OH) groups in $M(OH)_n$.

The soaps produced correspond to the carbon skeletal structure of the alcohols reacted, being of the formula $(RCOO)_n M$ wherein R is selected from normal alkyl and branched alkyl having from about 1 to 29 carbon atoms per molecule. Alcohols used range from substantially pure individual alcohols to various mixtures of alcohols such as those available in various commercial mixtures.

In the foregoing formula $(RCOO)_n M$, M (cation) is selected from the group consisting of alkali metal and alkaline earth metal elements. In the foregoing formula for the carboxylic acid soaps $(RCOO)_n M$, n is a conventional valence factor for the metal M being 1 for those molecules wherein M is an alkali metal such as sodium, lithium, potassium and being two where M is an alkaline earth metal such as calcium, magnesium and barium.

The liberation of hydrogen in the course of the caustic fusion reaction is a matter of a very definite and abrupt reaction threshold involving a fairly narrow transitional range of temperatures, for example, 5° to 20°F. In general, the threshold or transition is of such a sharp nature as to result in the virtual absence of liberation of hydrogen below the threshold whereas above the threshold the liberation of hydrogen is not an equilibrium proposition but continues even with the maintenance of autogenous pressures in excess of many thousands of pounds per square inch.

One important aspect of this forced liberation and release of hydrogen or of any other volatile material, even water, for that matter, is that the released material acts as a stripper gas to enhance removal of less volatile materials such as alcohols (and water) from the system.

Although the actual caustic fusion reaction of alcohol or of intermediate is described in the foregoing as involving a fairly sharp temperature threshold proposition, the heat treating reaction is more of the nature of a time temperature proposition which is accomplished at various rates for various temperatures which range from about ordinary room temperature up to a temperature just below that at which the fusion reaction begins as evidenced by a sharp increase in pressure for only a small change in temperature occasioned by the release of hydrogen. Thus, the pretreatment ranges from a temperature from about 60° to 500°F. for essentially pure normal alcohols in which the R groups are straight chain with a terminal link to (—CH_2OH), or somewhat higher up to about 520°F. where the alcohols are substantially all branched alcohols. The time aspect of the heat treatment involves either a short time basis of the order of 10 to 15 minutes for the elevated temperatures of the order of 480° to 500°F. or a longer term basis such as up to 24 or even 48 hours when using the lower temperatures such as those of the order of 60° to 120°F. A fundamental consideration for a most effective heat treatment with minimum loss of volatile alcohols is that the heat treatment system be closed, that is, that it operate under autogenous or moderate super pressure without release of either hydrogen or other gas or vapor material that may carry with it some of the volatile alcohols.

It is desired that the heat treatment in the preferred embodiments be performed in such a way as to remove residual quantities of oxygen and free oxygen-providing materials from the reactants prior to a time at which a significant proportion of the heat treatment reaction can occur. In some embodiments this preliminary removal of oxygen is accomplished by sweeping the system with nitrogen or by subjecting the alcohol and caustic reactants to vacuum treatment to remove part or all of copresent oxygen. Such a treatment is particularly effective, for example, where the caustic is employed in the form of a 50% by weight aqueous solution which has been handled or stored under such conditions as to permit the absorption therein of significant quantities of oxygen.

Example 1: 1,724 g. of dry NaOH, 304 g. of water and 5,000 g. of alcohols were added to an electrically heated, well agitated 5 gallon autoclave provided with a relief valve preset to 350 psig. The water used provided an 85 weight percent aqueous caustic system plus the alcohol. The alcohol used was equal weights of synthetic hexanol-1 and octanol-1.

The autoclave was closed, swept with nitrogen, pressurized to 10 psig, heated to 450°F. and held at that temperature for 60 minutes. Pressure was autogenous rising to about 70 psig at the conclusion of the 60 minutes treatment. At the conclusion of the heat treatment period, the temperature of the autoclave was raised to 530° to 540°F. in a 20 minute period and was maintained at that temperature for 180 minutes. The pressure of the autoclave rose rapidly at about 500°F., reaching the preset pressure of 350 psig at a temperature of 510°F.

After the 180 minute constant temperature operation, the temperature was raised gradually during an additional period of about 100 minutes duration reaching a concluding temperature of 650°F. after a total time of 285 min. of fusion reaction. Soaps were obtained corresponding to the alcohols. A portion of the soaps was converted to acid by reaction with 30% aqueous H_2SO_4. The acid phase was separated from the aqueous phase by decantation.

Example 2: A pretreatment was performed as in Example 1, however, the alcohols used were a mixture of 65 weight percent dodecanol-1, 25 weight percent tetradecanol-1 and 10 weight percent hexadecanol-1 which had an average molecular weight of 197. The mixture was stirred initially and the agitation stopped allowing the mass to remain in a dormant state for approximately 65 hours at room temperature. The system was then heated to caustic fusion temperatures of 560° to 580°F. providing a higher reaction rate as evidenced by rapid gas evolution and short reaction time in comparison to similar reactions without the pretreatment.

Oxidative Dehydrogenation in Presence of Carbon

H.L. Dimond and A.C. Whitaker; U.S. Patent 3,365,476; January 23, 1968; assigned to Gulf Research & Development Company provide an improved process for preparing organic acid salts by the oxidative dehydration of certain oxygen-containing organic compounds with an alkali or alkaline earth metal compound.

High yields of an organic acid salt are obtained by contacting at least one oxygen-containing compound reactant selected from the group consisting of primary alcohols, ethers having at least two hydrogen atoms on at least one of the carbon atoms adjacent to the ether oxygen atom, aldehydes, aldols and esters with an alkali or alkaline earth metal compound selected from the class consisting of their oxides and hydroxides under oxidative dehydrogenation conditions in the presence of at least 0.1 weight percent solid carbon based on the amount of oxygen-containing compound reactant employed, the solid carbon having a surface area between 25 and 1,700 square meters per gram.

The oxygen-containing compounds can have between 1 and 40 carbon atoms per molecule. The preferred oxygen-containing organic compound reactants are those having between 4 and 20 carbon atoms per molecule. It is understood that the oxygen-containing compound reactants defined above may be polyfunctional, if desired, and include compounds such as, for example, acetals and glycols where at least one of the oxygen atoms is directly connected to a carbon atom having two substituent hydrogen atoms. The oxygen-containing compound reactants can be either straight or branched chain in structure.

The reactants can comprise a mixture of straight and branched chain primary alcohols, straight and branched chain aldehydes, admixtures of primary alcohols and aldehydes, together with esters, aldols and ethers as defined above, if desired. The solid carbon which is employed in the process can be any of the commercially pure solid carbons having a surface area between 25 and 1,700 $m.^2/g$.

It is preferred that the surface area be between 300 and 1,200 m.^{2}/g. and more preferred that the solid carbon have a surface area between 400 and 800. Suitable solid carbons include the active carbons, carbon black, charcoals, lampblacks and cokes. The solid carbon is preferably in finely comminuted form. Carbon black and lampblack are normally in finely powdered form having a particle size between 50 and 5,000 A. Graphite, coke and active carbon (including charcoal) are usually available in larger sizes and are preferably ground to a mesh size between about 4 and 1,000 before use.

The amount of solid carbon to employ is at least 0.1 weight percent based on the oxygen-containing compound reactant. It is usual to employ between 0.1 and 10 weight percent solid carbon and preferably between 0.2 and 2.0 weight percent and more preferably between 0.5 and 1.5 weight percent. The alkali or alkaline earth metal compound for this reaction can be any of their oxides and hydroxides. The preferred alkali metal oxides and hydroxides are those of sodium and potassium.

The amount of metal compound to employ is substantially the stoichiometric requirement to oxidize all of the oxygen-containing compound reactants to the corresponding acid salts. The mol ratio of the metal compound to the oxygen-containing compound reactant can vary between about 0.5:1 and 4:1 and is preferably between 1:1 and 1.5:1.

The function of the reaction temperature is to promote the rate of reaction. The reaction temperature can generally vary between about 175° and 400°C. The preferred temperatures depend to some degree upon the type of oxygen-containing compound reactant employed. For the oxidative dehydrogenation of aldehydes, a preferred reaction temperature is between 175° and 260°C. For the other oxygen-containing compound reactants defined above, the preferred reaction temperature is between 240° and 350°C. with the most preferred temperatures being between 320° and 330°C.

The function of reaction pressure is to maintain the reactants in the liquid phase. The reaction pressure can vary over a wide range, for example, from 0 to 2,000 psig or higher, with preferred reaction pressures between 75 and 750 psig. The most preferred pressures are between 100 and 400 pounds per square inch gauge.

The reaction time can vary between 0.25 and 6 hours or more. Prolonged contacting times at elevated temperatures promote decomposition of the soap products into undesirable side products such as carbonates. In general, the higher the temperature the shorter the maximum contacting time. At temperatures of about 300°C., for example, the preferred contacting times are between 1 and 2 hours after preheating to reaction temperature.

Longer contacting times within the broad range defined above can be employed at the lower reaction temperatures. The organic acid salt can be separated from the reaction mass by any suitable means, such as solvent extraction.

Example 1: In this experiment, 390.5 g. (3 mols) of isooctyl alcohol and 124.0 g. (3.02 mols) of solid 97.5% NaOH pellets were charged to a 1 l., Inconel lined, turbo stirred autoclave. The autoclave was purged of air with nitrogen and the stirrer started. The reaction mixture was heated to about 285°C. and the pressure increased to 270 psig. The pressure was maintained at 270 psig by the gradual release of the H_2 formed and the temperature increased from 285° to 305°C.

After a 1 hour reaction period, evolution of H_2 appeared to cease, and the pressure was gradually reduced (a period of about 30 minutes) to 200 pounds per square inch gauge while the temperature remained at 290°C. The acid salt was converted to isooctanoic acid by reaction with aqueous HCl, and the products were separated and analyzed. The alcohol conversion was found to be 91.2 mol percent, while the yield of isooctanoic acid was 77.0 mol percent. The efficiency was, therefore, 84.4 mol percent.

Example 2: Example 1 was repeated except 316.8 g. (2.43 mols) of isooctyl alcohol and 82.1 g. (2 mols) of 97.5% NaOH pellets were employed together with 4 g. of Darco G-60 solid active carbon (1.26 weight percent based on the alcohol). The reaction time was 1.5 hours while the temperature was maintained at 286°C. and the pressure at 270 psig. The organic salt was converted to the acid by reaction with dilute aqueous HCl. Analysis of the product showed an alcohol conversion of 99.5 mol percent based on the stoichiometric amount of alcohol, a 96.6 mol percent yield of acid, and an efficiency of 97.1 mol percent.

In this example an excess of alcohol over the stoichiometric amount required to react with the sodium hydroxide was employed. The alcohol conversion figures in this and succeeding examples are based only on the stoichiometric amount of alcohol required. Thus, in this example, the 99.5 mol percent alcohol conversion is based on 2 mols of alcohol (the stoichiometric amount since 2 mols of sodium hydroxide were employed) rather than the actual 2.43 mols employed. A comparison of Example 2 with Example 1 shows the beneficial effect of the added solid carbon, for the conversion, efficiency and yield all increased.

Oxidative Dehydrogenation in Presence of Water

In the process of H.L. Dimond and A.C. Whitaker; U.S. Patent 3,370,074; February 20, 1968; assigned to Gulf Research & Development

Company high yields of an organic acid salt are obtained by the oxidative dehydrogenation of at least one oxygen-containing compound reactant selected from the group consisting of primary alcohols, ethers having at least 2 hydrogen atoms on at least one of the carbon atoms adjacent to the ether oxygen atom, aldehydes, aldols and esters by a process which comprises reacting under oxidative dehydrogenation conditions in the liquid phase a mixture consisting essentially of the oxygen-containing compound reactant, a substantially anhydrous alkali or alkaline earth metal compound selected from the group consisting of their oxides and hydroxides and between 0.5 and 8 mol percent water based on the metal compound employed.

The oxygen-containing compounds can have between 1 and 40 carbon atoms per molecule. The preferred oxygen-containing organic compound reactants are those having between 4 and 20 carbon atoms per molecule. The alkali or alkaline earth compound for this reaction can be any substantially anhydrous compound selected from the group consisting of their oxides and hydroxides. The preferred alkali metal oxides and hydroxides are those of sodium and potassium.

The amount of metal compound to employ is substantially the stoichiometric requirement to oxidize all of the oxygen-containing compound reactants to the corresponding acids. The mol ratio of the metal compound to the oxygen-containing compound reactant can vary between about 0.5:1 and 4:1, and preferably between 1:1 and 1.5:1.

It has been found that high yields of the desired organic acid salts are obtained when the water content of the reaction mixture is maintained within certain narrow limits, namely, between 0.5 and 8 mol percent based on the metal compound employed. The optimum water content is 5 mol percent based on the metal compound. Amounts of water above and below the described limits result in reduced yields of the desired organic acid salts. The function of the water is believed to be to inhibit the undesirable formation of the metal alkoxide.

If H_2O is to be effective to inhibit the formation of the metal alkoxide, the water content should be present in the oxygen-containing compound reactant phase rather than the metal compound phase since the alkoxide tends to dissolve in the alcohol phase. The manner in which the water is added to the reaction mixture is therefore critical.

The water can be added to the oxygen-containing compound reactant prior to the addition of the anhydrous metal compound or the water can be added to the mixture of the anhydrous metal compound and the oxygen-containing compound reactant just before reaction begins. It is preferred, however, to add the water last in the sequence of addition of reactants.

If the water is added with the metal compound, it will not be as effective in inhibiting the formation of the metal alkoxide. The amounts of water required are so small that, if added with the metal compound, they would be insufficient to prepare an aqueous solution. In addition, the metal compounds are known drying agents because of their excellent water retention properties. Consequently, the added water would remain in the metal phase. As a result, the desired water content in the organic phase would be produced in situ along with the undesired formation of the metal alkoxide. This would reduce the desired yields of the organic acid salts.

The metal compound employed is substantially anhydrous. It is normally added as a solid to the reaction zone. The water is added as a separate phase either in admixture with the oxygen-containing compound reactant or to the mixture of the metal compound and oxygen-containing compound reactant.

When the metal compound employed is substantially anhydrous and the water is added in the amount and manner indicated, there is no necessity to preheat the oxygen-containing compound reactant and the metal compound to reaction temperature before admixture since yields of the desired salts are very high with only minor amounts of undesired by-products. The reaction temperature can generally vary between about 175° and 400°C.

The reaction pressure can vary over a wide range, for example, from 0 to 2,000 psig, or higher, with preferred reaction pressures between 75 and 750 psig. The reaction time can vary between 0.25 and 6 hours or more. Prolonged contacting times at elevated temperatures promote decomposition of the soap products into undesirable side products such as carbonates.

Examples 1 through 6: A series of experiments were performed to determine the effect of added small amounts of water on the oxidative dehydrogenation of isooctyl alcohol in the presence of NaOH. In these experiments a 1 l. Inconel lined, turbo stirred autoclave, equipped with a cooling coil and external condenser was employed.

The procedure involved adding the isooctyl alcohol and anhydrous solid NaOH pellets to the autoclave followed by careful addition of the desired amount of water. The temperature was slowly raised over 1 3/4 hours to about 285°C. while the pressure increased to 270 psig.

The pressure was held at 270 psig by the gradual release of H_2 formed. The reaction time was 1 hour. The pressure was permitted to fall to 200 psig while the temperature was reduced to 230°C. The product was recovered as an acid by the careful, dropwise addition (about 2 mols of mineral acid per mol of salt per hour) to the molten salt at 230°C. of the stoichiometric amount of aqueous HCl having a concentration between 16 and 38%. Almost no steam or other vapor was observed. After addition of the acid, the product temperature was between about 100° and 150°C. The product was cooled further, withdrawn from the bomb, and the acid layer water washed to remove the excess HCl. The yield of organic acid was determined by titration. Results of this series of experiments are shown in the table below.

Effect of Traces of H$_2$O

Example No.	ROH/NaOH, Mol	Mol percent H$_2$O based on NaOH	Time, hours	Efficiency, Mol	Conversion, mol percent	Yield, mol percent
1	1.0	0.0	1.0	84.4	91.2	77.0
2	1.0	2.5	1.0	96.2	91.6	88.1
3	1.2	5.0	1.0	95.6	97.0 [1]	92.7
4	1.0	7.5	1.5	94.9	91.6	86.9
5	1.2	10.0	1.0	94.6	88.9 [1]	84.2
6	1.0	17.5	1.0	97.6	57.2	55.8 [2]

[1] This conversion is based on the stoichiometric amount of alcohol, that is, a 1.0 ROH:NaOH mol ratio rather than the 1.2 ROH:NaOH mol ratio actually employed.
[2] Example 6 indicates, by its poor yield and conversion, the deleterious effect of adding too much water.

OTHER STARTING MATERIALS

Phenyl Mercuric Salts Using Branched Chain Acid Salts

J. Geraci and S.V. Chodsky; U.S. Patent 3,304,316; February 14, 1967; assigned to Alcolac Chemical Corporation provide a process for the preparation of phenyl mercury salts of branched chain aliphatic carboxylic acids which acids have a total of from 4 to 18 carbon atoms. Thus, the process contemplates salts such as phenyl mercuric isobutyrate, phenyl mercuric 14-ethyl hexadecanoate and 2-propyl pentadecanoate.

The compounds may be produced by mixing phenyl mercuric acetate with an alkali metal salt of a branched aliphatic carboxylic chain acid in an aqueous alkaline medium. The mixture is heated and agitated for several hours until a suspension of the phenyl mercuric salt of the branched chain acid forms. The suspended solids are then separated from the suspending medium and the solid product washed and dried. It is possible to speed up the reaction and increase the reaction efficiency by the continuous removal from the alkaline medium of the product formed.

This is readily accomplished by the methods well-known to those skilled in the art. Further, as is known, not only will the reaction proceed more rapidly, but the reactants will be utilized more completely. The chemical reaction mechanism is as follows: a suitable phenyl mercuric salt, such as phenyl mercuric acetate, is reacted with an alkali metal salt of the desired branched chain acid; an ester interchange-type reaction occurs to produce the desired branched chain phenyl mercuric salt and an alkali metal salt such as sodium acetate. For complete reaction, the alkali metal salt reactant should be present in about stoichiometric quantities. However to increase the rate of reaction, amounts in excess of stoichiometric are suitably employed. In general, it has been found to be particularly advantageous to utilize a mol ratio of alkali metal salt reactant to phenyl mercuric compound reactant of the order of about 1.25 to 1.

The amount of alkali metal hydroxide dissolved in water to form the aqueous alkaline medium should also be such that the mol ratio of alkali metal hydroxide to phenyl mercuric compound reactant is about 1.25 to 1. It should be noted that as employed herein, the terms "alkali metal salt" and "alkaline metal hydroxide" are intended to include the corresponding ammonium compounds.

The alkali metal salt reactant may be formed in situ if desired. Thus, in addition to the alkaline medium, the reaction mixture can comprise phenyl mercuric salt, the desired branched chain aliphatic carboxylic acid and sufficient additional alkali metal hydroxide to form the desired alkali metal salt.

Temperatures and pressure are not critical and the reaction may be performed at ambient temperature and pressure. However, to complete the reaction in the shortest period of time, the reaction should be conducted at temperatures just below the melting point of the final product. Thus, for phenyl mercuric 2-ethyl hexanoate, the temperature should be about 70°C. or lower.

Reaction times required may vary considerably dependent upon the specific temperature chosen. In the case of preparation of the phenyl mercuric 2-ethyl hexanoate, the reaction time may vary from about 30 minutes up to about 15 or 20 hours. When the product is not removed during the reaction, it settles from the reaction mixtures as a crystalline solid and may be readily recovered by conventional separation methods, such as filtration, decantation, centrifugation and the like.

Phenyl mercuric 2-ethyl hexanoate is the preferred compound, although the isobutyrate also possesses exceptional properties. The former is a white, highly stable, crystalline material containing by titrimetric analysis, about 47.5% by weight of mercury. The phenyl mercuric 2-ethyl hexanoate has been found to be soluble in a wide variety of organic solvents and water-containing solvent systems.

Examples of these solvents include alcohols, chloroform, dioxane, acetone, naphtha, benzene, chlorinated hydrocarbons, aliphatic and aromatic hydrocarbons, aqueous ammonia, acetic acid and ammoniacal alcohol and acetone and dioxane. The compound dissolves readily and forms a stable solution containing from about 10 to 50% by weight of phenyl mercuric 2-ethyl hexanoate in all of the abovementioned solvents without the addition of any solubilizing agents. The compound is completely compatible with all of the abovementioned solvents and solutions thereof can be made on both the alkaline or slightly acid side.

Furthermore, all solutions have excellent stability and are useful in water-base or oil-base compositions for imparting bactericidal properties thereto. The stability, high solubility and excellent dispersibility of the phenyl mercuric compound of the process are very advantageous from a consumer standpoint. These attributes permit shipment of the compounds in the solid form and thus afford tremendous economic advantages over materials of the prior art.

Example 1: 50 g. of sodium hydroxide (1.25 mols) were dissolved in 460 grams of water. To the resulting alkaline solution were added 180 g. of 2-ethyl hexoic acid (1.25 mols); the mixture was agitated at ambient temperature until complete dissolution occurred. The pH ranged from 6.8 to 7.0. The mixture was cooled to room temperature (20° to 25°C.) and one mol of phenyl mercuric acetate was added. The mixture was then agitated at ambient temperature for about 3 hours, following which the temperature was raised to about 40° to 45°C. and the mixture was agitated at that temperature for an additional 3 hours.

During this period the product formed as a suspension of particles in the aqueous medium. The solids were separated by filtration, washed with water until free from sodium acetate and unreacted sodium 2-ethyl hexanoate and dried at 40° to 50°C. The white crystalline product contained, by analysis, 47.0% mercury; the theoretical mercury content is 47.66%. The melting point range of the white crystaline product was 71° to 74°C.

Example 2: The procedure of Example 1 was repeated using 1.25 mols of n-octanoic acid in place of the 2-ethyl hexoic acid. The phenyl mercuric n-octanoate product contained, by analysis, 46.9% mercury as compared to a theoretical content of 47.66%. The melting point range of the product was 77° to 80°C.

Aluminum Salts from Aluminum Trialkyls

In the process of N.R. Artman; U.S. Patent 3,244,735; April 5, 1966; assigned to The Procter & Gamble Company aluminum salts of organic carboxylic acids (aluminum soaps) are prepared in a high percentage yield of the theoretically obtainable value by the interaction, under temperature and pressure, of an aluminum trialkyl with excess carbon dioxide in the presence of a solvent which forms a complex with the aluminum trialkyl, the solvent-complexer being selected from the group consisting of ethyl ether, tetrahydrofuran, dioxane, ethylene glycol dimethyl ether, isopropyl ether, dibutyl ether and tetrahydropyran. The aluminum trialkyl starting compound has the general formula of:

$$\begin{array}{c} R_1 \\ \diagdown \\ R_2 - Al \\ \diagup \\ R_3 \end{array}$$

where each of the R's is the same or a different alkyl radical and contains from 2 to 30 carbon atoms. When admixed with the ether solvent-complexers used herein, the aluminum trialkyls form a complex with the ether. This aluminum trialkyl-ether complex in turn is reacted, under certain forcing conditions (time, temperature and pressure) with excess carbon dioxide, the molar ratio of carbon dioxide to alkyl aluminum being at least 3 to 1, and preferably 10:1 or higher. The product of this carbonation reaction is an aluminum soap.

The aluminum soap can be separated from the ether-aluminum soap mixture and recovered from solution. A preferred method is to heat the mixture of aluminum soap, ether, by-product hydrocarbons, and unreacted materials to drive off all of the undesired materials which are volatile, thereby leaving the nonvolatile aluminum soaps behind. Passing a stream of steam or inert gas such as nitrogen through the solution of reaction products will also aid in stripping out the volatile materials.

Another method of recovering the aluminum soaps in the form of a useful product is to add to the reaction mixture a material which, although volatile, is less volatile than the materials to be removed. This mixture can then be heated at atmospheric or reduced pressure to drive off all of the volatile undesired materials and that part of the added high-boiling material which codistills with the undesired materials, leaving a solution or suspension of aluminum soaps in the desired, high-boiling material. Such additive high-boiling material can be lubricating oil, in which case the final product is thickened grease.

The aluminum trialkyl compounds which can be used in the process can contain branched or normal alkyl radicals. It is preferred, however, to employ aluminum compounds containing the straight chain or normal alkyl substituents. Accordingly, the employment of straight chain aluminum trialkyl compounds will result in a production of straight chain aluminum soaps which can either be used as lubricants, for example, or can be used to produce straight chain organic monocarboxylic acids which are useful in producing detergent compounds. In the practice of this process, the aluminum trialkyl (liquid) and ether solvent-complexer in the desired mol ratio of solvent to aluminum trialkyl are placed in a reaction vessel and the vessel is sealed. It has been found that a standard glass lined autoclave is eminently suitable.

After the autoclave is sealed and while still cold, a molar excess (at least 3 mols carbon dioxide to 1 mol aluminum trialkyl) of carbon dioxide is added, then heat is applied. Though less convenient it would also be possible to heat the aluminum trialkyl ether complex in the autoclave and then add CO_2 from a cylinder. The pressure is maintained in the range of from about 500 to 20,000 psig and the temperature in the range of from about 150° to 250°C. The reaction is continued under these conditions for a period of from about 1 to 60 hours.

The preferred pressure is about 5,000 psig when the temperature is maintained at a level of about 200°C. If the pressure is lower than 800 psig the yield falls off considerably although it is still at a significantly increased level over that obtained using prior art processes. Thus the preferred pressure range is from 800 to 5,000 psig. The temperature of the reaction is quite important. Highest yields are obtained when the temperature of the reaction mixture is maintained at about 170° to 200°C.; thus this is the preferred temperature range.

Higher temperatures diminish the yield somewhat while lower temperatures diminish the yield greatly. The time of the reaction will, of course, depend on the particular aluminum trialkyl compound used, the pressure and the temperature. The shorter the reaction time, the less is the yield of aluminum soap because of incomplete carbonation reaction. The preferred reaction time is about 20 to 30 hours.

It is important that the proper mol ratio of aluminum trialkyl to the ether solvent-complexer be used. It has been found that a mol ratio of less than about 1:1 results in a low yield of aluminum soaps due to side reactions. Ratios ranging from about 1:1 to about 1:10 or higher give optimum results. The preferred mol ratio is 1 mol of aluminum trialkyl to 2.5 mols of ether.

The ether solvent-complexer used in this reaction is very important. It has been found that by using an ether solvent-complexer of the class mentioned supra, very high yields of aluminum soap can be obtained. The ethers used herein act not only as complexers of the aluminum trialkyl but they also act as solvent for the reactants and for the reaction products of the process. This complexing-solvent action aids in the completion of the reaction and in obtaining high yields. The preferred ether is ethyl ether. It is essential to get complete carbonation of the aluminum trialkyl compounds that excess carbon dioxide be present in the reaction vessel. The carbon dioxide is added to the reaction vessel before or after heat is applied in the form of a gas at cylinder pressure. Higher carbon dioxide pressures can be achieved by packing the free space of the reaction vessel with Dry Ice (solid CO_2) before sealing it and then pressuring in CO_2 at cylinder pressure into the still cold vehicle. It is desirable to agitate the reaction vessel during the period of the reaction.

Example: 20 ml. (0.04 mol) of tridodecylaluminum was cautiously mixed with 5 ml. (0.09 mol) of ethyl ether in a 300 ml. glass lined autoclave. The free space in the autoclave was packed with Dry Ice before sealing. After sealing, and before the application of heat, CO_2 gas was let into the autoclave at cylinder pressure, then heat was applied in the usual manner by means of an electric heating coil.

In this example the temperature was maintained at 200°C. and the pressure inside the reaction vessel was 1,600 psig. The reactants were agitated for 20 hours. The heating coil was then shut off and the autoclave was allowed to cool to room temperature, then the pressure was released. The solution containing the aluminum soap-ether mixture, unreacted starting materials, and by-products of the reaction, was then hydrolyzed by treatment with aqueous sodium hydroxide whereupon two phases were formed, the top layer containing the unreacted diluents, by-products and oil-soluble salt of tridecanoic acid.

The two layers were then separated and the sodium salt was then acidified with dilute sulfuric acid again forming two layers, the top layer containing the fatty acid and the bottom layer containing H_2O, Na_2SO_4 and H_2SO_4. The fatty acid was then separated. As the amount of organic carboxylic acid formed is directly proportional to the amount of aluminum soap formed by the carbonation reaction, it can readily be seen that the percentage yield of monocarboxylic acid as compared to theoretical obtainable value is the same as the percentage yield of aluminum soap as compared to the theoretical obtainable value.

The percent aluminum soap, aluminum tridecanoate, formed as compared to the theoretically obtainable value in this example was 53%. The aluminum tridecanoate is useful as a lubricant; or, as was seen above, it can be acidified with H_2SO_4 to form tridecanoic acid which in turn can be saponified with caustic soda to form a detergent compound. The acid can also be sulfonated with SO_3 to form a different type of detergent compound.

Instead of hydrolyzing and/or acidifying the aluminum soap formed in the carbonation reaction above to recover monocarboxylic acids, it is also possible to separate the aluminum soap as a pure compound by driving off the volatile materials with heat and recovering the residual aluminum soap. The soap can then be used as lubricating aids, grinding aids or for other purposes herein mentioned. In the above reaction the ethyl ether can be replaced by tetrahydrofuran or dioxane with comparable results. In addition, the tridodecyl aluminum can be replaced with tributyl aluminum, trioctyl aluminum, tritetradecyl aluminum or tridecyl aluminum, for example and comparable results are obtained thereby.

Lead, Cadmium and Divalent Tin Salts Using Acid Anhydrides

In the process of E. Ruf; U.S. Patent 3,546,263; December 8, 1970; assigned to Th. Goldschmidt AG, Germany lead, cadmium, and divalent tin salts of carboxylic acids having more than 6 carbon atoms, are prepared by reacting lead oxide, cadmium oxide or stannous oxide with carboxylic acid anhydrides at elevated temperatures that are above the melting point of the carboxylic acid anhydride.

According to a preferred form of the process the reaction is carried out with stoichiometric amounts of the reaction components, i.e., the metal oxide and carboxylic acid anhydrides. Provided the required reaction temperatures and reaction times are properly adhered to, the reaction, calculated on the stoichiometric amounts of the respective oxide and the carboxylic acid anhydride or anhydrides, proceeds essentially in quantitative manner. Further, the formed metal soaps are obtained in liquid form at the respective reaction temperatures. For these reasons the use of solvents is not absolutely required although, of course, the reaction may be carried out in a solvent medium.

Dependent on the particular metal soap to be produced, the reaction temperature should advantageously be in the range of between 80° to 250°C. If the bivalent metal oxides used in the reaction are contaminated by oxide moieties of higher valency, then these higher valency oxide portions do not take part in the reaction with the higher molecular carboxylic acid anhydrides. If the respective lead oxide, cadmium oxide or stannous oxide is supplied to the reaction in contaminated form the contaminant either being an oxide of different valency or another substance, separation of the contaminant from the reaction product may be readily effected since the contaminant remains as a solid residue.

Such separation can be effected by the addition of a suitable solvent as, for example, benzene, toluene, xylene, trichloroethylene, perchloroethylene or the like. The metal soap is then dissolved in the solvent but the residue remains in the reaction vessel. The reaction may be carried out with anhydrides of a wide variety of carboxylic acids of more than 6 carbon atoms.

Examples of anhydrides of acids with which the reaction is particularly advantageously carried out are those of the aliphatic saturated and unsaturated carboxylic acids, such as the fatty acids. A particular advantage of the procedure is that the reaction proceeds so smoothly and without requiring any substantial energy expenditure and that, considering the available space or volume of the reaction vessel, a maximum yield of metal soap is obtained.

Further, the reaction product needs no subsequent purification. This, of course, only applies to those instances in which the reactants are used in pure form. A further advantage is that the metal soaps, which are in liquid form at room temperature, can, from the very outset, be prepared with desirable physical characteristics and conditions by suitably choosing the reaction conditions with a view to the subsequent use of the metal soap.

Since the reactions are partly strongly exothermic it is oftentimes advantageous to interrupt the supply of energy to the reaction once the reaction has been initiated or to cool the reaction mixture. The metal soaps which are produced have manifold utilities. They can be used as separating agents, as agents for imparting hydrophobic qualities, as thickeners, catalysts and for many other purposes.

Example 1: 111.6 g. of lead oxide (litharge) and 135.2 g. of 2-ethylhexanoic acid anhydride were heated in a 500 ml. three-neck flask of glass to a temperature of 80°C. The mixture was agitated during the heating. Once the 80°C. temperature had been reached, the inner temperature of the product rose strongly without further extraneous heating, due to the occurrence of an exothermic reaction between the reaction components. The reaction proceeded for about 15 minutes and was thereafter complete. The reaction product is a yellow-brown colored lead octoate. The yield was 246.8 g.

Example 2: 22.3 g. of lead oxide and 55.2 g. of stearic acid anhydride, containing 70% of stearic acid anhydride and 30% of palmitic acid anhydride, were heated in a 250 ml. three-neck flask of glass under stirring for about 30 minutes and to a temperature of about 200°C. After termination of the reaction 77.5 g. of lead stearate were obtained.

Example 3: 22.3 g. of litharge and 54.7 g. of oleic acid anhydride were added to a 250 ml. three-neck flask of glass. Contact of the two reactants resulted in heat evolution. The reaction mixture was then heated for about 2 hours to about 90°C. resulting in the formation of 77 g. of lead oleate.

Example 4: 6.42 g. of cadmium oxide and 19.1 g. of lauric acid anhydride were heated in a 250 ml. three-neck flask of glass under stirring for about 15 minutes and to about 200° to 230°C.

The reaction resulted in the formation of 25.52 g. of cadmium laurate.

Example 5: 76.3 g. of technical grade stannous oxide having an SnO content of 88.1%, and 135.2 g. of 2-ethylhexanoic acid anhydride were heated in a 500 ml. three-neck flask of glass under stirring and in a nitrogen atmosphere. The heating was effected for about 12 hours and to a temperature of about 100°C. Upon termination of the reaction, the unreacted residue which remains in the reaction system can be recognized by the color change from black to light gray.

In order to separate the solid residue from the reaction product, the reaction product, upon finished reaction, was dissolved in a suitable solvent as for example toluene, of which 250 ml. were added to the flask. This resulted in dissolution of the reaction product and the solution was separated from the solid residue in any suitable manner. After removal of the solvent by distillation under vacuum conditions, 200 g. of tin octoate were obtained.

Alkali Metal Salts from Aldehydes

The process developed by R.B. Duke, Jr. and M.A. Perry; U.S. Patent 3,398,166; August 20, 1968; assigned to Eastman Kodak Company is based on the discovery that in certain aldehydes having a hydrogen atom attached to the alpha-carbon atom, atoms are dismutated to the corresponding alcohol and monocarboxylic acid when contacted with an alkali metal hydroxide or alkoxide at a temperature of 40° to 250°C. The method can be represented by the following equations,

$$2H-\underset{R^2}{\overset{R^1}{C}}-CHO + MOH \longrightarrow H-\underset{R^2}{\overset{R^1}{C}}-COOM + H-\underset{R^2}{\overset{R^1}{C}}-CH_2-OH$$

$$2H-\underset{R^2}{\overset{R^1}{C}}-CHO + MOR^3 \longrightarrow H-\underset{R^2}{\overset{R^1}{C}}-COOR^3 + H-\underset{R^2}{\overset{R^1}{C}}-CH_2-OM$$

R^1 and R^2 are straight or branched chain alkyl of 2 to 8 carbon atoms, R^3 is straight or branched alkyl of up to about 8 carbon atoms and M is an alkali metal. Preferably R' is ethyl, R^2 is alkyl of 2 to 4 carbon atoms, R^3 is lower alkyl and M is sodium. The best results are obtained when R^1 is an ethyl group and R^2 is a straight or branched alkyl of 2 to 4 carbon atoms. Examples of suitable aldehydes include 2-ethylbutanal, 2-ethylpentanal, 2-ethylhexanal, 2-ethyloctanal, 2-ethyldecanal, 4-methyl-2-ethylheptenal, and 2-ethylisohexanal.

Example 1: 2-ethylhexanal, 512 g. (4 mols) and 50% sodium hydroxide, 320 g. (4 mols) were weighed into a 3 l., three-necked flask equipped

with a stirrer, thermometer and reflux condenser and subsequently heated
to reflux (125° to 130°C.). Refluxing was continued for 5 hours. The mixture was allowed to come to room temperature and then transferred to a
separatory funnel. Two distinct phases separated. The lower layer (215 g.)
was separated and analyzed and was found to contain 36.9% sodium hydroxide and a trace (<1%) of sodium 2-ethylhexanoate. The upper layer,
containing alcohol and acid salt, was diluted with 2 to 3 volumes of water.

The diluted alcohol-acid salt solution was placed on a continuous organic
decanter and refluxed for 20 hours recovering 255 g. of organic material
which analyzed 95+% 2-ethylhexanol. Only a trace of unreacted aldehyde could be found. The aqueous salt solution (811 g.) was titrated
potentiometrically with standard hydrochloric acid and found to contain
3.7% sodium hydroxide and 40.6% salts as sodium 2-ethylhexanoate. The
yields were 97% to ethylhexanol and 98% to sodium 2-ethylhexanoate.
The aqueous salt solution was cloudy but a simple filtration gave a clear
solution. This solution was light yellow in color.

Example 2: Treated in same manner as described in Example 1, 2-ethyl-
butanal gave an 89% conversion to 2-ethylbutanol and a 91% conversion
to sodium 2-ethylbutanoate.

Example 3: Treated in the same manner as described in Example 1, only
employing potassium hydroxide rather than sodium hydroxide, 2-ethyl-
octanal gave a 92% conversion to 2-ethyloctanol and a 93% conversion to
potassium 2-ethyloctanoate.

Example 4: Treated in the same manner as described in Example 1, only
employing potassium hydroxide rather than sodium hydroxide, 2-ethyliso-
hexanal gave a 93% conversion to 2-ethylisohexanol and a 95% conversion
to potassium 2-ethylisohexanoate.

Salts from Tetravalent Alkoxides and Divalent Metal Carboxylates

In the process of J.H.W. Turner and S.E. Harson; U.S. Patent 3,461,146;
August 12, 1969; assigned to Hardman & Holden Limited, England metal-
organic compounds are prepared by reacting an alkoxide of a tetravalent
element, e.g., silicon, titanium, tin, hafnium and zirconium with a carboxylate of a divalent metal, e.g., a salt of two carboxylic acids having
together from 10 to 28 carbon atoms, or a basic salt.

The resulting compounds contain at least one divalent metal and at least
one tetravalent element, the divalent and tetravalent atoms being linked
together through oxygen atoms and their remaining valencies being occupied by carboxylic acid radicals and hydrocarbonoxy radicals.

Synthesis of Salts and Soaps   275

The compounds of the process can be represented by the following generic formulas:

(1)
$$P-\left(O-\underset{\underset{ODX}{|}}{\overset{\overset{ODX}{|}}{M}}-\right)_n-O-Q$$

(2)
$$P-O-\underset{\underset{OR}{|}}{\overset{\overset{ODX}{|}}{M}}-\left(O-S-O-\underset{\underset{OR}{|}}{\overset{\overset{ODX}{|}}{M}}-\right)_m-O-Q$$

where M is a tetravalent element selected from silicon, titanium, tin, hafnium and zirconium; D is a divalent metal selected from zinc, lead, magnesium, cadmium, calcium, strontium, beryllium, mercury, iron, barium, cobalt and nickel; X is a carboxylic acid radical of up to 24 carbon atoms; R is alkyl up to 12 carbon atoms, aryl or alkaryl up to 16 carbon atoms, or hydrogen; P is R or DX; Q is R or DX; S is D or alkylene up to 10 carbon atoms or diarylenealkyl up to 15 carbon atoms; O is oxygen; n is a whole number from 1 to 10 and m is a whole number from 1 to 10.

The process further comprises condensed products of these compounds, in which a number of atoms of a tetravalent element are linked together through oxygen atoms, or through oxygen-divalent metal-oxygen links, or through residues of di- or polyfunctional hydroxyl compounds, each tetravalent atom being also linked through oxygen atoms to two divalent metal atoms carrying carboxylic acid radicals.

The products may be prepared by the reaction of an alkoxide of a tetravalent element such as silicon, titanium, tin, hafnium, or zirconium with a carboxylic acid salt of a divalent element with the formation of volatile or nonvolatile ester. For example, two molecules of zinc acetate oleate may be reacted with one molecule of tetraethyl orthosilicate with the formation of 2 molecules of ethyl acetate which is distilled off during processing leaving a diluent-free condensate.

$$Si(OEt)_4 + 2\,\underset{\underset{Oleate}{|}}{\overset{\overset{Ac}{|}}{Zn}} \longrightarrow EtO-\underset{\underset{O}{|}\atop Zn\text{-oleate}}{\overset{\overset{Zn\text{-oleate}}{|}\atop O}{Si}}-OEt + 2EtAc$$

The preferred tetravalent element alkoxides are the ethoxides, propoxides or butoxides, but higher alkoxides having up to 12 carbon atoms in the alkyl groups can be used or mixed alkoxides may be formed by the substitution of some of the lower alkoxide groups by a higher alkoxide group. The divalent metal salts used in the processes may be made from one carboxylic acid of up to 24 carbon atoms or from a mixture of carboxylic acids having together from 10 to 28 carbon atoms.

For ease of handling in solvent-free preparations it is preferred to use two carboxylic acids having together about 16 to 18 carbon atoms, but where one of the lower acids C_2 to C_4 (which yield volatile esters) is used it is generally convenient to use it in conjunction with a higher C_8 to C_{24} carboxylic acid. In other cases, as for example with calcium and barium, preparation of the salt may be facilitated by the inclusion of a low boiling solvent which can subsequently be removed by distillation before or during the condensation reaction. Salts of lead, magnesium, cadmium, beryllium mercury, iron, cobalt or nickel may also be used.

The divalent metal salts can generally be prepared from the oxides, hydroxides or carbonates or in some cases from the acetates by replacement of one acetic radical by a higher carboxylic acid. Preferred carboxylic acids are acetic, propionic, isobutyric, natural fatty acids, tall oil fatty acids, naphthenic acids and synthetic liquid or low melting point carboxylic acids, such as Versatic acid which consists principally of tertiary carboxylic acids which are fully saturated and highly branched.

The products prepared according to the processes and equations are obtained as oily liquids, greasy waxy resinous or amorphous solids depending on the choice of organic components and on the degree of condensation. Many of them are soluble in hydrocarbon solvents including mineral lubricating oil and in oxygenated solvents (excluding the lower alcohols and ketones) and in esters and are compatible with various synthetic resins, polymers and elastomers.

They are capable of reacting with acids and for this and other reasons they can be used, for example, as stabilizers for PVC or as lubricants or as lubricant additives. The processes and products are illustrated by the following examples in which T stands for a tallate group.

Example 1: $(TZnO)_2Si(OEt)_2$ — This compound was prepared in two stages. Stage 1 is the preparation of anhydrous zinc acetate tallate and Stage 2 is the reaction of zinc acetate tallate with ethyl orthosilicate. Stage 1 is prepared as follows. 812 g. of tall oil fatty acid were transferred to a 3 necked bolt head flask fitted with a reflux condenser, stirrer and an adaptor for dropping funnel and thermometer. While stirring 228 g. of zinc oxide were added giving a slurry. The temperature was raised to 70°C. and 176 g. of glacial acetic acid were added slowly.

The mixture was then stirred under reflux for 15 minutes. The condenser was changed to the distillation position and water and excess acetic acid was distilled off to a flask temperature of 154°C., applying vacuum in the later stages. A total distillate of 62 ml. was obtained.

Stage 2 is prepared as follows. The zinc acetate tallate in the flask was cooled to 130°C. and 291.4 g. of ethyl orthosilicate were slowly added. The flask temperature was slowly raised to distill off the ethyl acetate produced. 275 ml. of distillate were obtained by slowly raising the flask temperature to 225°C. Product yield is 1,198 g. The product was obtained as an oily liquid soluble in hydrocarbons and in mineral lubricating oil.

Example 2: 613.5 g. of $(TZnO)_2Si(OEt)_2$ prepared as in Example 1 was transferred to a three-necked bolt head flask fitted with a stirrer, reflux condenser and an adaptor for thermometer and dropping funnel. The temperature was raised to 100°C. and 186.5 g. of isooctyl alcohol were added. The product was refluxed at 120°C. for 1 1/2 hours and then the ethyl alcohol produced was distilled off. Distillation was continued to a flask temperature of 225°C. when 78 ml. of distillate had been collected. Product yield 727 g. The product was obtained as a stable low viscosity oily liquid soluble in mineral lubricating oil in all proportions.

Example 3: $(TMgO)_5Si_2(OR)_3$ — 725 g. of tall oil fatty acid were transferred to a three-necked two liter reaction flask and while stirring an addition was made of 240 g. of magnesium carbonate (2 1/2 mols). The mixture was heated and 160 g. of glacial acetic acid were run in during 25 min. The product temperature was raised to 170°C. in 2 hours and 115 cc of water and excess acetic acid distilled off, using vacuum in the final stage. Tetraethyl orthosilicate 208.3 g. were weighed out and slow addition started. The product became viscous and solidified and stirring was stopped.

Heating was continued with distillation of ester and the product softened and liquefied about 190°C. The first ester fraction (100 cc) was found to contain some tetraethyl orthosilicate. It was therefore returned slowly to the product through a separating funnel and ester (ethyl acetate) distilled slowly from a reaction temperature of 180°C. to a reaction temperature of 200°C. which was held for 1 hour. Vacuum was used to assist distillation of the ethyl acetate in the final stages and a distillate of 200 cc was obtained. The final product was a mobile oily liquid at 200°C. but solidified quickly and set to a tough transparent hard solid at room temperature.

Example 4: 580 g. of tall oil fatty acid were transferred to a three-necked stirred reaction flask and an addition made of 192 g. of light industrial magnesium carbonate (2 mols). The mixture was heated and an addition made of 128 g. of glacial acetic acid.

The product was heated and dehydrated to a reaction temperature of 160°C. using vacuum in the final stages of drying. A total of 85 cc of water and excess acetic acid was obtained. Condensed ethyl orthosilicate (Monsanto Silester, SiO_2 content 41.2%) 300 g. was added fairly quickly. The product solidified at 50% addition but softened again on complete addition.

Stirring was stopped and heating continued. The product thinned considerably and became easily stirrable at 205° to 210°C. The temperature was raised to 235°C. in 3 1/2 hours and held at 235° ±5°C. for a further 2 hours when a total distillate of 182 cc was obtained. 200 g. of the product were removed and on cooling yielded a greasy solid which skinned on contact with air.

Example 5: The remainder of the product from Example 4 was cooled to 140°C. and 38.5 cc of water was added rapidly while stirring. Hydrolysis of residual Si—Or groups occurred rapidly and the product solidified. The final product was a hard waxy substance which could be granulated.

Diorganoantimony Compounds Using Carboxylic Acid Salts

J.R. Leebrick and N.L. Remes; U.S. Patent 3,367,954; February 6, 1968; assigned to M & T Chemicals, Inc. provide a process to produce high yields of high purity diorganoantimony carboxylate compounds of the formula $R_2SbOOCR'$ wherein R is selected from the group consisting of alkyl, aryl and alkenyl and R' is hydrocarbon. It comprises mixing together as reactants R_2SbX where in X is halogen having an atomic weight greater than 19, and $M(OOCR')_a$ wherein M is a cation selected from the group consisting of ammonium, alkali metals and alkaline earth metals, and a is the valence of M, in the presence of an inert solvent for at least one of the reactants, thereby forming and recovering the product.

Typically, both R and R' may be selected from the group consisting of alkyl, aryl and alkenyl. Typical alkyls may include methyl, ethyl, n-propyl, isobutyl, tert-butyl, dodecyl, cyclohexyl, etc. Typical aryls may include phenyl, naphthyl, phenanthryl, etc. Typical alkenyls may include vinyl, allyl, 1-propenyl, 2-butenyl, etc. The radicals R and R' may be inertly substituted alkyl, aryl or alkenyl radicals, i.e., chlorophenyl, nitrophenyl, benzyl, tolyl, phenylethyl, ethoxyethyl, methylcyclohexyl, etc.

Preferably, R may be aryl and most preferably it may be phenyl. Preferably R' may be selected from the group consisting of alkyl containing at least 3 carbon atoms, aryl and alkenyl. In the reactant R_2SbX, X may be halogen, e.g., chlorine, bromine and iodine, most preferably chlorine. Typical R_2SbX reactants, which may be employed include diphenylantimony chloride, dibenzylantimony bromide, diallylantimony iodide, as well as dichlorophenylantimony bromide and dicyclohexylantimony chloride, etc., but preferably diphenylantimony chloride. In the reactant $M(OOCR')_a$ wherein R' is independently selected from the same group as R, M is a cation selected from the group consisting of ammonium, alkali metals and alkaline earth metals; and a is the valence of M. Preferably M may be ammonium, sodium or potassium. Typical illustrative $M(OOCR')_a$ reactants may include: ammonium acetate, sodium acetate, potassium caprylate, etc.

The product $R_2SbOOCR'$ may be recovered as a liquid, oil or solid, depending upon the particular reactants and conditions chosen. It may be recovered from the reaction in high yields, typically approaching theoretical yields. The reaction may give product of high purity, which may be further purified, if desired by distillation, recrystallization from an organic solvent such as toluene cyclohexane, etc.

Illustrative products which may be prepared in accordance with this process include: diphenylantimony acetate, butyrate, valerate, linoleate, p-chlorobenzoate, etc. The products prepared by the process have a high degree of biological activity and may be used as bactericides, fungicides, etc. For example, diphenylantimony butyrate may control the growth of such organisms as Staphylococcus aureus, Aerobacter aerogenes, Candida albicans, etc., on a wide variety of substrates.

Example 1: Diphenylantimony acetate, $\phi_2SbOOCCH$ — 233.4 g. (0.75 mol) of diphenylantimony chloride was dissolved in one liter of methanol in a 2 liter beaker and 102 g. (0.75 mol) of sodium acetate trihydrate was added thereto. The resulting slurry was placed on a steam bath and heated for 6 hours. The slurry was filtered hot to remove precipitated sodium chloride (42.5 g., 98%).

The filtrate was cooled whereupon a first crop of diphenylantimony acetate (138 g., MP 130° to 132°C.) was obtained and filtered off. A second crop (112 g.) was obtained by evaporation of the solvent from the filtrate. The combined crops represented a yield of 99.5% of theory. The product was recrystallized from toluene and analyzed. Calculated for $C_{14}H_{13}O_2Sb$: Sb, 36.35%; Acid No. 167.5. Found: Sb, 36.92%; Acid No. 163.

Example 2: Diphenylantimony p-chlorobenzoate, $\phi_2SbOOCC_6H_4Cl$ — A mixture of 15.6 g. (0.05 mol) of diphenylantimony chloride, 8.9 g. (0.05 mol) of sodium p-chlorobenzoate and 250 ml. of water was refluxed with stirring for 30 minutes, after which 50 ml. of methanol was added and refluxing continued for an additional 4 hours. At the end of this time, the resultant slurry was filtered to recover the product, which had precipitated during the reaction. The yield after drying, was 21.5 g. (100% of theory).

The product, as further purified by recrystallization from cyclohexane and isopropyl alcohol, had a melting point of 124° to 126°C. Analysis showed Calculated for $C_{19}H_{14}O_2ClSb$: Sb, 28.22%; Cl, 8.22%. Found: Sb, 28.10%; Cl, 8.35%.

Example 3: Di-n-octylantimony 2-ethylhexanoate, $(C_8H_{17})_2SbOOCC_7H_{15}$
A mixture of 38.4 g. (0.1 mol) of di-n-octylantimony chloride, 16.1 g. (0.1 mol) of ammonium 2-ethyl-hexanoate and 500 ml. benzene may be heated to reflux and refluxed with stirring for 5 hours. At the end of this time, the ammonium chloride which precipitates during the reaction may be removed by filtration and product di-n-octylantimony-2-ethylhexanoate may be recovered in high yield from the filtrate by stripping off benzene under reduced pressure.

PREPARATION OF OTHER DERIVATIVES

ESTERS

Neoalkylpolyol Esters

Neoalkylpolyol esters of mixtures of straight chain fatty acids or branched chain fatty acids which are not neo acids, and neoalkyl fatty acids are prepared by a process which results in a product having superior low temperature properties and oxidation stability. The process comprises partially esterifying a neoalkylpolyol with a mixture of straight chain or branched chain carboxylic acids and a neoalkyl fatty acid, removing unreacted acid from the mixture before the esterification is complete, and adding straight or branched chain fatty acid sufficient to complete the esterification.

T.S. Chao and M. Kjonaas; U.S. Patent 3,562,300; February 9, 1971; assigned to Sinclair Research, Inc. describe the procedure for the preparation of these neoalkylpolyol esters.

This process is concerned with liquid synthetic esters, which are useful, for instance, as base fluids for lubricants, and functional fluids such as plasticizers. Improved low temperature storage stability has important bearing on the use of esters in jet aircraft lubricants and in functional fluids and plasticizers which are subjected to low temperature environments.

In accordance with the process, the esters are prepared by esterifying a neoalkyl polyol of up to 10 or 12 and preferably not more than 7 carbon atoms and 2 to 4 hydroxy groups, such as, for example, pentaerythritol, dipentaerythritol, or 1,1,1-trimethylolalkanes of 5 to 7 carbon atoms with straight chain alkanoic carboxylic acids having from 4 to 12 carbon atoms or branched chain alkanoic carboxylic acids of 4 to 12 carbon atoms other than neo acids and a neo alkanoic acid having preferably 5 to 10 carbons, and the general formula:

$$R_1-\underset{R_3}{\overset{R_2}{C}}-COOH$$

in which R_1, R_2, and R_3 are alkyl groups of 1 to 6 carbon atoms and R_2 and R_3 are preferably 1 to 4 carbons, particularly methyls. Examples of suitable neoalkyl acids are 2,2-dimethylpropanoic, 2,2-dimethylbutanoic, and 2,-dimethyloctanoic acids. The esterification of the neoalkyl polyol with the neo and straight or branched chain acids is carried out using a mol ratio of neoalkyl polyol to straight or branch chain acid to neo acid of 1:1.5 to 2:3 to 8 and is allowed to proceed until 80 to 90% completion as judged from the quantity of water formed. At this point the remaining unreacted acids are removed by distillation, preferably under reduced pressure. Following removal of the unreacted acids, sufficient straight chain alkanoic carboxylic acid of from 4 to 12 carbon atoms is added to complete the esterification.

The esterification is preferably carried out in the presence of an inert gas such as N_2 and at temperatures of 150° to 210°C. and in the presence of a solvent to facilitate mixing during the earlier stages of esterification and to aid water removal via azeotropic distillation. Suitable solvents include xylene, toluene, ethylbenzene and aliphatic hydrocarbons having comparable boiling points.

Purification, if desired, of the reaction mixture can then be accomplished by distillation under vacuum to remove any excess acid, and washing successively with aqueous Na_2CO_3, or other suitable alkali reagents, and water, drying under vacuum, and filtering to give a clear liquid ester.

The reaction is usually carried out in the absence of a catalyst. However, catalysts which do not interfere with the suitability of the finished ester for the intended use can be used. Sulfuric acid, p-toluene sulfonic acid and other sulfur-containing acids are generally avoided in the preparation of esters intended for use as base fluid for synthetic lubricants. These acids can be used, however, if the ester is to be used as a plasticizer and a functional fluid. Other catalysts which may be used include phosphoric acids, organotin compounds, titanium esters, acidic ion exchange resin, acidic clay and crystalline alumino silicates.

The esterification may be carried out using conventional esterification equipment which may consist of a reaction vessel made of materials resistant to organic acids (such as glass or stainless steel), a stirrer, a reflux condenser, and an azeotrope trap.

Example 1: The preparation of pentaerythritol neoheptanoate n-valerate (Ester A) is as follows. A mixture of 272 g. (2.0 mols) of pentaerythritol, 408 g. (4.0 mols) n-valeric acid, 1040 g. (8.0 mols) of neoheptanoic acid and 200 g. of xylene was placed in a 2-liter, 4-necked flask equipped with a mechanical stirrer, a reflux condenser and a Dean-Stark azeotrope trap. The mixture was refluxed at 156° to 178°C., with constant stirring and under the protection of N_2, for a period of 22 hours. During this period a total of 115.5 ml. (80% of theory) of water was collected from the trap. The mixture was distilled under vacuum to remove the unreacted acids, the final temperature and pressure being 175°C. and 1 mm. Hg. To the residue was added 204 g. (2 mols) of n-valeric acid and 200 g. of xylene. Esterification was continued at 173° to 180°C. for another 33 hours during which an additional 28.5 ml. (20% of theory) of water was collected.

The reaction mixture was vacuum distilled to remove remaining acid and then washed twice with 5% Na_2CO_3 solution. The ester was then stirred with 6 g. of $NaBH_4$ and 100 ml. of 0.1 N NaOH at 50° to 60°C. for about 20 hours under a N_2 atmosphere. Upon cooling and settling, the aqueous layer was removed and the ester layer was diluted with xylene and washed twice with water. The washed solution was vacuum distilled and the residue was treated with 50 g. of Attapulgus Fines (a decolorizing clay) for 2 hours at 100° to 110°C. and filtered through Hyflo Super-Cel (A diatomite filter aid). There was obtained about 750 g. of a light yellow clear viscous liquid which will be called Ester A.

Example 2: The preparation of pentaerythritol neopeptanoate n-caproate (Ester B) is as follows. A mixture of 2 mols of pentaerythritol, 4 mols of n-caproic acid, 8 mols of neoheptanoic acid and 200 g. of xylene was similarly refluxed at 160° to 176°C. until 122 ml. (84.6%) of water was collected in the Dean-Stark trap (43 hours). After removal of unreacted acids by vacuum distillation 116 g. (1 mol) of n-caproic acid and 100 g. of xylene were added. Esterification was continued at 175° to 177°C. until no more water was collected (18 hours). The reaction mixture was worked up in the same manner as described in Example 1, yielding 940 g. of light yellow clear liquid which will be called Ester B.

Example 3: The preparation of a liquid pentaerythritol ester (Ester C) from a mixture of neoheptanoic, n-valeric, isovaleric, n-caproic and n-heptanoic acids is as follows. A mixture of 1 mol (136 g.) of pentaerythritol, 3 mols of neoheptanoic acid and 0.5 mol each of n-valeric, isovaleric, n-caproic and n-heptanoic acids was refluxed with 125 g. of xylene in the same manner as described above. After 39.5 hours at 173° to 182°C., a total of 58 ml. (80% of theory) of water was collected in the trap. After removal of the unreacted acids and xylene, 163 g. (1.5 mols) of n-valeric acid and 125 g. of xylene were added and esterification was completed after another 31.5 hours at 171° to 181°C. The reaction mixture was worked up in the same manner as described in Example 1, yielding a light yellow clear liquid which will be referred to as Ester C. The yield before the $NaBH_4$ and clay treatment was 507 g.

Physical Properties of Pentaerythritol Neo-Acid Esters Prepared by Different Methods

Identity	Ester A	Ester B	Ester C
Acids other than neo C_7	n-C_5	n-C_6	n-C_5, i-C_5, n-C_6, n-C_7
Method of preparation	New	New	New
Kinematic vis., c.s.:			
210° F	4.744	4.988	4.854
100° F	25.29	30.14	29.12
0° F	980.4	1,429.0	1,303.1
−40° F	18,325	42,414	27,498
Pour point, °F	−70	−75	−70
Flash point, °F	470	*475	*450
Fire point, °F	520	*540	*540
Appearance after 60 hrs	Clear liquid	Clear liquid	Clear liquid
20° F	do	do	do
0° F	do	do	do
−30° F	do	do	do
−60° F	do	do	do

*Micro-scale

Dehydrogenation of Alcohols

According to A.C. Hecker and M.W. Pollock; U.S. Patent 3,188,330; June 8, 1965; assigned to Argus Chemical Corporation alcohols having one or two labile hydrogen atoms on the carbon atom bearing the hydroxyl group are converted in a one step reaction to ketones or esters, respectively, by reaction in the presence of a salt of an organic acid and a metal of Group IIB of the Periodic Table, preferably, cadmium or zinc. Hydrogen is liberated in the course of the reaction, and a portion of the metal of the catalyst is reduced to the free metal, probably by way of a side reaction with hydrogen, because the major proportion of catalyst is unchanged, and can be reused.

In the case of primary alcohols, the overall reaction proceeds as follows:

$$2RCH_2OH \longrightarrow R\underset{O}{\overset{\|}{C}}OCH_2R + 2H_2$$

Preparation of Other Derivatives

In one mol of the alcohol, the two hydrogens of the carbon bearing the hydroxyl group are replaced by oxygen, and the resulting radical is found attached to another mol of alcohol in the final ester. The reaction can be characterized as a dehydrogenation, due to the loss of two hydrogen atoms from one mol of alcohol, and this is verified by the liberation of hydrogen gas in an amount of roughly one mol per mol of ester produced.

In the case of a secondary alcohol, the reaction proceeds as follows:

$$\underset{R}{RCHOR} \longrightarrow \underset{R}{RC=O} + H_2$$

In this case, a ketone is formed, by direct dehydrogenation.

Esters are obtained from any primary alcohol of the formula RCH_2OH, wherein R is a straight or branched chain alkyl group, or an aryl, alkylaryl, arylalkyl, cycloalkyl or heterocyclic radical. In general, R will contain from one to about fifty carbon atoms, but there is no real upper limit on the size of the molecule, inasmuch as the reaction occurs at the CH_2OH group.

The process is applicable not only to monohydric alcohols but also to polyhydric alcohols, such as the glycols and higher polyhydric alcohols, so that R can contain additional primary hydroxyl groups. If two or more primary alcohol groups are present, a polymeric ester can be formed. Glycols produce a linear polyester having repeating alcohol and acid units. Polyhydric alcohols containing three or more primary alcohol groups such as pentaerythritol and trimethylolpropane, form three dimensional or cage type polymers.

The catalyst employed is a salt of an organic carboxylic acid having from about two to about thirty carbon atoms, and a metal of Group IIB of the Periodic Table, preferably cadmium or zinc. Any organic acid can be employed, and typical salts are the acetates, propionates, butyrates, oxalates, laurates, 2-ethyl hexoates, isooctoates, benzoates, cyclohexanoates, naphthenates, naphthoates, and phthalates of cadmium and zinc.

The reaction will proceed in the presence of a small amount of the salt. As little as 0.25% salt by weight of the reaction mixture is effective.

In carrying out the reaction, the alcohol itself serves as the reaction solvent. If the alcohol is extremely reactive, the reaction will proceed at a satisfactory rate at room temperature.

The time required for the reaction to reach completion will depend upon the alcohol involved, the reaction temperature, and the amount of catalyst.

The reaction conditions are readily adjusted so as to complete the reaction within about one-half to about ten hours.

Example 1: Decanol and 20% by weight of cadmium isooctoate were refluxed at temperatures from the boiling point initially to a final temperature of about 280°C. under a reflux condenser, and the reaction halted when hydrogen gas evolution had ceased. This required about six hours. Analysis of the reaction mixture showed that it was composed of 89.8% decyl decanoate, 4.28% decanal, 2.23% decanoic acid, and 4.5% decene.

Example 2: Benzyl alcohol and 20% by weight cadmium 2-ethyl hexoate were refluxed at temperatures ranging from the boiling point initially up to about 280°C. Hydrogen gas was evolved throughout the reaction. Analysis of the reaction mixture showed that it was composed of 89.6% benzyl benzoate, 1.61% 2-ethyl hexoic acid, 2.08% benzoic acid, and 6.1% benzaldehyde.

Example 3: Cadmium acetate (0.0377 mol) and isooctanol (0.69 mol) were refluxed under a reflux condenser for eight hours. By the end of this time, 0.089 mol of hydrogen gas had been liberated, free cadmium was formed, and the main reaction product was isooctyl isooctoate.

Example 4: A solution of cadmium-2-ethyl hexoate in isooctanol (0.42 equivalent of cadmium, 1.3 mols isooctanol) was refluxed at 157°C. for five hours. At the conclusion of this time, 0.0895 equivalent of cadmium metal was recovered from the reaction mixture, and 0.75 mol of hydrogen gas had been liberated.

Distillation of a 100 gram portion of the reaction mixture gave 44 grams of distillate, corresponding to crude isooctyl isooctoate, boiling at 279°C.

Polymeric Esters

In the process of G.A. Silverstone; U.S. Patent 3,661,956; May 9, 1972; assigned to Victor Wolf Limited, England alkyl esters of dimeric and polymeric fatty acids are produced by heating an alkyl ester of a hydroxy acid in a liquid hydrocarbon solvent which forms an azeotrope with water and in the presence of a dehydration catalyst selected from acid and alkaline clays, inorganic oxides, ion exchange resins and acid sulfates, thereby simultaneously dehydrating and polymerizing the ester.

The polymerized esters are achieved by the production of an ester of the hydroxy acid, particularly ricinoleic acid as the free acid or as castor oil by ester interchange techniques using an alcohol containing from 1 to 8 carbon atoms, for example, methanol and a suitable esterification catalyst after which the esters so produced, are treated with dehydration catalyst.

The dehydration catalyst is a heterogeneous catalyst selected from acid and alkaline clays, inorganic oxides, ion exchange resins and acid sulfates. Examples of suitable catalysts are $NaHSO_4$ and the so-called Surrey Powder. The process is carried out in the presence of an organic liquid hydrocarbon solvent which forms an azeotrope with water, e.g., xylene. A suitable amount of catalyst is from 1 to 30% by weight of the ester. The esters are dehydrated to esters of the corresponding dienoic acid, which in the case of ricinoleic acid is linoleic acid. In the presence of the catalyst, the dienoic acid dimerizes and polymerizes to give a good yield of a polymerized fatty acid ester. The fatty acid ester undergoes scarcely any saponification during the reaction since the water of dehydration is constantly removed from the reaction by the azeotroping solvent.

The reaction is carried out at a temperature within the range of 120° to 300°C., particularly between 150° and 250°C. As water is removed as an azeotrope the boiling point rises and ultimately the liquid refluxes at the boiling point of the solution which is in excess of that of the solvent alone.

The mixture of dimerized, polymerized and unchanged monomeric esters together with the azeotroping solvent, is freed from the catalyst, for example, by filtration or washing, and distilled to remove solvent and monomeric esters. The residue consists mainly of dimerized fatty acid esters, together with some residual monomer and some more highly polymerized esters. The monomeric esters recovered from the reaction are of industrial value and may be used as such or reprocessed to give more polymer. The products may, if desired, be hydrolyzed to the free acids.

Hydroxy acids which may be used in the process are the various dihydroxy carboxylic acids such as 10,12-dihydroxy stearic acid so long as they produce a dienoic acid on dehydration. However, the preferred hydroxy acid is a monohydroxy monounsaturated aliphatic carboxylic acid, such as ricinoleic acid, used either as pure acid or as castor oil.

Example 1: 100 g. of the methyl esters of castor oil fatty acids were stirred in 50 ml. of xylene containing 10 g. of dried Filtrol 13 at a temperature of 180°C. for 1 hour during which the water of reaction was continuously removed as an azeotrope with the boiling xylene which was returned to the reaction. The product was freed from catalyst by filtration and from xylene by distillation after which monomer was stripped from the product by distillation at 0.2 mm. pressure until the kettle temperature was 270°C. The polymerized residue consisted of 48.4% of the product and had a ratio of dimer to more highly polymerized esters of 3.9 (as determined by the method of Paschke et al, J. Am. Oil Chem. Soc., 1954, 31,5).

The acid value (AV) of the polymerized fraction was 7.9 and of the recovered monomer 4.4 and both had zero hydroxyl value (a sample of residue was reesterified to AV of less than 1 prior to analysis for dimer and polymer).

Example 2: This example illustrates the ability to vary dimer/polymer ratio in the product by modification of the technique of mixing the ingredients. If the ester of ricinoleic acid is added to the stirred and refluxing suspension of catalyst in the azeotroping solvent, an improvement in dimer/polymer ratio comes about.

To a stirred suspension of 100 g. of dried Filtrol 13 in 200 ml. of xylene under reflux at 140°C. was added 500 g. of technical methyl ricinoleate over a period of 53 minutes during which the theoretical quantity of water of reaction was removed and the temperature of the mixture rose to 184°C. After a further 5 minutes stirring and refluxing the mixture was cooled, filtered and the filter cake washed with xylene to remove absorbed product. The combined filtrates were distilled first to remove solvent and then at 0.2 mm. pressure until the kettle temperature was 270°C. to remove unreacted monomer. The yield of polymerized ester was 51.8% and contained some monomeric esters and had a dimer to polymer ratio of 5.6. The AV of the residue was 7.1 and of the recovered monomer 3.8.

LACTONES

Oxidation of Ketones

K. Sennewald and H. Rehberg; U.S. Patent 3,483,222; December 9, 1969; assigned to Knapsack Aktiengesellschaft, Germany presents a process for the simultaneous manufacture of aliphatic hydroxycarboxylic acid lactones and of aliphatic or aromatic carboxylic acids by catalytic oxidation of a mixture comprising a cycloaliphatic ketone and an aliphatic or aromatic aldehyde with oxygen or an oxygen-containing gas, in the presence of an iron compound.

The process for the simultaneous manufacture of aliphatic hydroxycarboxylic acid lactones of the general formula:

$$H_2\underset{|}{C}-(CH_2)_n-\underset{|}{C}=O$$
$$\underset{O}{\underline{\qquad\qquad}}$$

in which n stands for a number of 2 to 30, preferably 2 to 10, and of aliphatic or aromatic carboxylic acids of the general formula: R—COOH in which R means hydrogen or an alkyl group having 1 to 30 carbon atoms or means an optionally alkyl-substituted phenyl group, comprises reacting a mixture consisting of (A) a cycloaliphatic ketone of the general formula

$$\underline{CH_2-(CH_2)_n-C}=O$$

in which n has the meaning given above and (B) of an aliphatic or aromatic aldehyde of the general formula: R—CHO in which R has the meaning given above, in a molar ratio of at least 1:1, with an excess of oxygen or an oxygen-containing gas at a temperature of about 0 to 100°C., optionally under pressure and in the presence or absence of an inert solvent. The starting mixture is mixed with a soluble iron compound which serves as a catalyst and is added in a proportion sufficient to obtain an iron concentration of 0.3 to 3 parts by weight per 1 million parts by weight of starting mixture, then completing the reaction and thereafter distilling off resulting ω-hydroxycarboxylic acid lactone and resulting carboxylic acid.

Suitable starting products include, for example: cyclobutanone, cyclopentanone, cycloheptanone or cyclododecanone as the ketone component and include formaldehyde, acetaldehyde, propionaldehyde, or benzaldehyde as the aldehyde component.

It is especially advantageous to use the ketone in a slight molar excess proportion with respect to the aldehyde, preferably 1.1:1 to 3:1. Basically it is possible to oxidize a proportion of ketone equivalent to the proportion of aldehyde present. It would therefore be uneconomic to use a molar ratio greater than 3:1.

The temperatures at which the reaction can be carried out should conveniently be limited to a range of about 30° to 60°C., as the reaction proceeds too reluctantly at lower temperatures, while higher temperatures promote the formation of polymers and undesirable carboxylic acids. The oxidizing reaction can be realized with pure oxygen or an oxygen-containing gas, e.g., air, at atmospheric pressure or under elevated pressure of up to about 10 atmospheres (gauge pressure). All that must be done is to ensure good distribution of the oxygen in the reaction liquid by means of a suitable mechanical device in the reaction vessel.

As the ketone to be oxidized is a relatively costly material, it is advantageous to use the ketone in a proportion not greater than that which corresponds to the absolutely necessary minimum excess with respect to the aldehyde, and to dilute the starting mixture by means of an inert organic solvent, such as ethyl acetate or acetone. When used in an appropriate excess, the ketone itself may serve as a solvent for the other components.

An essential feature comprises using a catalyst for accelerating the oxidizing reaction. Iron compounds soluble in the reaction mixture, such as ferric chloride, ferric acetate or iron acetonyl acetate, have proved especially suitable for this. The catalytic effect obtainable with these compounds is especially favorable for a concentration of about 1 to 3 parts by weight iron per 1 million parts by weight starting mixture.

The reaction of the process takes place more especially in two phases. In the first phase, the catalyst incurs the accelerated formation of a peroxidic compound which produces the lactone in the second phase. The end of the first phase is reached when the starting mixture ceases to absorb oxygen, and the end of the second phase is reached when the reaction mixture no longer includes the peroxidic compound. The presence of any peroxidic compound in the reaction mixture can be detected by adding a potassium iodine solution which results in iodine being separated.

The first process stage comprising peroxide formation is complete when oxygen ceases to be absorbed, whereupon the reaction mixture obtained is conveyed from a first reaction vessel to a second reaction vessel to undergo post-reaction therein. In order to avoid undesirable side-reactions, it is advantageous to stabilize the reaction mixture in the second processing stage by admixture of an agent, such as an ammonium pyrophosphate or a polyphosphate, known to be a stabilizer for percarboxylic acid solutions.

For discontinuous operation, the reaction can be carried out in a single reaction vessel. In this latter case, the reaction mixture is allowed, once oxygen ceases to be absorbed, to stand for some time in the same reaction vessel to undergo post-reaction therein.

Example 1: 210 grams cyclobutanone (3 mols) and 106 grams benzaldehyde (1 mol) were reacted with oxygen in a heatable shaking means at a temperature of 30°C. and under a pressure of 2 atmospheres (gauge pressure) in the presence of $FeCl_3$ as a catalyst. The reaction mixture contained 2 parts by weight iron per 1 million parts by weight. After 8 hours, oxygen ceased to be absorbed. After a further 12 hours, the reaction mixture could not be found when treated with a potassium iodide solution to still include peroxidic oxygen, and the reaction was complete.

Distilling the reaction mixture under a pressure of 10 mm. mercury resulted in 189 grams cyclobutanone, 18.5 grams γ-butyrolactone boiling at a temperature of 78° to 83°C., and 122 grams benzoic acid. For a 20% cyclobutanone conversion rate, the yield of γ-butyrolactone was 72%, related to the quantity of ketone transformed. For further identifying the γ-butyrolactone, the hydrazide was prepared which melted at 89°C.

Example 2: A stainless steel flow reactor in upright position and having a capacity of 5 liters was charged per hour with 9 kg. of a solution of 15% acetaldehyde in cyclohexanone and oxygen was introduced concurrently therewith through a gas distributing plate in a proportion such as absorbed by the reaction solution, a pressure of 4.5 atmospheres (gauge pressure) being maintained. The temperature prevailing in the reactor was maintained at 47°C. by cooling. The reaction solution was continuously removed from the reactor as its upper end and introduced into a container having a capacity of 100 liters to undergo post-reaction therein. The reaction solution leaving the post-reactor was free from peroxides and was continuously distilled. 1.84 kg. acetic acid, 6.18 kg. cyclohexanone, 1.54 kg. monomeric ε-caprolactone and 0.17 kg. distillation sump were obtained per hour. Monomeric lactone was obtained in a yield of 90% related to the cyclohexanone conversion rate. There were also obtained 8% polymeric lactone in the sump phase of the distilling means.

ANHYDRIDES

Symmetrical Anhydrides of Hydroxy Acids

It is known in the art that certain acids may be converted into their symmetrical anhydrides by reacting (1) a tertiary amine salt of the acid with (2) a mixed (carboxylic-carbonic) anhydride of the same acid. A typical synthesis in this field (Shipper and Nichols, Jour. Am. Chem. Soc., 80, pp. 5714 to 5717) involves preparation of symmetrical oleic anhydride by reaction of (1) the triethylamine salt of oleic acid with (2) a mixed oleic-carbonic anhydride of the formula

$$CH_3-(CH_2)_7-CH=CH-(CH_2)_7-\overset{O}{\underset{\|}{C}}-O-\overset{O}{\underset{\|}{C}}-OC_4H_9$$

prepared by reacting oleic acid triethylamine salt with isobutyl chloroformate.

T.H. Applewhite and J.S. Nelson; U.S. Patent 3,247,231; April 19, 1966; assigned to U.S. Secretary of Agriculture describe the products and the preparation of symmetrical anhydrides of hydroxy aliphatic carboxylic acids containing at least eight carbon atoms. Depending on the acid from which they are derived, the products may be saturated or unsaturated and may contain two or more hydroxy groups per molecule.

Among the preferred compounds of the process are symmetrical anhydrides derived from the C_{18} hydroxy fatty acids, saturated or unsaturated, typically the mono- or polyhydroxy substituted stearic, oleic, or linoleic acids.

The products of the process are generally solid materials, crystalline in a pure state, and are stable when stored at room temperature or below. When heated at temperatures well above their melting points they are slowly decomposed, giving polymeric esters and an acidic material of unknown composition. The compounds are eminently useful as starting materials for the preparation of esters and amides by application of conventional syntheses. Typically the amides, especially the morpholides, are useful as plasticizers for vinyl chloride, vinyl acetate copolymers, and cellulose acetate.

The compounds are prepared by reacting (1) a tertiary amine salt of the selected hydroxy acid with (2) a mixed (carboxylic-carbonic) anhydride of the same hydroxy acid. The reaction is generally carried out at ordinary (room) temperature for convenience, however, lower or higher temperatures can be used if desired. For example, the reaction temperature may be as low as about minus 10°C., although it is obvious that at such temperatures the reaction rate will decrease and it may require more solvent to keep the reactants in solution. Generally, temperatures over about 40°C. should be avoided to prevent decomposition of the mixed anhydride or the product. The reactants are generally employed in the equimolar proportions as involved in the reaction, i.e., one mol salt plus one mol mixed anhydride yields essentially one mol of symmetrical anhydride product. To promote good contact between the reactants the reaction is carried out in a conventional inert solvent, for example, tetrahydrofuran, benzene, toluene, xylene, etc.

After the reaction is completed the products may be recovered in various different ways. A suitable plan involves evaporation under vacuum of the solvent from the reaction mixture followed by extraction of the residue with a solvent such as ether or chloroform. The resulting solution is washed with dilute acid, dilute base, then with water. After this solution is dried over a desiccant the solvent is evaporated, leaving the pure symmetrical anhydride.

The course of the synthesis in accordance with the process is shown by the following equation:

$$CH_3-R-COOH \cdot Z \quad \text{(Tertiary amine salt of hydroxy acid)} \; +$$
$$\underset{(OH)_a}{|}$$

$$CH_3-R-\overset{O}{\underset{|}{\underset{(OH)_a}{C}}}-O-\overset{O}{\overset{\|}{C}}-OR' \quad \text{(Mixed anhydride of hydroxy acid and carbonic acid half-esterified with lower alkanol)} \longrightarrow$$

$$\left[CH_3-R-\overset{O}{\underset{|}{\underset{(OH)_a}{\overset{\|}{C}}}}- \right]_2 O + CO_2 + R'OH + Z$$

Symmetrical anhydride (product)

In the above formulas, R stands for an aliphatic hydrocarbon chain containing at least 7 carbon atoms, R' is a lower alkyl radical, Z is a tertiary amine, and n is an integer from 1 to 4.

A consideration of the above equation demonstrates the unexpected nature of the particular process. Thus it would be expected that the mixed anhydride would react with the hydroxy (alcohol) group on the tertiary amine salt, forming an ester. Such reaction does not, in fact, occur and the desired symmetrical anhydrides are produced in high, virtually quantitative, yields.

Example: (A) Preparation of Mixed Anhydride — A solution containing triethylamine (1.53 ml., 0.011 mol) and 12-hydroxy-cis-9-octadecenoic acid (3.3 g., 0.011 mol) in 100 ml. tetrahydrofuran was cooled to minus 5°C. and ethyl chloroformate (1.05 ml., 0.011 mol) was added slowly while maintaining the temperature below 0°C. The mixture was held at about 0°C. with stirring for 20 minutes. This product contained the mixed carboxylic-carbonic anhydride,

$$CH_3(CH_2)_5-\underset{\underset{OH}{|}}{CH}-CH_2-CH=CH-(CH_2)_7-\underset{\underset{O}{\|}}{C}-O-\underset{\underset{O}{\|}}{C}-OC_2H_5$$

plus by-product triethylamine hydrochloride.

(B) Production of Symmetrical Anhydride — Triethylamine (0.011 mol) and 12-hydroxy-cis-9-octadecenoic acid (0.011 mol) were dissolved in 50 ml. of tetrahydrofuran. This solution was added from a dropping funnel into the product of part A above, while stirring and maintaining the temperature at or near 0°C. with an ice-salt bath. Following the addition, the system was allowed to come to room temperature with stirring and let stand overnight.

The solution was then filtered to remove precipitated triethylamine hydrochloride and the precipitate washed with additional tetrahydrofuran. The filtrate and washings were combined and the solvent removed in vacuo at room temperature on a rotary evaporator. The product was taken up in ether or chloroform and the resulting solution washed with dilute hydrochloric acid, 1 M sodium carbonate, followed by water until the washes tested neutral to pH paper. The organic solution was dried over $MgSO_4$, filtered, and returned to the rotary evaporator for removal of solvent at room temperature. The product, symmetrical 12-hydroxy-cis-9-octadecenoic anhydride, is shown on the following page. It was obtained in 95% yield.

$$\left[CH_3-(CH_2)_5-\underset{OH}{CH}-CH_2-CH=CH-(CH_2)_7-\underset{O}{\overset{\parallel}{C}}-O \right]_2$$

KETO ACIDS

From Dicarboxylic Dihalides and Organic Aluminum Halides

γ-Keto acids are useful in the fat industry as raw material for the production of taste-forming γ-hydroxy fatty acid-lactones.

These compounds are also valuable as surface active agents and find particular application as starting products in the wetting agent and washing agent industries.

γ-Keto acids of various structures are also necessary in the plastics industry.

H. Reinheckel, K. Haage, and R. Gensike; U.S. Patent 3,412,116; November 19, 1968; assigned to Deutsche Akademie der Wissenschaften zu Berlin, Germany describe γ-keto acids which are prepared by reacting dicarboxylic dihalides with organic aluminum chlorides or bromides in solutions in partially halogenated hydrocarbons at temperatures of +20° to -50°C. and hydrolyzing the product of this reaction.

The process comprises the preparation of a γ-keto acid of the formula:

$$R-CO-\underset{Y}{\overset{U}{C}}-\underset{Z}{\overset{W}{C}}-COOH$$

wherein R is an aliphatic, araliphatic, cycloaliphatic or aromatic radical and wherein U, W, Y and Z are each independently selected from the group consisting of hydrogen, aliphatic radicals, arylaliphatic radicals, cycloaliphatic radicals and aromatic radicals, and U, W, Y and Z together with the carbon atoms to which the same are attached are selected from the group consisting of homocyclic and heterocyclic ring systems, by reacting dicarboxylic dihalides of the formula:

$$X-CO-\underset{Y}{\overset{U}{C}}-\underset{Z}{\overset{W}{C}}-CO-X$$

wherein U, W, Y and Z represent the same groups as above and X stands for halogen in the presence or absence of solvents with alkylaluminum compounds of the formula: R_nAlX_{3-n} wherein R and X have the same meaning as above and wherein n is 1 to 3.

Example 1: Production of γ-Ketocaproic Acid — 49.5 g. of aluminumethyl sesquichloride (0.4 mol) dissolved in 70 g. of methylene chloride are added slowly under vigorous stirring at -30°C. to -25°C. to 77.5 g. of succinic acid dichloride (0.5 mol) in 250 g. of methylene chloride so that the heat of reaction is carried off by cooling from the outside. After bringing the reaction components together, the abovementioned temperature is maintained for an additional 3 hours while stirring.

Up to the beginning of the hydrolysis the reaction must be carried out under the strict exclusion of air and moisture, and this is accomplished by the passing of a dry inert gas (pure nitrogen) over the reaction mixture.

The reaction product is, for hydrolysis purposes, added under stirring to 200 g. of approximately 15% sulfuric acid at a temperature of -20°C., whereby as a result of careful cooling care is taken that the temperature of the hydrolysis mixture during the introduction does not increase to above -10°C. The mixture is then permitted to warm to room temperature and the organic phase (reaction product plus methylene chloride) is subsequently separated from the aqueous phase after the addition of 100 g. of ether. The aqueous phase is extracted with ether. The total yield is 59 g. of γ-keto caproic acid (equivalent to 90.8% of the theoretical): BP at 15 mm. Hg is 145° to 147°C.; MP is 35° to 37°C.

Example 2: Production of α,β-Dimethyl-γ-Phenyl-γ-Ketobutyric Acid — 97 g. of phenylaluminum sesquibromide (0.37 mol) dissolved in 100 g. of methylene chloride are slowly added under vigorous stirring at a temperature of -20°C. to -15°C. to 91.5 g. of α,α'-dimethyl succinic acid dichloride (0.5 mol) in 250 g. of methylene chloride. The working up of the reaction product proceeds as in Example 1, however in order to complete the hydrolysis of the formed ketocarboxylic acid chloride the separated organic phase is vigorously stirred with pure water for an additional 3 hours. The aqueous phase is then again extracted with ether. The yield is 87 g. of α,β-dimethyl-γ-phenyl-γ-ketobutyric acid, which is equivalent to 84.2% of the theoretical.

Example 3: This example describes the production of a mixture of aliphatic-γ-keto fatty acids from the product of ethylene addition onto aluminum trialkyl. 233 g. of succinic acid dichloride (1.5 mol) are added to 134 g. of water-free aluminum chloride (1.0 mol) in 750 g. of methylene chloride and to this mixture is added slowly under stirring at -15°C., 280 g. of a product of ethylene addition on aluminum triethyl with an average chain length of C_{10}, which product contains, besides hydrocarbons, 80% by weight of pure aluminum alkyl compound. The addition is dropwise. The further working up of the reaction product proceeds in analogy to Example 1. The yield is 254 g. (= to 73.3% of the theoretical) of a mixture of γ-keto fatty acids ($C_{2n}H_{4n-2}O_3$), wherein n is an integer greater than 2 and statistically averages 7. The reaction product is subjected to pressure hydrogenation with Raney nickel at 100 atmospheres pressure at 165°C. to provide a 90% yield of a mixture of γ-hydroxy fatty acid lactones.

HALO ACIDS

Halooxidation of Aldehydes

Alpha-haloaliphatic acids can be prepared directly by halooxidation of enolizable aldehydes in a one-step process by contacting the aldehyde with a halide in an aqueous medium and the absence of light.

Particularly the alpha-chloroaliphatic acids are useful intermediates for the preparation of numerous useful end products. These haloacids are readily esterified, and the esters can be subjected to dehydrohalogenation to form monomers which polymerize and find use as lube oil viscosity improvers. The most widely used haloacid is the alpha-chloroisobutyric acid.

P.H. Washecheck; U.S. Patent 3,661,986; May 9, 1972; assigned to Continental Oil Company describes the process with particular reference to the preparation of the alpha-chloroisobutyric acid.

The aldehydes to which this process is applicable are enolizable aliphatic saturated aldehydes, e.g., having at least one hydrogen in the alpha position, and therefore must contain at least two carbon atoms. Preferably the maximum number of carbon atoms will be about twenty carbon atoms; however, the only upper limit is the availability of the aldehyde. The normal aldehydes are useful for production of useful alcohols; e.g., n-butyraldehyde is used in the production of 2-ethyl hexanol; however, the isobutyraldehyde, when reduced to isobutyl alcohol, is useful only as a solvent or other low value use. On the other hand, if such isobutyraldehyde were converted to methacrylate derivatives, the value would be greatly increased.

The temperature and pressure can vary over a wide range; however, atmospheric or only slight pressure will ordinarily be employed. Heat favors the yield of chloroacids up to about 65°C.; thus, a temperature in the range of 45° to 65°C. is preferred. The chlorooxidation of the saturated aldehyde can be carried out as a one-step or a two-step process. In general, increased acidity results in an increase in the selectivity of chlorination in the alpha position; however, acid appears to adversely effect the oxidation portion of the reaction.

Thus, the reaction can be carried out as a one-step process in which the acidity is chosen to balance the advantage of acidity in the chlorination reaction and the disadvantage of the acidity in the oxidation reaction. The reaction can also be carried out as a two-step process in which the acid used to an advantage in the chlorination portion of the reaction is diluted to minimize the disadvantage of acidity in the oxidation portion.

The process can also be operated in a third manner which is similar to the two-step process. The α-haloaldehyde can be prepared separately by some other method of the prior art. In this case, the chlorination portion of the reaction has already been accomplished and no acid is then required. Thus, the oxidation can be simply accomplished in an aqueous medium with no acid present. With no acid present the oxidation occurs in very high selectivity. In all three of the above cases, the exclusion of light is an essential part of the process.

METAL-CONTAINING DERIVATIVES

Magnesium Oxide Adducts

R.A. Patton; U.S. Patent 3,362,970; January 9, 1968; assigned to Morton International, Inc. describes magnesium oxide compositions and more specifically, organically modified magnesias, and methods of producing them.

The compositions have utility as reinforcing fillers for elastomeric products, particularly synthetic elastomers such as neoprene and the like; as readily dispersible turbine hydrocarbon fuel oil additives which furnish MgO to combine with vanadic oxide formed in the fuel combustion process to form infusible vanadium compounds (magnesium vanadates) and thereby reduce corrosion of the turbine alloy parts; and as ingredients of metal working and metal drawing compositions.

It has been found as an unexpected phenomenon that many of the lightly calcined magnesias of commerce have unusual properties which are not common to the hard calcined periclase or the starting materials from which magnesias are prepared, namely, the hydroxide or the carbonate. One characteristic of these lightly calcined magnesias is the ability to adsorb iodine. The compositions of the process are prepared by reacting a lightly calcined magnesium oxide having an iodine adsorption number of from 10 to 300, preferably 15 to 200, with a fatty acid selected from the group consisting of monobasic fatty acids containing up to 26 carbon atoms, dimerized unsaturated C_{18} fatty acids, trimerized unsaturated C_{18} fatty acids, such as oleic, linoleic, linolenic, licanic and ricinoleic acids, and mixtures thereof.

Dimerization results in a dibasic 36 carbon atom acid and trimerization results in a tribasic 54 carbon atom acid. Ordinarily the dimerization and trimerization results in mixtures of monomeric C_{18} unsaturated acid, as well as the dimer and trimer.

The monobasic fatty acids which are operative in the process are: butyric acid, isovaleric acid, caproic acid, caprylic acid, capric acid, lauric acid, myristic acid, palmitic acid, stearic acid, arachidic acid, behenic acid, lignoceric acid, and cerotic acid. In addition, unsaturated monobasic fatty acids, as exemplified by oleic acid, are operative.

The mixtures of dibasic and tribasic fatty acid reactants referred to above are known commercially as "dimer" and "trimer" acids. Dimer acids which may be employed in this process, contain from 75 to 95% by weight of dibasic acids containing 36 carbon atoms, and from about 4 to 25% by weight of tribasic acids containing 54 carbon atoms, and up to 3% by weight of monobasic 18 carbon atom acids. The trimer acids consist essentially of approximately 90% by weight of tribasic acids containing 54 carbon atoms and approximately 10% by weight of dibasic acids containing 36 carbon atoms.

The products of the process may be prepared by reacting a lightly calcined magnesia with a fatty acid in an inert organic solvent selected from the group consisting of aromatic hydrocarbons, aliphatic hydrocarbons and chlorinated hydrocarbons. The temperature ranges from ambient to the reflux temperature of the particular solvent employed. The reaction may be carried out by admixing the reactants at ambient temperature in an inert solvent such as benzene, toluene, petroleum ether or trichloroethylene, and thereafter separating the product from the solvent.

Alternately, the reaction may be effected by dissolving the fatty acid in the solvent, adding magnesia and refluxing the admixture for from 1 to 3 hours, filtering and drying the solid product. The quantity of solvent used is not critical as the solvent does not enter into the reaction and merely serves as a convenient medium for the reaction. Generally, in the procedure in which the admixture is refluxed, approximately 500 to 700 cc. of solvent are adequate for about 100 to 200 grams of reactants. The time of reaction is not critical and times of about one-half hour to about twenty-four hours or more may be used depending upon the mode of reaction. In those instances where the magnesia and fatty acid are reacted under reflux conditions, the course of the reaction may be followed by the evolution of water, the end of the reaction being indicated by the cessation of water evolution. The water produced in the reaction may be collected and measured in a Dean-Stark trap or similar apparatus.

When the reaction is complete, the reaction product is removed by filtration and washed with a volatile solvent to remove any excess organic reactant. Solvents for washing may be any inert material substantially of the same type as are used for the reaction medium. After washing, the filter cake is dried, preferably at temperatures of from between about 65° and 100°C. and pulverized into a powder. Alternately, the reaction product may be freed of its solvent by a vacuum technique followed by subsequent drying and pulverization. The adducts have an organic content of from about 1 to 25% by weight.

Example 1: Into a 3-liter, 3-necked flask, equipped with a thermometer, stirrer and reflux condenser with attached Dean-Stark trap, are placed 550 milliliters of dry toluene solvent and 25 grams of caproic acid. To this are added 100 grams of magnesium oxide having an iodine adsorption number of 128. This reaction mixture is then refluxed at a temperature of 110° to 112°C. for a period of approximately 1 1/2 hours. At the end of this time, the solvent is removed by vacuum and the product dried overnight at a temperature of from 70° to 80°C. to constant weight. This procedure yields a caproic acid-magnesia adduct weighing approximately 123.7 grams and having an organic content of 17.7% by weight. The following examples illustrate the production of similar products by the method of Example 1 using various fatty acids:

Example	Magnesium Oxide Amount (grams)	Iodine Number	Fatty Acid	Amount (grams)	Product (grams)	Solvent	Solvent Removal	Weight Percent Organic in Product
2	100	128	Caprylic	25	123.2	Toluene	Vacuum	19.6
3	100	128	Capric	25	123.4	Toluene	Vacuum	20.0
4	115	119	Lauric	25	139.3	Trichloroethylene	Vacuum	17.9
5	100	128	Palmitic	25	123.8	Toluene	Vacuum	21.4
6	115	114	Stearic	20.3	133.4	Trichloroethylene	Vacuum	15.2
7	230	119	Oleic	50	278.6	Trichloroethylene	Vacuum	17.9

Example 8: Into a 3-liter, 3-necked flask, equipped with a thermometer, stirrer and reflux condenser with attached Dean-Stark trap, are placed 500 milliliters of dry toluene solvent and 50 grams of a dimer acid hereinbefore described and sold under the tradename of Empol 1018. To this are added 230 grams of magnesium oxide having an iodine adsorption number of 100. This reaction mixture is then refluxed at a temperature of from about 110°C. to about 115°C. for approximately 2 to 3 hours. At the end of this time, the mass is cooled, filtered, washed and dried to constant

weight at a temperature of from about 70° to about 80°C. This procedure yields a magnesium oxide dimer acid adduct having an organic content of about 18.2% by weight. The following examples illustrate the production of various other dimer and trimer adducts of magnesium oxide by the process of Example 8:

Example	Magnesium Oxide Amount (grams)	Iodine Number	Fatty Acid	Amount (grams)	Percent by Weight of Organic Component in Product
9	230	107	Dimer acid*	41.5	15.4
10	340	116	Dimer acid**	75.0	17.8
11	258	119	Dimer acid**	57.2	17.8
12	230	116	Trimer acid***	50.0	18.0

*Empol 1014   **Empol 1022   ***Emery 3162-D

As hydrocarbon fuel oil additives, these compositions have the capability of reducing corrosion of turbine alloy parts with which fuel oil comes into contact. Fuel oils typically contain approximately 200 to 500 parts per million of vanadium which is converted to vanadic oxide (V_2O_5) upon combustion. This oxide is fusible at the temperatures generally attained within a gas turbine or boiler. Impingement of the fused vanadic oxide on the turbine blades or boiler tubes leads to spot solution of the metal by the molten oxide with subsequent deterioration of the equipment. In addition, these fuels also contain appreciable amounts of sulfur which is oxidized in the combustion process to acidic gases having corrosive properties.

Incorporation of magnesia in the fuel oil provides a reagent which combines with or scavenges the vanadic oxide to produce harmless magnesium vanadate which is readily conveyed out of the combustion chamber by the fuel gases. If excess magnesia is incorporated, it serves to render harmless the acidic sulfur oxides by combination therewith to form magnesium sulfate. For example, 7.5 grams of a stearic acid-magnesium oxide adduct, prepared as described in Example 6, is added to 742.5 grams of carbon tetrachloride.

This forms a suspension which is stable for from 3 to 5 weeks and which may be incorporated into a fuel oil which normally contains a few hundred parts per million of vanadium with the end result that the adduct effectively inactivates the vanadium and thereby alleviates the corrosion problem. Unmodified magnesium oxide settles rapidly when added to carbon tetrachloride.

Werner Complexes of Chromium and Fatty Acids

J.W. Trebilcock; U.S. Patent 3,375,263; March 26, 1968; assigned to E.I. du Pont de Nemours and Company describes Werner complexes of trivalent nuclear chromium atoms coordinated with omega(ethenyl carboxy)-aliphatic carboxylic acids such as methacryloxyundecanoic acid. These are prepared by bringing together a water-soluble chromium salt such as basic chromic chloride, an alcohol such as isopropanol, and an omega(ethenyl carboxy)aliphatic carboxylic acid and heating the mixture at reflux for about 15 minutes.

The Werner complexes are useful as glass-treating agents in the preparation of glass fiber-plastic laminates. It has been found that an improvement is obtained in wet strength of glass fiber-plastic laminates when the glass fibers have been treated with the chromium complex.

The carboxylic acids of the process can be prepared generally by the reaction of a hydroxy carboxylic acid with an anhydride or acid chloride of acrylic or methacrylic acid as shown in U.S. Patent 2,141,546. They can also be prepared generally by the reaction of an acrylate or methacrylate alkali-metal salt and an omega-halo alkanoic acid as shown in the examples. The most preferred acid is methacryloxyundecanoic acid, because of the particularly high wet and dry strengths exhibited by glass laminates made using the Werner type chromium complex prepared with this acid. The molar ratio of chromium to acid in the complexes varies generally from about 1:1 to 5:1, although complexes having ratios outside of this range can be prepared with some decrease in effective properties. The molar ratio is preferably from 2:1 to 3:1.

The salt of the basic chromium ion can be any salt of such metal ionizable in aqueous solution, such as the chlorides, bromides, chlorates, iodides, nitrates, acetates, formates and the like. For convenience and economy, the chloride salts are generally preferred. The water content of the basic chromium salt solution can vary from substantially anhydrous to large amounts of water. The water content of the chromium complex of the carboxylic acid will therefore range from very small amounts of water to substantial amounts of water, usually from 3 to 30%. The reaction of the acid with the basic chromium salt can be carried out in any medium in which the reactants are mutually soluble, preferably an organic solvent, such as ethanol, n-propanol, isopropanol or butanol. Isopropanol is the most preferred solvent.

Aqueous solutions or dispersions of the chromium complexes are best obtained by adding an alcoholic solution of the complex to water. The alcoholic solution and the water are thoroughly mixed. The alcoholic solution can be prepared directly or by dissolving the solid complex in the alcohol. The pH of aqueous solutions of the chromium carboxylic acid complexes, which normally contain at least 0.5% of an alcohol arising from the alcohol in which the complex is dissolved, can be adjusted if and as desired by the addition of a dilute alkali such as amines, ammonia or various inorganic bases. A 1% solution of ammonia works quite well to obtain a pH of from about 2.6 to 6.0. The reaction is generally complete after the reactants have remained in contact with each other for a period of about twenty-four hours at a temperature of about 20°C. At a temperature of about 100°C., the complex is formed in about twenty minutes or less.

Example: To prepare the chrome complex 64.0 grams of basic chromic chloride solution containing 7.88% Cr are prepared according to the procedure described in U.S. Patent 2,683,156 and are dissolved in 19.0 g. of isopropanol. 7.0 g. of methacryloxyacetic acid are added to the basic chromic chloride solution. The reactants then are heated to reflux for 15 minutes and allowed to cool. The resulting solution contains a chrome complex of methacryloxyacetic acid with a 2/1 Cr/acid mol ratio and 5.6% Cr.

A treating solution is prepared by diluting 40 grams of the chrome complex solution made above with 1,960 ml. of water with agitation and adjusting the pH to 6.0 with a 1% aqueous ammonia solution. Pieces of heat-cleaned 181-style glass cloth are then immersed in the treating solution for a period of 1 minute. The glass fabric is then passed through a rubber rolled hand wringer and dried in an oven at 125°C. for 10 minutes. After the fabric is removed from the oven it is allowed to cool and then is washed in 1,500 ml. of distilled water and redried at 125°C. for 10 minutes.

A laminate is prepared from the treated glass cloth by impregnating pieces of the cloth with a polyester resin, such as Paraplex-P-43, containing 1% benzoyl peroxide as a curing catalyst. A sandwich containing 12 layers of glass fabric and approximately 60% glass is formed and cured under a pressure of 90 psi in a press at 175°F. for 15 minutes, 225°F. for 20 minutes, and 275°F. for 20 minutes. The laminate is then allowed to cool and is removed from the press and cut into flexural strength samples. The samples, as shown by standard testing procedure Federal Specification L-P-406a, exhibit high flexural strength before and after boiling in water for two hours.

PURIFICATION AND SEPARATION

PURIFICATION PROCESSES

Using Acid Activated Crystalline Clay

The object of a process described by B.L. Hampton; U.S. Patent 3,052,701; September 4, 1962; assigned to The Glidden Company is to improve the color and heat-stability of distilled tall oil fatty acids. The procedure used to attain this objective was to heat 500 grams of the fatty acids to the desired temperatures in a 1 liter, 3 neck round bottom flask fitted with a stirrer, a thermometer and a nitrogen gas inlet tube. The desired amount of clay was then added all at once and the mixture stirred vigorously for the desired time.

The clay was then removed by filtration using a Büchner funnel at a temperature not greater than around 90°C. The filtrate was then distilled at 1 to 3 mm. absolute pressure (a range of from 1 to 25 mm. can be used) with no fractionation. To insure removal of most of the volatile acids a flame was played over the top of the flask toward the end of the distillation.

Example: The table below records an experiment on a relatively fresh sample of a fatty acid, that is the sample was only 24 hours old when used after taking from a regular plant sampling connection. This sample had the specification color of 5 to 6 (Gardner). The Gardner color was 8 to 9 after a heat test in which the fatty acids were added to a 1" x 8" test tube and immersed in an oil bath at 205°C. The level of the acids is adjusted to the level of the oil bath. Remove from the bath after one hour, cool, fill a Gardner color tube and read the color on a Gardner Comparator (1933 varnish scale).

The sample was treated with 2% of an acid-activated crystalline clay for the specified time at 90°C.

Time, minutes	Color After Filtering	Color After Heat Test on Filtrate	Color of Distillate	Color After Heat Test on Distillate
5	2 to 3	7	2 to 3	4
10	2 to 3	7	2 to 3	4
20	2 to 3	7 to 8	1 to 2	3 to 4
30	2 to 3	7 to 8	1 to 2	3 to 4
45	2 to 3	8 to 9	1 to 2	3 to 4

Good initial color is had rather quickly, but there is some improvement by allowing the reaction to continue. It will be noted that the heat-stability appears to be poorer after the longer period of heating, but the distilled product is superior to the product obtained after the shorter period. By distillation alone, without clay, the color of the tall oil fatty acid is improved very little, color 5 to 6.

Using Organic Aldehyde and Acidic Crystalline Clay

B.L. Hampton; U.S. Patent 3,066,160; November 27, 1962; assigned to The Glidden Company has developed an improved tall oil fatty acid product which yields, upon epoxidation or upon use in alkyds, a product of improved color. This can be accomplished by a process which comprises heating a tall oil fatty acid in the presence of an acidic crystalline clay mineral and an organic aldehyde under conditions of agitation and thereafter recovering the thus-treated fatty acids from the treated mixture. The treated fatty acids can then be distilled for use in epoxidation reaction and in the plasticizer or alkyd field.

Examples: The procedure used was to heat 500 grams of the fatty acids to the desired temperature in a 1 liter, 3 neck round bottom flask fitted with a stirrer, a thermometer and a nitrogen inlet tube. In all examples the fatty acids were covered with nitrogen. The desired amount of clay and paraformaldehyde was added and the reaction mass stirred vigorously for the desired time. The clay was then removed by filtering using a Büchner funnel at a temperature not greater than around 90°C. The filtrate was then distilled at 1 to 2 mm. Hg absolute with no fractionation.

The distillation step greatly improves the product and the color of the epoxidized solution is greatly improved over that of a tall oil fatty acid which has been similarly treated but not distilled. For example, in a typical experiment the color of the original tall oil fatty acid was 5 to 6 Gardner.

The color of the product after treating and filtering out the clay but not distilling was 5 to 6. The color of the epoxidized solution was 6 to 7 with no red versus a 14 and deep red for an untreated but epoxidized tall oil fatty acid. On distilling the filtrate of the treated tall oil fatty acid the color of the distillate was 2 to 3 and the epoxidized solution was also 2 to 3. Thus in these examples it was found that (a) an untreated tall oil fatty acid, that is, a commercial fatty acid of color 5 to 6 Gardner if epoxidized, yields a product of 14 Gardner color and deep red; (b) a similar fatty acid treated with clay and an aldehyde but not distilled, yields on epoxidation a 6 to 7 Gardner color product and no red color; (c) a similar fatty acid treated with clay and an aldehyde, recovered and distilled, yields on epoxidation a 2 to 3 Gardner color and almost water white.

Thus, by this process ordinary commercial fatty acids can be treated with clay and an aldehyde and a product suitable for use in many fields can be obtained. If a high quality product is desired, the treated fatty acids can be further distilled under a good vacuum. A simple method for epoxidizing the treated tall oil fatty acids is as follows: to 266 grams of glacial acetic acid there is added 38 grams of 90% hydrogen peroxide and 3 grams of reagent grade sulfuric acid. This mixture is then allowed to stand at 24° to 28°C. until ready for use [Analytical Chemistry, 20, 1061 (1948)].

In testing tall oil fatty acids with this epoxidizing solution, 5 ml. of the treated acids are treated with 5 ml. of the peracetic acid solution prepared above and the solution is then shaken well and cooled on an ice water bath. The solution is then removed from the bath and graded on a Gardner colorimeter. The table records the results of experiments using a tall oil fatty acid which was treated according to the method described and distilled under vacuum.

Ex.	"Filtrol," percent	CH$_2$O, percent	Temp., °C.	Time, Hours	Distillate	
					Gardner Color	Color of Soln. after Peroxidation
1	1.0	0.3	90	1.5	3	6
2	1.0	0.5	90	1.0	3-4	7
3	1.0	0.5	90	4.0	3-4	4
4	1.0	0.5	120	4.0	3-4	2-3
5	2.0	0.5	90	1.5	2-3	2-3
6	2.0	1.0	90	1.5	2-3	2-3
7	2.0	0.5	60	16.0	2-3	4
8	2.0	0.5	70	4.0	2-3	4
9	2.0	0.5	80	4.0	2-3	2-3
10	2.0	1.0	90	4.0	2-3	2

An examination of the table reveals that by using 1% of an acid activated clay and 0.5% paraform at 120°C. (Example 4) a very good product can be produced. However, at 90°C., 2% clay is desirable (Example 5). It is also desirable, that as low a temperature as practical be used. The table also adequately demonstrates the effect of time on heating. By the process about half of the unsaponifiables ordinarily present in tall oil fatty acids can be removed. As an example of the improvement of the overall grade of tall oil fatty acids accomplished by this process reference is made to Example 4. The tall oil fatty acid raw material had an acid number of 197.0; unsaponifiables 0.94%; rosin acids, 1.12%; and color, 5 to 6. After treatment the acid number was 199; unsaponfiables, 0.5%; rosin acids, 1.03%; and color 2 to 3. By this treatment of tall oil fatty acids the product appears to have very little conjugated rosin acids present as the Libermann-Storch color test is negative after such treatment.

Stilbene Removal with Boron Trifluoride Etherate

A.F. Wicke, Jr., H.E. McLaughlin and J.H. Stump, Jr.; U.S. Patent 3,257,438; June 21, 1966; assigned to Tenneco Chemicals, Incorporated describe a method for treating tall oil fatty acids to remove most of the impurities including most of the stilbene compounds. Removal of these stilbene compounds eliminates or greatly reduces the development of the red color upon epoxidation of the tall oil fatty acids. In addition, the product is lighter in color, is free of rosin acids, has a higher saponification value, a higher acid value, better color stability, and a lower unsaponifiable content than the original material.

The tall oil fatty acids are treated with a catalytic amount of boron trifluoride to convert at least a major portion of the original stilbene compounds to one or more stilbene derivatives which boil at a higher temperature, the catalyst is then removed, and the treated tall oil fatty acids are distilled to separate the tall oil fatty acids from a residue containing a major portion of the stilbene impurity originally present in the starting material.

The stilbene present in the original fatty acids are derivatives having absorption maxima at 298 mμ and 305 mμ, tentatively identified as 3,4- and 3,5-disubstituted stilbene derivatives including 3-hydroxy-5-methoxy-stilbene. The process converts most of the original stilbene impurity to material having a boiling point higher than the boiling point of the fatty acids so that fatty acids of high purity can be separated by distillation from a residue containing most of the stilbene derivatives originally present. The boron trifluoride catalyst may be boron trifluoride, as such although it is preferred to use boron trifluoride in the form of a molecular compound with an organic compound such as an alcohol, ether, ester, acid, amine, or phenol.

Best results have been obtained with boron trifluoride etherate, a molecular compound of boron trifluoride and diethyl ether containing 45 to 50% boron trifluoride. The amount of catalyst may be varied considerably. As little as 0.25% of catalyst, based on the weight of tall oil fatty acid starting material will produce a noticeable effect. Preferably a minimum of 0.50% of catalyst is used. The chemical reaction or reactions involved in the presence of the catalyst take place readily at room temperature. The catalyst is mixed with the tall oil fatty acids and the mixture held until a major amount, preferably at least 90%, of the stilbene originally present has been converted to a material which will remain in the residue at 290° to 300°C. when the treated tall oil fatty acids are distilled under partial vacuum. Good results have been obtained when the tall oil fatty acids and catalyst were agitated at 30° to 100°C. for 2 to 25 hours.

The catalyst must be removed prior to distillation to avoid formation of an undesirably large residue as the results of side reactions. The catalyst can be removed by washing the tall oil fatty acids-catalyst mixture with water. Removal of the catalyst is facilitated by the use of hot water at a temperature of at least 60°C. with best results being obtained when the wash water is at a temperature in the range of 75° to 100°C. To facilitate complete removal of the catalyst, it is preferable that the wash water be alkaline and contain a water-soluble alkaline compound of sodium or potassium. Excellent results are obtained with 10 to 100% of sodium hydroxide based on the amount of catalyst.

Prior to separation of the alkaline wash water from the treated fatty acids, it is preferable that a small amount of acid be added. Any strong acid may be used that will neutralize any free alkali and will convert any saponified fatty acid back to the acid form. The washed fatty acids are heated and distilled under partial vacuum to separate the distillate of tall oil fatty acids from the stilbene-containing, higher boiling fraction. Distillation is carried out under partial vacuum (3 to 6 mm. Hg) to avoid heating to a maximum temperature above 310°C.

Example: Five hundred grams of a commercially available refined tall oil fatty acids having a low rosin content were charged into a 1,000 ml. flask equipped with a stirrer and thermometer. The charge was stirred at ambient temperature and 5 grams (1% by weight of the fatty acids) of boron trifluoride etherate was added. Agitation was continued for 21 hours with the reaction mixture at room temperature. The treated tall oil fatty acids were washed twice with separate 125 ml. portions of water at 90°C. and the wash water separated.

The fatty acids were then washed with 125 ml. of water at 90°C. containing 1.25 grams of sodium hydroxide. After thorough agitation of the fatty acids and the wash water containing the sodium hydroxide, 2.5 grams of acetic acid was added and the mixture agitated to break the slight emulsion which formed. The wash water was then separated. In each instance the wash water was separated by allowing the mixture to stand and separating the layer of wash water which formed readily. The treated fatty acids from which the catalyst has been removed was charged to a still at the bottom of an 8 plate distillation column. The charge was heated and distilled under a pressure of 3 to 6 mm. Hg until the residue in the still reached a temperature of 295°C.

During distillation 10 cuts of the distillate from the top of the column were taken and these cuts were substantially equal in volume. The residue weighed 48.5 grams, 9.7% by weight of the original charge so that each cut constituted 45 grams or 9% of the charge. These percentages are based on the 500 grams of fatty acids charged originally which also is the amount charged to the still. The residue and various cuts were analyzed using an ultraviolet spectrophotometric method. The results are set forth in the table.

Cut Number	Stilbene, %
1	0.042
2	0.021
4	0.019
6	0.015
8	0.012
9	0.018
10	0.031
Residue	2.40

The tall oil fatty acids originally charged contained 0.35% stilbene. It will be noted that most of the stilbene remains in the residue and that the first cut contains more stilbene than the other cuts. Without the catalyst treatment, the distillate would contain substantially all of the stilbene. The catalyst treatment causes the original stilbene derivatives to react in some manner to form a higher boiling compound or compounds which boil at a temperature higher than the monomeric fatty acids.

A large portion of these higher boiling compounds are stilbene derivatives retaining the conjugated double bond system characteristic of stilbene and substituted stilbenes as shown by their detection by the UV analytical method. Some of original stilbene also is converted to higher boiling compounds, possibly polymers, which do not have the characteristic conjugated double bond system of 3-hydroxy-4-methoxystilbene. Regardless of the particular chemical reactions involved, all of the above distillate contains less than 10% of the stilbene impurity originally present in the tall oil fatty acids so that over 90% of the stilbene originally present has been converted to material boiling at a temperature higher than the fatty acids in the starting material. Combined cuts 2 to 10 contain slightly less than 0.02% stilbene. The addition of the head cut, cut No. 1, would increase the stilbene content. However, the composite of cuts No. 1 through 10 would have a stilbene content below 0.025%, a commercially satisfactory product.

Stilbene Removal with Boron Trifluoride Etherate and Activated Carbon

W.C. Doyle, Jr.; U.S. Patent 3,433,815; March 18, 1969; assigned to Tenneco Chemicals, Incorporated describes a method of treating tall oil fatty acids containing stilbene impurities to improve the color of the fatty acids and remove a substantial portion of the stilbene impurities which impart a reddish color to the fatty acids upon epoxidation. The method involves treating the tall oil fatty acids with both a boron trifluoride catalyst and activated carbon. An aldehyde, for example, formaldehyde also may be used during the treatment with the catalyst and carbon.

Thereafter, the catalyst and the carbon are removed by filtration through acid-activated clay. The filtrate is subjected to a distillation treatment and a distillate of tall oil fatty acids is collected that contains a much smaller amount of stilbene impurities than the starting material. The carbon-catalyst treatment converts the stilbene impurities to derivatives having a higher boiling point than the fatty acids so that the derivatives are separated upon distillation and remain in the pot residue. The activated carbon is essential to prevent the catalyst from causing a large change in the relative amounts of oleic and linoleic acids present in the treated tall oil fatty acids as compared to the tall oil fatty acids in the starting material.

Example 1: In a flask fitted with stirrer and thermometer, 250 grams of tall oil acids containing 14% resin acids, 0.5% stilbenes and having a Gardner color of 6 to 7 was heated to 80°C. In rapid succession there was added 2.5 grams of activated carbon (pulverized) and 2.5 grams of boron fluoride etherate. The mixture was stirred at 80°C. for 1/2 hour and then filtered by suction through a 1 cm. bed of acid activated clay. The filtrate (213 grams, color 6 to 7) was pot distilled to 250°C. pot temperature at 0.6 mm. through a short entrainment separator, giving 197 grams of clear distillate having a Gardner color of less than 1 and containing 0.09% stilbenes.

The residue (14 grams) amounted to 7% of the charge to the distillation. Distillations of untreated tall oil acids under the same conditions have given 4 to 6% residue. The treated material remaining on the filter cake may be partially recovered by washing with benzene or by reuse of the cake in subsequent runs.

Example 2: To 250 grams of tall oil fatty acids containing 10% resin acids and 0.51% stilbene impurities at 80°C. was added 1.25 grams of activated carbon, 1.25 grams of boron fluoride etherate and 3.4 grams of 37% aqueous formaldehyde. After stirring at 80°C. for 1/2 hour the mixture was filtered and distilled as in Example 1. The filtrate (208 grams, Gardner color 5) gave, on distillation, 182 grams of distillate having 0.04% stilbenes and Gardner color 1 to 2 and 22 grams (10.6%) residue.

Using Amino Compounds

J. Klere and R. Gadefaix; U.S. Patent 3,471,536; October 7, 1969; assigned to Lever Brothers Company describe a process in which impurities present in a fatty acid which, when the acid is used to make soap, engender color instability. This is accomplished by contacting the fatty acid with an amino compound that is a hydrazine having a free amino group (hydrazine or phenylhydrazine), a primary aliphatic amine with 12 to 18 carbon atoms in the molecule such as laurylamine, or reaction products of the amino compound. The impurities are subsequently removed by distilling the fatty acid.

Example: To a crude fatty acid of groundnut oil, obtained by hydrolysis of an acid oil obtained as a by-product during the neutralization of crude groundnut oil with caustic soda, was added 0.4% by weight of a 24% aqueous solution of hydrazine hydrate; the mixture was stirred at 60°C. and subjected to distillation under normal conditions used in the production of a technical fatty acid.

The temperature during the distillation was 225° to 230°C., the pressure 3 to 4 mm. of Hg and a conventional vacuum distillation column (Lurgi column) was used, the fatty acid being introduced in the middle of the column after preliminary heating. The residue was recovered at the bottom and the improved fraction was recovered in the upper part of the apparatus, the distillation treatment being continued until the yield of the upper fraction was 80%. The acid obtained was converted to soap with potassium hydroxide.

The color of the soap was determined by means of a spectrophotometer (Jobin Yvon type) at a wave length of 470 millimicrons with a cell of 4 cm., using a 5% aqueous alcoholic solution of the soap. The optical density was determined as a measure of the color of the soap, a value of 0.200 indicating that the fatty acid is unsuitable for the preparation of soap while a value below 0.100 generally indicates an excellent quality of fatty acid. The presence of carbonyl compounds in the treated fatty acid was determined by thin layer chromatography. The adsorbent used was silica gel G, the film had a thickness of 250 microns and was activated for 2 hours at a temperature of 110°C. The mobile phase consisted of a mixture of light petroleum (80%) and ether (20%), containing a small amount of acetic acid, and the elution front was 15 cm. long. The chromatogram was treated with a 0.4% solution of 2,4-dinitrophenylhydrazine in 2 N hydrochloric acid in order to develop any spots due to the presence of carbonyl compounds: such spots have a yellow, orange or yellow-orange color. The groundnut oil fatty acid treated as described above gave a soap of color 0.080 and no carbonyl compounds were detected. The distillation process was repeated without using the hydrazine and the final product had a soap color of 0.100 and was shown to contain carbonyl compounds.

Using a Solvent Mixture

S. Serota and H.E. Kenney; U.S. Patent 3,429,902; February 25, 1969; assigned to the U.S. Secretary of Agriculture describe a process by which stearic acid is purified by crystallizing at ambient room temperatures from a solvent mixture consisting of 97 to 96% petroleum ether and 3 to 4% methylene chloride. The process eliminates the need for low temperature crystallizations and large volumes of solvent. Petroleum ether is a poor solvent for stearic acid, and, when used as such, is inefficient and impractical for purposes of purification. Methylene chloride is such a good solvent for most of the fatty acids that it is not suitable for recrystallization of stearic acid.

The combination of 3 to 4% by volume of methylene chloride with petroleum ether, however, not only provided an excellent solvent for recrystallizing stearic acid, but, at ambient (room) temperatures, retained in solution on the first recrystallization a major portion of the other fatty acids contained in commercial grade stearic acid. Subsequent recrystallization from the solvent removed a progressively smaller proportion of impurities, but three crystallizations gave a product of 98.5 to 99% stearic acid. The purified stearic acid can thus be obtained in just a few hours instead of several days.

Since the process indicates that the impurities in commercial grade stearic acid are more soluble in the petroleum ether-methylene chloride solvent than the stearic acid, the primary consideration is to prepare a solution saturated with stearic acid at a temperature above that to which the mixture will be cooled or allowed to cool for collection of crystallized stearic acid. The desired collection temperature is ambient temperature (21° to 24°C.), the volume of solvent needed is that at least sufficient to dissolve all the stearic acid at the temperature above ambient to which the mixture is heated. Typically, a volume of solvent having a ratio of 6 to 8 times the weight of stearic acid (a weight ratio of solvent to stearic acid in the range of 5:1 to 6:1) was used.

As the process is conducted at existing atmospheric pressure, the upper limit of heating is the temperature at which the mixture boils.

Example: Two kilograms of a commercial stearic acid product containing 94% stearic acid, 4+% palmitic acid, and the remainder a mixture of C_{14}, C_{20} and C_{22} fatty acids, was combined with 16.5 liters of a solvent consisting of 16.0 liters redistilled petroleum ether (BP 38° to 55°C.) and 0.5 liter methylene chloride. The fatty acid-solvent mixture was heated until all the fatty acids were in solution. The solution was allowed to cool to room temperature, 23°C. The resulting solid mass of crystals was broken up by vigorous stirring with a wooden paddle. The crystals were collected by filtration and the filter cake rinsed with cold petroleum ether. The cakes were removed, triturated with cold petroleum ether and again collected by filtration. Yield: 1,800 grams by weight.

The 1,800 grams was crystallized from 15 liters of the same solvent mixture in a manner similar to the first crystallization except that it was a very hot day and room temperature was 30° to 32°C. during the filtering, washing and triturating steps and yield was only 1,200 grams. The dry silvery flakes were indicated by gas-liquid chromatography to be 98% stearic acid. The twice crystallized product was recrystallized from 7.75 liters solvent (7.50 liters redistilled petroleum ether, 0.25 liter methylene chloride), filtered, the filter cake triturated with cold petroleum ether, and the crystals collected and air-dried. The large silvery plates, weight 950 grams, had a melting point of 70° to 71°C. and analyzed 98.7% stearic acid, comparable in purity to the best products obtained by low temperature recrystallization from acetone.

Neocarboxylic Acid in Two Stages with H_2SO_4

R. Bearden, Jr.; U.S. Patent 3,489,779; January 13, 1970; assigned to Esso Research and Engineering Company describes a process which is directed to the refinement or purification of neo acids by removal of close boiling olefinic impurities, which greatly devalue the economic value of these acids by developing objectionable coloration on exposure to air and/or sunlight. The term "neo acids" refers to branched chain C_5 to C_{30} carboxylic acids produced from olefins, e.g., by the Koch synthesis. These acids can be visualized as having the representative formula:

$$R-\underset{\underset{R''}{|}}{\overset{\overset{R'}{|}}{C}}-\overset{\overset{O}{\|}}{C}-OH$$

where R, R' and R'' are the same or different alkyl groups. The neo acid purification process is conducted in essentially two stages. In the first stage, the raw product neo acid containing unreacted olefin trace metal(s), principally iron and oxygenated by-products, as impurities is contacted with concentrated sulfuric acid containing at least 85+ weight percent H_2SO_4. Usually the sulfuric acid strength is 90+% to preferably 95+%. This acid contact renders the neo acids and olefinic and other impurities mutually soluble in a homogeneous solution.

In the second stage of the process, the homogeneous neo acid-impurities solution is contacted with a phase separation agent such as a paraffinic hydrocarbon capable of effecting phase separation of the neo acid and olefinic impurities. By rendering the neo acid and olefinic and other impurities mutually soluble in a homogeneous sulfuric acid phase, a more complete separation of impurities is rendered possible during the second stage treatment (phase separation). This is the case because far better contact of impurities with sulfuric acid results in more complete reaction of impurities to form materials, viz, sulfates, capable of separating from neo acid in the second stage.

Both of these stages are essential for the advantageous results of this process. Conducting the second stage without performing the first, does not produce the desired purification.

Example 1: A mixture of isomeric neo decanoic acids (commercial product) prepared from C_9 UOP olefins via the Koch reaction was found to exhibit poor color stability, primarily as a result of contamination by close boiling olefins. Trace metals, chiefly iron (50 to 100 ppm), were also found present. An attempt to remove these impurities and improve color stability by fractional distillation proved ineffectual. Although virtual elimination of the metal contamination was achieved the olefin impurity was found to boil within the boiling range of the C_{10} neo acid mixture, i.e., 266° to 278°F. (7 mm.) and could not be removed. Color stability of neo acid mixture (measured by Acid Crea color) was not improved.

Neo Decanoic Acid	Gardner Color [1]	Acid Crea No.[2]	Iodine No.[3]
Untreated commercial product	9	2+	2.5
Distilled product	6	2+	2.2
Target specification	<2	<1.0	<1.0

[1] Undiluted acid samples rated against the 0-16 Gardner color scale.
[2] Sample darkening by concentrated H_2SO_4 absolute centimeters at 470 mmµ. Found to predict color stability. Maximum Crea value=2.
[3] Measure of unsaturation. Expressed as gms. iodine/100 g. sample.

Example 2: The untreated acid mixture of Example 1, 100 parts, was diluted with 150 parts (by weight) of n-heptane and stirred with 50 parts of 96% sulfuric acid for 30 minutes at ambient temperature (77°F.). The hydrocarbon layer was then separated and washed with water to remove traces of sulfuric acid. Heptane was removed by flash distillation; maximum pot temperature was 266°F. at 150 mm. A simple one-plate distillation of the residue gave 95 parts of the neo decanoic acids BP 263° to 268°F. (7 mm.), which analyzed as follows:

	Gardner Color	Acid Crea No.	Iodine No.
Neo Decanoic Sample:			
Untreated	9	2+	2.5
Acid washed	10	2+	2.3
Target specification	<2	<1.0	<1.0

As will be noted from the above data, essentially no removal of impurities occurs if the paraffin is added prior to sulfuric acid contact.

Example 3: The untreated neo acid of Example 1, 100 parts, was treated with 70 parts of concentrated (96%) sulfuric acid at ambient temperature (77°F.). There resulted a homogeneous solution of deep red coloration and an accompanying rise in temperature from 77° to 110°F. After 30 minutes time the solution was extracted twice with fresh n-heptane (100 parts used for each extraction). The combined extracts were then water-washed free of sulfuric acid, and the neo acids were recovered according to the procedure described in Example 2. The purified product, 85 parts, gave the following analyses.

Neo Decanoic Acid Sample	Gardner Color	Acid Crea No.	Iodine No.
Untreated	9	2+	2.5
H_2SO_4 paraffin treated	1	0.178	0.4
Target specification	<2	<1.0	<1.0

The removal of color forming impurities by this process is clearly apparent.

Using Alkyl Ester of Titanic Acid

In the process described by S.S. Naskar, H.L. Hülsmann, and G. Renckhoff; U.S. Patent 3,526,649; September 1, 1970; assigned to Dynamit Nobel AG, Germany discoloration and subsequent darkening of fatty acid forerunnings are prevented by heating the fatty acids with at least one alkyl ester of titanic acid and/or polytitanic acid at a temperature of approximately 180° to 250°C., and then distilling the resultant mixture to recover the fatty acids. The heating step is carried out for 0.5 to 4 hours.

Example 1: (A) The untreated fatty acid forerunnings used were derived from the hydrolysis of acid oil obtained during refining. Gas chromatographic analysis showed, in percent by weight, that the fatty acid forerunnings were composed of: C_6 acid, 0.5; C_8 acid, 58.2; C_{10} acid, 28.5; C_{12} acid, 10.1; C_{14} acid, 1.8; C_{16} acid, 0.6; and 0.3% each of methyl heptyl and methyl nonyl ketones. 3,000 parts by weight of this fatty acid forerunning containing 2% of water, were dehydrated under agitation and mixed, at a sump temperature of 220°C., with 0.5% by weight of butyl titanate. The treatment time was 2.5 hours. During this period, a temperature of 220°C. was maintained. Thereupon, the sump temperature was lowered to 90°C. by cooling, and the contents of the flask were distilled over a distillation column under a vacuum of 1 to 2 torr within 2 hours. Three fractions were withdrawn. As fraction I, 7.8% by weight was obtained; as fraction II, 81.2% by weight, and as fraction III, 5.1% by weight, based on the amount of anhydrous fatty acid forerunnings employed. The amount of residue was 5.9% by weight. The values obtained are set forth in the table.

(B) For comparison purposes, 3,000 parts by weight of untreated fatty acid forerunnings were distilled under the same conditions, the resultant data also given in the table.

Example 2: (A) 3,000 parts by weight of fatty acid forerunnings from the pressure dissociation of coconut oil and palm nut oil were dehydrated at 450 torr and mixed with 0.6% by weight of the ethyl ester of polytitanic acid at a sump temperature of 210°C. During the treatment time of 3 hours, a temperature of 220°C. was maintained. Thereafter, the sump temperature was lowered by cooling to 90°C., and the contents of the flask were distilled under a vacuum of 1 to 2 torr over a distillation column within 2 hours. As fraction I, 7.2% by weight was obtained; as fraction II, 81.5% by weight; as fraction III, 6.1% by weight. The residue was 5.2% by weight.

(B) For comparison purposes, 3,000 parts by weight of untreated fatty acid forerunnings from the pressure-hydrolysis of coconut oil and palm nut oil were distilled under the same conditions. The values are also indicated in the table.

Example	Fraction I				Fraction II				Fraction III			
	Amount, percent by weight	Acid No.	Iodine Color No.	Iodine Color No. after 6 hours at 200° C.	Amount, percent by weight	Acid No.	Iodine Color No.	Iodine Color No. after 6 hours at 200° C.	Amount, percent by weight	Acid No.	Iodine Color No.	Iodine Color No. after 6 hours at 200° C.
1(a)	7.8	381	<1	28.5	81.2	368	<1	7.8	5.1	305	1.2	24
1(b)	7.9	382	5.4	108	81.3	367	2.1	52	5.2	307	2.6	62
2(a)	7.6	365	1	16.3	81.4	358	<1	5.3	5.6	295	1.1	14
2(b)	7.8	366	2.2	33	81.1	359	1.1	20	5.2	294	1.0	20

Generally, the alkyl groups in the alkyl esters have from 1 to 4 carbon atoms (methyl, ethyl, n-propyl, isopropyl, n-butyl, isobutyl, sec-butyl and tert-butyl).

Using Alkyl Ester of Silicic Acid

S.S. Naskar, H.L. Hülsmann and G. Renckhoff; U.S. Patent 3,531,506; September 29, 1970; assigned to Dynamit Nobel AG, Germany describe another method for purification and prevention of the formation of unsaponifiable compounds in fatty acid forerunnings. In this case the discoloration and subsequent darkening is prevented by heating the fatty acids with at least one alkyl ester of silicic acid, polysilicic acid and/or carbonic acid at a temperature of approximately 180° to 250°C., and then distilling the resultant mixture to recover the fatty acids. The heating step is carried out for 0.5 to 8 hours.

Example 1: The untreated fatty acid forerunnings employed had the following composition, according to gas chromatographic analysis (numerical data in percent by weight): C_6 acid, 0.2; C_8 acid, 68.4; C_{10} acid, 23.5; C_{12} acid, 7; C_{14} acid, 0.5; C_{16} acid, 0.2; methyl heptyl ketone, 0.2 and methyl nonyl ketone, 0.2.

2,400 parts by weight of this fatty acid forerunning, containing approximately 2% water, were dehydrated with agitation and mixed at a sump temperature of 240°C. with (b) 0.5% by weight of silicic acid tetrabutyl ester or (c) the dibutyl ester of carbonic acid. The treatment time was 3 hours. During this time, a temperature of 240°C. was maintained. Thereafter, the sump temperature was lowered to 100°C. by cooling, and the contents of the flask distilled over a small distillation column under a vacuum of 3 to 5 torr (mm. Hg) within 2 hours, 3 fractions being withdrawn. For comparison purposes, 2,400 parts by weight of untreated fatty acid forerunnings were distilled under the same conditions [Example 1(a), no additive].

As fraction I, 8 to 10% by weight was obtained; as fraction II, 76 to 78% by weight; as fraction III, 5 to 7% by weight all based on the initial charge of anhydrous fatty acid forerunnings. The amount of residue was 7 to 9% by weight. The values are compiled in the table.

Example 2: The procedure of Example 1 was repeated with the exception of the treatment time which amounted to 8 hours. The table also shows these results.

Fraction	Example	Amount % by wt.	Acid Number	Iodine Color		Unsaponifiables % by wt.
				Initial	After 6 hrs. at 200°C.	
I	1(a)	8.8	380	5.2	104	--
	1(b)	9.0	378	1.0	38	--
	1(c)	9.8	377	1.5	48	--
	2(a)	8.6	381	<1	33	--
	2(b)	8.1	379	1.3	42	--

(continued)

				Iodine Color		
Fraction	Example	Amount % by wt.	Acid Number	Initial	After 6 hrs. at 200°C.	Unsaponifiables % by wt.
II	1(a)	77.5	376	2.1	51	--
	1(b)	77.8	375	<1	6.4	--
	1(c)	76.7	376	<1	9.6	--
	2(a)	76.0	376	<1	7.0	--
	2(b)	77.5	375	<1	9.3	--
III	1(a)	5.5	315	3.5	60	--
	1(b)	5.8	318	2.6	15.2	--
	1(c)	5.9	317	2.3	18.3	--
	2(a)	6.7	314	2.4	17.0	--
	2(b)	5.6	318	2.7	21.6	--
Residue	1(a)	8.2	--	--	--	3.2
	1(b)	7.4	--	--	--	3.8
	1(c)	7.6	--	--	--	3.5
	2(a)	8.7	--	--	--	3.4
	2(b)	8.8	--	--	--	3.3

Using Alkali Metal Borohydride

J.D. Craske and C. Szonyi; U.S. Patent 3,542,823; November 24, 1970; assigned to Lever Brothers Company describe a process by which objectionable colored compounds present in low grade fatty acids used in making soap can be successfully removed. The means by which this is accomplished is the treatment of a soap-containing system at any stage during production with an alkali metal borohydride at a pH of at least 9.5.

The color of the soap obtained from this process is conveniently measured on a 5.84% wt./vol. aqueous solution of the soap (dry basis) with the aid of a Lovibond Tintometer using a Lovibond 13.3 cm. cell. The acceptable standard of color depends on the purpose to which the soap is to be applied. The color is determinable in terms of Lovibond red and yellow units, these units being combined to form one value (here referred to as the "soap color") by use of the formula:

$$\text{soap color} = 10 \times (\text{yellow reading}) + 30 \times (\text{red reading})$$

The term "soap charge" refers to the material obtained by saponification of a suitable charge of fat and alkali. The term "fat" may refer to an animal tallow, a vegetable oil such as palm oil, palm kernel oil or coconut oil, a fish oil or to the fatty acids obtained from such materials by a conventional splitting technique. Mixtures of these fats may be used, a convenient mixture, for example, being based on tallow and up to 20% wt./wt. of coconut oil. These fats are referred to as the "fat charge." When the fat charge is of a low grade, it is desirable that it be given a pretreatment with an activated earth or other adsorbent bleaching agent (standard bleaching treatment) before saponification, as the color thus removed will not then compete with the unsorbed material for the borohydride. The color of a bleached low grade tallow may vary from 4.0

yellow, 0.8 red to 15.0 yellow, 2.5 red (when measured in a 0.635 cm. cell of a Lovibond Tintometer). The alkali metal borohydride preferably is added as a solution in aqueous alkali, suitable alkalies being sodium hydroxide or potassium hydroxide.

The alkali metal borohydride is conveniently added either towards the end of the saponification stage of the soap manufacture or after the saponification has been completed, as, at these points, the pH of the saponification system does not vary so widely as during the initial period of saponification. If the borohydride is added during the saponification stage, boiling of the saponification system should be continued for a further period of 30 minutes to ensure complete dispersion of borohydride and maximum reduction of color and odor of the soap charge. The total color and odor reduction is dependent on the effectiveness with which the borohydride is spread through the saponification system as well as the level used.

A preferred amount of borohydride for the treatment of a soap obtained from a toilet grade standard bleached tallow lies within the range 0.02 to 0.10% by weight of the fat charge. Borate ion is readily removable from the treated soap by aqueous washing although its presence has no deleterous effect on the soap or any material (such as perfume) that is to be added to the soap at a later stage in its preparation.

A feature of the process is that it is so readily incorporated into a normal soap manufacturing process. Flame-proofing of the soap-making machinery may be necessary in view of the possible hazard associated with the evolution of small volumes of hydrogen. The amount of adsorbent agent used in the standard bleaching treatment of a low grade fat charge is preferably 6% by weight of the fat charge. Fuller's earth is a preferred bleaching agent.

Example: A fat charge containing 92.5% wt./wt. tallow (that had been bleached by treatment with 6% wt./wt. adsorbent earth) having a Lovibond Yellow reading of 11.7 and a Lovibond Red reading of 1.4 in a 5.1 cm. cell and 7.5% wt./wt. coconut oil was saponified at 95°C. in a conventional soap pan. The soap thus prepared was separated from the lye and washed, in a conventional washing unit, with brine containing 1% wt./vol. sodium hydroxide.

As the washed soap passed out of the washing unit it was treated with an amount of aqueous 5.0% wt./vol. sodium hydroxide solution containing 10 wt./wt. sodium borohydride, sufficient to provide 0.1% sodium borohydride based on the weight of the fat charge originally saponified. The boronhydride treated soap was subsequently fitted, neutralized, heated and dried according to standard practice. The soap color of the soap was

37, while the soap color of a soap prepared from a similar fat charge which was not treated with borohydride, was 60. In a further experiment the soap was washed with brine containing 2% wt./vol. sodium hydroxide. The soap color of the untreated soap was 54. The color of the soap that had been treated with 0.1% wt./wt. sodium borohydride was 43. Hydrogen evolution inflated the 20 tons of soap that were prepared in each of the above experiments where borohydride was used, to the volume that would have been occupied by 35 tons of soap.

SEPARATION PROCESSES

Using Aliphatic Hydrocarbon and Furfural

R.E. Beal; U.S. Patent 3,052,699; September 4, 1962; assigned to the U.S. Secretary of Agriculture describes a process in which mixed fatty acids derived from vegetable oils, such as safflower and linseed oils, are separated by liquid-liquid extraction to produce substantially pure linoleic and linolenic acids. To effect such a separation to obtain substantially pure linoleic and linolenic acids, closely controlled conditions of operation are required.

A vegetable oil, preferably one such as safflower oil which has a high content of linoleic acid and little or no linolenic acid, or an oil such as linseed oil which has a high content of linolenic acid, is used as the respective sources of these two acids. The oil is first hydrolyzed to free the fatty acids from the glycerol. Since it is important to the subsequent extraction process that the fatty acids undergo the least possible amount of oxidation because oxidized fatty acids are more soluble in the polar solvent used in the extraction than are unoxidized acids, the hydrolysis of the oil to fatty acids should be conducted using oil which has been deaerated under vacuum, and the mixed fatty acids should be used quickly or stored under an inert atmosphere until they are subjected to liquid-liquid extraction.

The liquid-liquid extraction is conducted using two solvents, namely an aliphatic hydrocarbon and furfural, the latter containing 1 to 3% water. When these solvents are passed countercurrently through an extraction column or centrifugal extractor and the deaerated mixed fatty acids derived from safflower oil are introduced to the midpoint of the column or extractor, the fatty acids become distributed between the two solvents, the more unsaturated fatty acids being found in the furfural, and more saturated fatty acids in the hydrocarbon solvent phase. When the deaerated feed mixed fatty acids comprised 75% linoleic acid (domestic safflower oil) the fatty acids recovered from the furfural phase issuing from the countercurrent extraction device, after evaporation of the solvent, comprised over 95% linoleic acid, providing the additional following conditions are met:

(1) the countercurrent extraction device is designed and operated to provide at least 30 equilibrium extraction stages;
(2) the extraction temperature is between 60° and 120°F.;
(3) the water content of the furfural is between 1 and 3%, or water in an equivalent amount is introduced into the extractor with dry furfural;
(4) the weight ratio of furfural to fatty acids fed to the extractor is greater than 10;
(5) combined feed rates of furfural, hydrocarbon solvent, and deaerated fatty acids is less than the minimum amount which will produce a flooding condition in the extractor; and
(6) the hydrocarbon solvent feed rate to the extractor is an amount such that the percentage of the deaerated feed fatty acids which were dissolved in the furfural phase issuing from the extractor (the percent extract) does not exceed the linoleic acid content of the feed acids.

The same conditions apply to the extraction of linolenic acid, in a purity of over 95%, from deaerated mixed linseed fatty acids.

Example: Deaerated safflower fatty acids containing 76% linoleic acid were subjected to liquid-liquid extraction using furfural (containing 2.5% water) and hexane as the immiscible solvents. The extractor was a centrifugal type Podbielniak having 36 actual mixing and settling stages, with provision for introducing the fatty acids into the extractor midway between the solvent feed points.

All feed streams to the extractor were preheated to 100°F. and cooling water was sprayed on the rapidly revolving centrifugal extractors to overcome heat build-up which results from liquid-flow friction and mixing and to hold the product streams issuing from the extractor at 100°F. Feed rates to the extractor in pounds per hour were furfural 30, hexane 6, safflower fatty acids 2. Seventy-four percent of the fatty acids fed to the extractor were recovered in the extract phase from the extractor. After evaporation of the solvent, the fatty acids were found to comprise 95% linoleic acid, the balance being equal amounts of oleic and palmitic acids.

10-Hydroxydecanoic Acid by Acetylation

G.I. Fray, R.H. Jaeger, and E.D. Morgan; U.S. Patent 3,084,178; April 2, 1963; assigned to Shell Oil Company describe a process for recovering 10-hydroxydecanoic acid both from the oily reaction products obtained by heating ricinoleic acid in the presence of aqueous alkali metal hydroxide and also under the conditions under which the 10-hydroxydecanoic acid is obtained as 10-acetoxydecanoic acid. 10-hydroxydecanoic acid is recovered as 10-acetoxydecanoic acid from the oily, 10-hydroxydecanoic acid-containing residue obtained by the sequential steps of (a) heating ricinoleic acid with aqueous alkali metal hydroxide, (b) removing lower boiling components comprising octanol and octanone from the resulting reaction mixture, (c) acidifying the resulting reaction mixture now freed of lower boiling components, and (d) extracting the acidified reaction mixture with hot water, by acetylating the oily 10-hydroxydecanoic acid-containing residue, and separating 10-acetoxydecanoic acid from the resulting acetylation products.

The recovery process is applied to oily 10-hydroxydecanoic acid-containing residues obtained by interaction of ricinoleic acid, as such or in the form of its salt or ester, with alkali metal hydroxide in a homogeneous liquid medium in the presence of an alkali metal phenoxide, or mixture of phenoxides, for example, those derived from commercial cresol or xylenol mixtures.

The 10-hydroxydecanoic acid-containing residue starting material should preferably be in anhydrous, or substantially anhydrous, state before being subjected to the acetylation treatment of this process. Any water present is removed by treatment with a dehydrating agent such as anhydrous magnesium sulfate with or without the aid of a volatile solvent or diluent, which if used, are removed after the drying step. Acetylation of the 10-hydroxydecanoic acid-containing oily residue is effected with acetylating agent such as acetic anhydride. The acetylation is effected by heating the oily residue starting material, in admixture with the acetylating agent, at a temperature from 50°C. to the boiling temperature of the mixture.

The mixture is heated under reflux conditions. The heating is continued for a period of time which varies with the specific temperatures employed, in general, from 3 to 7 hours is satisfactory. Under these conditions the 10-hydroxydecanoic acid will react with the formation of reaction products comprising 10-acetoxydecanoic acid.

After the heating step the reaction mixture is cooled, by quenching with cold water, i.e., discharged into water or onto ice. Decomposition of unreacted acetic anhydride will take place. The resulting reaction products comprising 10-acetoxydecanoic acid are separated from the aqueous phase by liquid phase extraction with an organic solvent such as diethyl ether, hydrocarbon solvents of aromatic or nonaromatic character, lower boiling paraffinic hydrocarbons, petroleum ether, etc. The product of the acetylation treatment may be washed with water prior to the extraction. In a preferred procedure the acetylated product is washed in the form of its solution in the organic solvent employed to extract it from the acetylation reaction mixture. The solution is then dried and freed of solvent. The oily acetylation product, after the removal of the solvent, may be subjected to further distillation to separate therefrom a product of high purity from it. Pure 10-acetoxydecanoic acid having a boiling temperature in the range of 140° to 142°C. at 0.2 mm. pressure is thus readily obtained as a final product.

Example 1: A mixture of 115 parts by weight sodium hydroxide, 40 parts by volume water, 45 parts by weight tricresol and 150 parts by weight castor oil was heated under reflux in an oil bath at 180° to 195°C. with vigorous stirring. Violent frothing occurred in the earlier stages of the reaction but was controlled by stirring at high speed. After 3 hours, the volatile products were removed by distillation, the oil bath being maintained at the same temperature. Stirring was continued during the distillation. The distillation residue was then dissolved in 1,500 parts by volume water, acidified to Congo red with 50% sulfuric acid (190 parts by volume) and the mixture brought to the boil. The aqueous layer which contained sebacic acid was separated while still hot from the oily upper layer. The remaining oily layer was diluted with ether and dried with anhydrous magnesium sulfate.

After removing the drying agent and the ether, the oily residue (175 parts by weight) containing cresols, 10-hydroxydecanoic acid and other acids was refluxed with 350 parts by volume acetic anhydride for 5 hours and the reaction mixture was then poured on to ice and left to stand at room temperature overnight. The product was collected in ether. The ethereal extract was washed with water and dried over anhydrous magnesium sulfate.

After removal of the ether solvent the residue was subjected to careful fractional distillation, the fraction of BP 136° to 160°C. at 0.2 mm. pressure (56 parts by weight) being collected; refractionation of this gave a fraction of BP 140° to 146°C. at 0.2 mm. pressure (48 parts by weight) and from this a final fractionation isolated pure 10-acetoxydecanoic acid (45 parts by weight) BP 140° to 142°C. at 0.2 mm. pressure. The infrared spectrum of this material had peaks at 5.76μ (C=O of acetate) and 5.87μ (C=O of carboxyl). A small sample was crystallized from petroleum ether (BP below 40°C.); this had a melting point of 36°C.

Example 2: The oily residue, obtained and dried as described in Example 1, was dissolved in hot petroleum ether (BP 60° to 80°C; 300 parts by volume) and allowed to cool to room temperature. The supernatant liquid was decanted from the precipitated material, and the latter was then refluxed with acetic anhydride (300 parts by volume) for 5 hours. The resulting reaction mixture was worked up as described in Example 1. Forty parts by weight of 10-acetoxydecanoic acid was isolated by fractional distillation.

Using a Fatty Acid Distillation Residue

A improved selective crystallization process for the separation of higher fatty acids is described by K.T. Zilch and R.H. Plantholt; U.S. Patent 3,235,578; February 15, 1966; assigned to Emery Industries, Incorporated. The method is of particular utility for recovering commercial stearic and oleic acids from fatty acid mixtures obtained from glyceride materials of animal origin such as tallow or one of the many available oils and greases.

Oleic acid is a liquid which normally contains approximately 75% oleic acid, the balance of the product being made up of other unsaturated acids together with a small percentage of saturated acids, primarily palmitic acid. Commercial stearic acid, on the other hand, is a waxy solid comprised of approximately equal parts of palmitic and stearic acids, the palmitic acid component normally being somewhat in excess. In this method of separation the fatty acid mixture obtained on the high pressure splitting of the glyceride is dissolved in a water-miscible polar solvent such as methyl or ethyl alcohol, acetone or similar solvent which normally contains from 5 to 15% by weight of water for best results.

The resulting fatty acid solution (heated, if necessary, to effect complete solution of the acids) is then cooled to a temperature, usually ranging from 0° to 10°C., at which the "stearic acid" fraction crystallizes out of solution and can be separated from the oleic acid fraction which remains in the filtrate. In commercial operations chilling of the acid solution is normally conducted in a continuous operation, with the crystalline phase also being continuously separated from the liquid phase, usually by means of a rotary filter.

The filter cake obtained is given a preliminary washing with cold solvent to remove occluded oleic acid, following which it is passed to a solvent still where it is stripped of its solvent content. The residual solids, melted if necessary for easier handling, are passed to an acid still, usually operated under high vacuum, from which the stearic acid product is distilled overhead, a representative distillate temperature being 200°C. at 5 mm. Hg. A residual, or bottoms fraction of unknown composition is also recovered from the acid still. This bottoms fraction probably contains acid polymer and a substantial portion of methanol-insoluble components. This residual stream, identified here as "stearic acid residue," is that portion of the crystallized fatty acid fraction which boils above the stearic acid distillate and is recovered as a bottoms stream from the acid still.

In an alternate stearic acid recovery method, the crystallized, stearic acid fraction, on being freed of its solvent content, is given a hydrogenation treatment before being distilled in vacuo to separate the stearic acid from the less volatile residual fraction. The still residue recovered on distilling off the stearic acid from a hydrogenated stearic acid product (which residue is believed to contain acid polymer along with trace amounts of nickel soaps) is referred to as "hydrogenated stearic acid residue."

The oleic acid fraction is usually worked up in a fashion similar to the stearic acid fraction with regard to the steps of solvent removal and acid distillation. Here again there is recovered a bottoms fraction boiling above the oleic acid distillate which is referred to as "oleic acid residue." The oleic acid is sometimes subjected to a hydrogenation treatment as described above to saturate the oleic acid. The residue obtained on distillation is called "hydrogenated oleic acid residue."

Improved results can be obtained in solvent separation operations which are so conducted that a small percentage of one or more of the residues is mixed with the fatty acid/solvent solution prior to chilling it to effect crystallization of a portion of the dissolved fatty acid mixture. Use of a residue component permits an increase in the concentration of the mixed fatty acid solution. As indicated above, the mixture of fatty acids to be separated into component fractions by selective crystallization is first dissolved in an appropriate organic polar solvent.

However, the crystal-forming characteristics of the resulting solutions are such that, with tallow acids at least, the concentration of acids in the starting solution may not exceed 25% by weight if good results are to be obtained during the crystallization and, more particularly, the crystal separation and washing steps. Thus, as the fatty acid concentration materially exceeds 25% the crystal mass formed on cooling the solution takes on a slimy character and is difficult to handle. Filtering of the crystals is slow, as are subsequent washing steps. Moreover, the washed filter cake tends to occlude an unduly large proportion of oleic acid. This represents not only a net loss of oleic acid, but also necessitates additional hydrogenation if the I.V. of the product is to be reduced to a low level.

Separation, by selective crystallization from solution, of fatty acids from fatty acid mixtures can be achieved by adding to the solution of fatty acids to be separated into component fractions, a small percentage of one or more of the residual fractions obtained on distilling off the separated acid components. The residues are those defined above as stearic acid residue, hydrogenated stearic acid residue, oleic acid residue or hydrogenated oleic acid residue. The amount of residue will normally range from 0.25 to 3% based on the weight of fatty acid present, a preferred range being from 0.75 to 2%.

Example: The acid separation runs for which data are presented in the table were made using 90.5% methanol (9.5% water content) and a mixture of fatty acids as obtained on the high pressure splitting of tallow, which mixture contains 3% myristic acid, 27% palmitic acid, 47% oleic acid, 17% stearic acid and 5% linoleic acid along with small amounts of various other fatty acids. Crystallization of the stearic acid was conducted at -10°C.

As indicated in the table, some runs were made without adding any tallow or residue as a crystal modifier, while on others a material of the latter character was employed. The residues added had been obtained by starting with the same mixture of fatty acids, separating them into respective stearic and oleic acid fractions using the same crystallization technique as used in this example, and distilling off the solvent-free oleic and stearic acid fractions so obtained. This distillation was effected in the case of both fractions at a pressure of 5 mm. Hg absolute, and at a distillate temperature of approximately 200°±10°C.

The one stearic acid residue was obtained without using a preliminary hydrogenation step, whereas the other stearic acid residue and the oleic acid residue had been subjected to a preliminary hydrogenation step to reduce the I.V. of the resulting hydrogenated acid to a level below 1.0, the hydrogenation having been effected at 160° to 200°C. and at 150 to 400 psi hydrogen pressure in the presence of 0.1 to 1% of a nickel catalyst and 0.1 to 2% of an acid-activated montmorillonite clay (Filtrol) as a filter aid. The resulting products were filtered before being distilled in vacuo to distill off the fatty acids and leave the residues here utilized as bottoms.

In conducting the various runs shown in the table the fatty acid mixtures and any crystal modifier used were dissolved in the methanol. The resulting solution was then cooled to -10°C. in a stirred, scraping crystallizer. The resulting slurries were then filtered using a Büchner funnel while maintaining a 15 psi vacuum until no liquid layer was visible above the crystalline layer. The latter was then washed under these same conditions using 200 parts by weight of the 90.5% methanol at -10°C. for each 100 parts of the solid cake in the funnel. Observations were made as to the character of the slurry which was first poured into the funnel. Those indicated in the table as being thin had unusually good (rapid) filtering characteristics; those described as medium (minus) or medium were also quite satisfactory, while those designated as medium (plus) were filtered only with considerable difficulty. Tests were run on the washed filter cake to determine (1) its content of solids and (2) the I.V. of the solid fraction of the cake as later freed of solvent (and water) by heating on a steam bath followed by drying on a hot plate. A high solids content in the cake is desirable, for this indicates a correspondingly low content of solvent to be evaporated and returned to the crystallizer unit. The I.V. should also be as low as possible, indicating a low content of occluded oleic acid in the washed and dried solids fraction. In these runs an I.V. of approximately 8 or below is regarded as satisfactory.

Crystal Modifier	Concentration of Tallow Acids in MeOH, Percent	Slurry Character	Washed Cake	
			Percent Solids	I.V.
None	25	Med	37.8	6.3
Do	30	Med	30.4	14.4
0.5% Tallow	25	Med	35.0	8.7
1% Tallow	30	Med.+	43.6	7.1
Do	35	Med.+	32.1	7.5
Do	40	Med.+	38.6	9.0
2% Tallow	40	Med	42.6	9.3
0.5% Hydrog. Stearic Aicd Residue	40	Med	50.1	6.9
1% Hydrog. Stearic Acid Residue	40	Med	47.5	6.7
Do	45	Med	58.5	7.5
Do	50	Med.+	46.7	8.8
2% Hydrog. Stearic Acid Residue	40	Med.−	46.5	6.6
Do	45	Med.−	51.7	8.1
1% Stearic Acid Residue	35	Thin	48.4	6.9
Do	40	Thin	44.7	7.4
Do	45	Med.+	42.2	9.9
1% Hydrog. Oleic Acid Residue	45	Med.+	44.4	7.3

From the data presented in the table, it will be seen that use of an appropriate residual material promotes the formation of crystals having good filtering characteristics and other desirable attributes. At the same time, use of the residue makes it possible to employ solutions having a far greater concentration of fatty acid than would otherwise be possible while still obtaining a solid phase which filters well, is high in solids content and has a low I.V.

Using a Halofluoroalkane

E.J. Bennett; U.S. Patent 3,320,230; May 16, 1967; assigned to E.I. du Pont de Nemours and Company describes a process for separating unsubstituted aliphatic monocarboxylic acids and haloaliphatic monocarboxylic acids from polycarboxylic acids and hydroxy, keto, mercapto and sulfo substituted aliphatic mono- and polycarboxylic acids.

The process consists of treating a mixture of carboxylic acids with certain halofluoroalkanes, removing the halofluoroalkane solution containing the dissolved soluble acids, thereby recovering the insoluble acids, and then evaporating or otherwise removing the halofluoroalkane to recover the soluble acids. The insoluble acids comprise unsubstituted aliphatic polycarboxylic acids containing from 2 to 22 carbons and having at least two carboxyl groups and hydroxyaliphatic, aminoaliphatic, ketoaliphatic, mercaptoaliphatic or sulfoaliphatic mono- and polycarboxylic acids containing from 2 to 22 carbons and having at least one carboxylic acid group.

Example: Treatment of oleic acid with ozone and then cleavage of the resulting ozonide gives a mixture of oleic acid, pelargonic acid and azelaic acid. In a typical procedure ozonolysis of oleic acid is 90% complete, resulting in a mixture consisting of 0.1 mol oleic acid (5.26 mol percent), 0.9 mol pelargonic acid (47.3 mol percent) and 0.9 mol azelaic acid (47.3 mol percent). One hundred parts of such mixture were added to 100 parts of 1,1,2-trichloro-1,2,2-trifluoroethane and the resulting mixture was agitated for 15 minutes at room temperature. The undissolved solids were collected by filtration. The solids proved to be essentially pure azelaic acid. Evaporation of the solvent gave a mixture of oleic and pelargonic acids containing less than 0.6 mol percent azelaic acid.

Using 2-Nitropropane

K.T. Zilch; U.S. Patent 3,345,389; October 3, 1967; assigned to Emery Industries, Incorporated describes a process which relates to the separation of glycerides and of fatty acids and particularly to the separation of mono- from polyunsaturated fatty acids using 2-nitropropane as the solvent for the fatty material to be separated into fractions of varying melting point. This compound has a low vapor pressure, thus reducing solvent losses and danger of explosion. In addition, it has the ability to dissolve from 15 to 25% by weight of the various fatty materials at room temperatures, this solvent action being coupled with the ability to retain these materials in solution at temperatures down to that at which the particular material being separated crystallizes out without giving rise to a second liquid phase.

Solutions of fatty materials in 2-nitropropane crystallize from the solution at significantly higher temperatures than is the case with many other solvents. At the same time, the crystalline phase which does form is characterized by a coarse, granular structure which permits the liquid phase to be readily drawn off as the crystalline product is washed and suction filtered. The fatty material, glyceride or fatty acid, is dissolved in 3 to 4 times its weight of 2-nitropropane and the solution cooled.

After cooling the solution to bring about precipitation or crystallization to the desired degree, the solution is filtered to remove the precipitated fatty material and the solids on the filter washed with fresh solvent to displace the retained solvent and the fatty material in solution. The solids are removed from the filter, melted and the solvent content removed by distillation. The filtrate containing the more unsaturated fat or fatty acids may either be further cooled to remove a second fraction or subjected to distillation to recover the solvent and its content of fatty material.

Example: 100 parts of refined cottonseed oil was dissolved in 400 parts of 2-nitropropane. The solution was cooled in a jacketed vessel, the walls of which were scraped continuously to maintain a clean cooling surface. At a temperature of -9°C. crystallization commenced. Cooling was continued to -20°C. The crystallized solids were removed by filtration and the filter cake washed with 250 parts of solvent. The filter cake amounting to 39.9 parts was melted and the solvent removed by distillation. 19.3 parts of solid glyceride was recovered. The filtrate was evaporated and 80.7 parts of liquid glyceride recovered. This "winterized" cottonseed oil showed no clouding when held at 0°C. for over 18 days.

Using Column Chromatography

The process described by J.E. Pike; U.S. Patent 3,405,151; October 8, 1968; assigned to The Upjohn Company is concerned with the separation of pure γ-linolenic acid lower alkyl esters from associated isomers of substantially the same molecular weight by column chromatography on an adsorbent impregnated with silver nitrate.

After alkaline hydrolysis, the corresponding free acid can be obtained. An important feature of this purification method is the high ratio of fatty acid esters applied to the column (a 1 to 3 to 1 to 10 ratio). The use of a low percentage of adsorbent in the process facilitates the rate at which the column can be operated and lowers the time during which the relatively unstable polyunsaturated acids and/or their esters are exposed to the atmosphere.

Diatomaceous earth (Celite), synthetic magnesium silicate (Florisil) and silicic acid (silica gel) impregnated with 25% by weight of silver nitrate can be used in the chromatographic column. Eluants that can be used include increasing percentages of ethyl acetate, chloroform, ether or benzene in cyclohexane, methyl cyclohexane or Skellysolve A (pentanes), Skellysolve B (hexanes) or Skellysolve C (heptanes). γ-Linoleic acid obtained from borage seed is preferred for this process.

Example: A batch of borage seeds (Borago officinalis L.) weighing 3.74 kg. was ground in a mill to give a sticky, black semisolid material, which was suspended in 4 liters of Skellysolve B and heated to boiling for 30 minutes with stirring. The suspension was filtered and the collected solids washed with 1 liter of hot Skellysolve B and the washings added to the filtrate. The filtrate was evaporated in vacuo to give 1,310 grams of oil, which was stored under nitrogen at 0°C. Eighty grams of hydrogen chloride was dissolved in 1,600 ml. of methanol while cooling and excluding moisture from the solution, 160 grams of the oil obtained was added to this. This mixture was heated to reflux for 6 hours while stirring under nitrogen, then allowed to stand at room temperature for 16 hours. Most of the methanol was removed in vacuo, the residue poured into 1 liter of ice water and extracted 3 times with 700 ml. of ether. The combined extracts were washed with 500 ml. of saturated sodium bicarbonate solution, then with 250 ml. of 5% aqueous potassium hydroxide and finally with water until the washings were neutral. The washings were back extracted with ether and the extracts added to those obtained above.

The organic ethereal material was dried with sodium sulfate and the ether evaporated in vacuo to give 159 grams of crude methyl esters. Thin-layer chromatography (TLC) of this material dissolved in 10% ethyl acetate to 90% cyclohexane and applied to silica gel impregnated with silver nitrate, when developed with vanillin:phosphoric acid spray shows three main clearly-separated spots. The desired γ-linoleic acid, methyl ester (methyl γ-linoleneate) is the most polar material.

A batch of 477.5 grams of crude methyl esters (obtained as above) was dissolved in 450 ml. of 10% ethyl acetate:90% cyclohexane and applied to a column (protected from light) of 2,250 grams of silica gel impregnated with 560 grams of silver nitrate made up in 10% ethyl acetate:90% cyclohexane. The column was eluted with 14 liters of 10% ethyl acetate:90% cyclohexane, collecting eighteen 1,500 ml. fractions. Further elution was with 10 liters of ethyl acetate followed by 10% methanol:90% ethyl acetate.

(1) Fractions 1 through 12 (weight 296.4 grams). These contained the esters of C_{18} monounsaturated acid and C_{18} diunsaturated acid; these esters correspond to the two less polar spots on TLC.
(2) Fractions 13 through 15 (weight 63.6 grams). These were mainly esters of C_{18} diunsaturated acid.
(3) Fractions 16 and 17 (weight 18.3 grams). These contained a mixture of the esters of C_{18} diunsaturated acid and the desired C_{18} triunsaturated acid.
(4) Remaining fractions (weight 102.7 grams). These showed only one TLC spot corresponding to the most polar ester of the desired C_{18} triunsaturated acid, i.e., γ-linoleic acid methyl ester.

Since the methanol:ethyl acetate eluates tend to remove some inorganic material from the column, after evaporation of the solvents the oil should be dissolved in Skellysolve B and the insoluble material removed by filtration. As these polyunsaturated fatty acids and their derivatives are readily autooxidized they should be stored under nitrogen at 0°C. When evaporating the later column fractions containing the ester of the desired C_{18} triunsaturated acid it is preferable to effect this in vacuo or in a nitrogen stream. Structural proof of the authenticity of the γ-linolenic acid methyl ester obtained is furnished by comparisons of its infrared and nuclear magnetic resonance spectra with standard samples of the compound.

Following the procedure of the example but substituting for the methanol: ethanol which yields γ-linolenic acid, ethyl ester; propanol which yields γ-linolenic acid, propyl ester; isopropanol which yields γ-linolenic acid, isopropyl ester; and butanol which yields γ-linolenic acid, butyl ester. Substituting for the silica gel: diatomaceous earth (Celite) and synthetic magnesium silicate (Florisil) also yields γ-linolenic acid methyl ester and the corresponding ethyl, propyl, isopropyl and butyl esters.

Using Aryl Sulfonates

In the process described by A. Koebner and T. Thornton; U.S. Patent 3,506,695; April 14, 1970; assigned to Marchon Products Limited, England a mixture of fatty acids of high polarity and fatty acids of low polarity may be separated by dissolving the mixture of fatty acids in an aqueous solution of aryl or alkaryl sulfonates of sufficient concentration to dissolve the mixture of acids. The solution is then cooled to crystallize out the acids of low polarity which are recovered relatively free from the fatty acids of high polarity.

When the bulk of the acids of low polarity has crystallized out, the acids of high polarity together with a residue of the low polarity acids remain in solution. The acids left in solution can be recovered by diluting the solution with water until the acids separate out as an oily layer. The dilution is usually such that the concentration of sulfonate falls below 40%, or about 20% in the case of cumene sulfonates. To improve the purity of crystallized acids, the product obtained on the first crystallization can be recrystallized using further quantities of the same solvent.

Example 1: An aqueous solution of 50% by weight of sodium xylene sulfonate (SXS) was prepared and divided into three equal parts. In each of these was dissolved at 70°C. a proportion of tallow fatty acid as shown in the table. Each solution was allowed to cool for several hours to room temperature (20°C.). Saturated fatty acids crystallized and were filtered off. Water was then added to the filtrate until the unsaturated acids separated as an oily layer, which took place at a concentration of SXS to water of below 40% by weight. The oily layer was run off and the SXS solution was concentrated by evaporation to 50% strength for reuse.

Purification and Separation

The separated acids were washed free of traces of SXS and dried. The iodine values and yields of the saturated and unsaturated fractions are given in the following table:

Percent tallow fatty acid	10	20	30
Saturated acid fraction:			
Yield, percent	63	66	65.6
Iodine value	19.1	21.9	21.1
Unsaturated acid fraction:			
Yield, percent	37	34	34.4
Iodine value	89.0	89.8	90.6

Example 2: The procedure of Example 1 was repeated using a 30% solution of tallow fatty acid. The saturated acids fraction was then recrystallized by the same procedure. The iodine values and yields of the various fractions were as follows:

	Iodine value	Yield, percent
1st crystallisation:		
Saturated fraction	16.7	56.6
Unsaturated fraction	82.0	43.4
2nd crystallisation:		
Saturated fraction	4.6	83.2
Unsaturated fraction	76.8	16.8

Example 3: The procedure of Example 1 was repeated using a 30% solution of tallow fatty acid, but the solution was cooled in 1 hour. In this case the saturated fraction yielded 43.5% and had an I.V. of 6.8; the unsaturated fraction yielded 56.2% and had an I.V. of 74.8. This shows that quick cooling gives a purer saturated acid fraction, but in smaller yield.

Using Reactive Extraction with Amines

Separation of organic acids by reactive extraction with amines is accomplished in a process described by J.W. Crandall and R.C. Grimm; U.S. Patent 3,541,121; November 17, 1970; assigned to Union Carbide Corp. The method is one in which higher organic acids (4 to 16 carbon atoms) are separated from the products of partial oxidation of aliphatic hydrocarbons containing 1 to 16 carbon atoms. These partial oxidation products (known as "oxidate") are first washed with water to remove the lower acids (those containing 1 to 3 carbon atoms). The water washed oxidate is then contacted with an amine or ammonia to form the corresponding amine-acid (or ammonia-acid) complexes. These complexes are then thermally decomposed to liberate the acids.

The process broadly comprises contacting the aqueous solution of the amine with the oxidate in any suitable contacting zone such as a tray column or any other contacting device. This operation may be conducted continuously, semicontinuously or batchwise although, continuous operation is preferable. When operating in a continuous manner the aqueous solution of the amine is generally introduced near the top and the oxidate is introduced near the bottom of the contacting zone. The two streams will then flow in a countercurrent manner in the contacting zone and the amine-acid complexes are formed upon contact of the two streams. The complexes are simultaneously extracted by water and an aqueous phase containing these complexes is removed from the bottom of the contacting zone and an oil-phase containing the remaining partial oxidation products of the oxidate is removed overhead.

The reaction of the amine with the acid to form the corresponding amine-acid complexes and the simultaneous extraction of these complexes in water makes this a reactive extraction process. The aqueous phase which is withdrawn from the contacting zone is subjected to thermal decomposition at a suitable decomposition temperature to liberate the acids from the amine. Thus the acids are recovered in high quality and essentially free from other contaminating materials and the amine which is thus recovered is recycled to the contacting zone for further use. Suitable amines for the process are the primary, secondary and tertiary aliphatic, heterocyclic and aromatic amines. The order of the effectiveness of these amines is tertiary amine, secondary amines and primary amines, respectively.

The amines are generally dissolved in water or other suitable solvent, although water is preferred. When using solvents other than water, the solvent must be inert toward all the components in the oxidate and must be capable of preferentially dissolving the amine as well as the amine-acid complexes rather than the other partial oxidation products or the paraffins. The optimum concentration of the amine in the solution generally depends upon the particular amine which is employed, preferably ranging from 5 to 30 weight percent of the solution. The relative amounts of the amine and the acids in the contacting zone are not per se critical in this process.

The temperature and pressure are selected so that the materials in the contacting zone remain essentially in the liquid phase, in general, ranging from 10° to 60°C. and the pressure from 15 to 50 psia. Since the amine-acid complexes can be thermally decomposed to liberate the acids and the amine recovered for recycle to the contacting zone, the aqueous phase which is withdrawn from the contacting zone is subjected to a temperature from 100° to 200°C. in a distillation zone in which the acids are liberated from the amine and withdrawn from the bottom of this zone. The amine together with the solvent are distilled overhead and recycled to the contacting zone. The pressure in this thermal decomposition-distillation zone may vary from 15 to 50 psia.

Example 1: Approximately 4 liters of a mixture (oxidate) containing aliphatic hydrocarbons, organic acids, ketones, alcohols and esters, each containing 6 to 16 carbon atoms in the carbon chain, together with 500 ml. aqueous ammonia (28 weight percent) and 1,500 ml. water were charged to a large kettle. The mixture was agitated at room temperature (25° to 30°C.) and 14.7 psia for approximately 3 minutes and separated into two layers, a lower aqueous phase and an upper oil phase. The lower aqueous phase (approximately 2,620 ml.) was charged to a 3 liter kettle and distilled at atmospheric pressure to remove the ammonia and water. The overhead temperature during this distillation was 85° to 102°C., rising rapidly to 150° to 200°C. after removal of the ammonia and water.

Approximately 457 grams of residues (regenerated acids) was recovered from this kettle and its acid number determined to be 150 as compared to an acid number of 44 of the original feed, thus indicating that the acids were concentrated approximately 3.4 fold in this operation. "Acid number" refers to the milligrams of potassium hydroxide required to neutralize the free acid in a one gram sample.

Example 2: This example illustrates the continuous, countercurrent reactive extraction of the higher acids with trimethylamine. Approximately 11,124 grams of a mixture of aliphatic hydrocarbons, acid, ketones, alcohols and esters, each having 6 to 16 carbon atoms in its carbon chain was introduced at the rate of 930 grams per hour to the bottom of a multistage, York-Scheibel extraction column having 1 inch inside diameter and equipped with 11 equidistantly spaced paddles. Approximately 4,355 grams of an aqueous solution of trimethylamine (containing 12 weight percent of the amine) was introduced to the top of the column at the rate of approximately 365 grams per hour, and the two streams were contacted countercurrently at a temperature of 25° to 30°C.

A raffinate stream (oil-rich phase having an acid number of 0.41) was withdrawn from this column as compared to an acid number of 33 for the feed, indicating that approximately 99 weight percent of the acid in the fee has been removed. The extract (aqueous phase) from this column which amounted to approximately 6,024 grams was distilled batchwise in a laboratory distillation column equipped with five actual trays, at atmospheric pressure and to a reflux-to-make ratio of 1.0 until the overhead temperature reached 160°C. Approximately 1,408 grams of residues (regenerated acids) having an acid number of 254 were recovered from this distillation column. This indicates that the acids have been concentrated 7.7 times and that the regenerated acid represents 12.7 weight percent of the original feed.

Using Selective Crystallization

G.R. Payne, W.B. Campbell, and N.S. Yanick; U.S. Patent 3,541,122;

November 17, 1970; assigned to Kraftco Corporation describe a method for separating mixtures of fatty acid in which the mixture of fatty materials is formed at a temperature at which the mixture is substantially fluid. The mixture will include fatty materials having fatty acid residues with carbon chain lengths greater than 10 and may comprise glyceride materials, fatty acids or esters.

The mixture is then cooled by placing it under vacuum conditions and evaporating a lower boiling fluid in the presence of the fatty materials. The lower boiling fluid may or may not be in a mixture with the fatty materials. The cooling conditions are selected to establish a temperature in the mixture so that at least a part of the mixture forms a solid phase. The liquid portion of the mixture is then emulsified with an aqueous solution of a surface active material by adding the solution to the mixture. The liquid emulsion of fatty materials and the aqueous solution is then separated from the solid phase by any suitable solid-liquid separation technique, such as filtration or centrifugation.

The mixture of fatty materials to be separated is heated to a temperature such that the higher melting of the components of the mixture substantially loses its crystal structure. However, it is not necessary to heat the mixture to a temperature at which each of the components of the mixture is completely melted. For example, where a mixture of stearic acid and oleic acid is to be separated, the mixture of acids is preferably heated to a temperature of at least 90°F., but does not have to be heated to a temperature in excess of 120°F. at which temperature the stearic acid is substantially melted.

After the mixture of fatty materials has been heated to the desired temperature, the mixture is transferred to a chamber equipped to draw a vacuum. Vacuum equipment is provided for establishing a vacuum sufficient to effect desired cooling under the conditions of the system, the rate of cooling being dependent on the level and capacity of vacuum, i.e., the lower the absolute pressure the more rapid the rate of cooling will be to the extent that the vacuum producing means is capable of withdrawing the evaporated fluid. The rate of cooling is also related to the rate of evaporation of the lower boiling fluid from the mixture of fatty materials and the latent heat of vaporization of the fluid. In general, it is desirable to provide an absolute pressure of less thn 10 mm. Hg.

A suitable fluid is then evaporated in the presence of the mixture. The fluid may be introduced into the mixture of fatty materials prior to introduction of the mixture into the chamber or the fluid may be introduced separately into the chamber while the chamber is under vacuum. It is preferred that the fluid have a latent heat of vaporization of at least

150 calories per gram at standard conditions of temperature and pressure and a boiling temperature at atmospheric pressure of less than 200°C. A preferred fluid is water, however, other fluids having suitable evaporation characteristics in terms of the latent heat of vaporization and atmospheric boiling temperature may be used so long as the fluid is substantially immiscible with and does not react with the fatty materials.

Preferably, a fluid is selected and vacuum conditions are established which permit the fluid to be evaporated at a rate sufficient to effect a temperature drop in the mixture of from 25° to 120°F. per hour. Evaporation of fluid is continued until the mixture is cooled to the desired temperature which is selected so that at least part of the mixture forms a solid phase. The mass or total weight of the mixture of fatty materials which is to be cooled is not important. The rate of cooling depends on the rate at which fluid is evaporated per pound of mixture, consequently, large volumes of fatty materials may be rapidly cooled by this method which provides a solid phase with a crystal form which is readily adaptable to separation by filtration. Filtration or separation of the mixture of organic compounds now containing a solid phase and a liquid phase may be readily effected without further treatment.

However, a higher degree of separation of the liquid phase of the mixture from the solid phase may be effected by first forming an emulsion with an aqueous solution of a surface active material. During formation of the emulsion, the solid phase crystals are dispersed throughout the emulsion.

It is also desirable to limit the emulsifying action of the aqueous solution of a surface active material to provide an emulsification effect that is not so strong as to cause difficulty in the subsequent separation of the liquid phase from the aqueous solution. The emulsifying properties of the solution of surface active material can be influenced by the addition of electrolytes which are inert to the fatty materials of the mixture. Electrolytes in the form of magnesium, calcium, aluminum or other soluble metal salts are suitable.

As previously stated, the cooling method provides a solid phase of the higher melting components of the mixture of fatty materials that are suitable for separation by conventional solid-liquid techniques such as vacuum filtration or filter presses. The conditions of separation, such as temperature, level of aqueous solution of surface active material, method of separation, and other variables affect the properties of the liquid and the solid fatty material that are obtained.

Example: One thousand grams of tallow fatty acids were heated to a temperature of 115°F. to provide a liquefied mixture of fatty acids. The tallow fatty acids contained 49% saturated fatty acids and 51% unsaturated fatty acids. The liquefied fatty acids at a temperature of 115°F. were introduced into a glass container equipped with ports to permit drawing a vacuum and to introduce a liquid while vacuum was maintained in the container. A vacuum of 6 mm. Hg pressure was drawn in the chamber. Water was then introduced into the container through a port in the bottom of the container. The water was added at a level of 0.3 gram per gram of fatty acid over a period of 1.5 hours. During this time period the temperature of the fatty acids was reduced to 43°F.

One thousand grams of an aqueous solution containing 50 grams of magnesium sulfate and 1 gram of sodium lauryl sulfate was then added to the container after the vacuum had been broken. The aqueous solution had been chilled to the same temperature as the fatty acids, i.e., 43°F. prior to introduction into the container. The water was added slowly with constant stirring to provide an emulsion.

After the aqueous solution had been added, the mixture was stirred for 5 minutes to complete wetting of the solid crystals of saturated fatty acids. The emulsion, containing a dispersion of the solid crystals, was then transferred to a Büchner funnel lined with coarse filter paper. The aqueous emulsion containing the liquid unsaturated fatty acids was then separated from the solid crystals over a period of minutes, using a vacuum of 15 inches. The aqueous emulsion broke immediately after filtration. The liquid phases obtained from the filtration step were then allowed to set overnight in a steam bath. A liquid phase which was rich in oleic acid was then removed from the aqueous phase by means of a separatory funnel.

The titer of the liquid oleic acid rich phase was then determined by the procedure described in AOCS Method Tr-la-64. Titer is an arbitrary designation for the solidification temperature of a fatty material. The titer of the liquid oleic acid rich phase obtained was 2.5°C. The titer of commercially available oleic acid is not usually lower than 15° to 20°C.

Using Detergent Fractionation

In prior processes for the separation of liquid and fatty acid compound mixtures, the fatty acids which are to be separated are usually first completely melted and then chilled to the separating temperature. For the cooling of the fatty acid mixtures, scraper coolers (Votator) are generally employed. These involve cylindrical cooling devices through which the fatty acid mixture flows and in which the cooling surfaces which come into contact with the fatty acid material are kept free of deposits of solid fatty acids by means of moving or rotating scrapers. A crystalline mass is thus formed, and the further the starting material is cooled, the stiffer the resultant crystalline mass. Consequently, in order to carry out the separation, relatively sturdy scraper coolers are required because these mixtures are very stiff at the separating temperature, and also because the heat transfer between the coolant and the fatty acid mixture becomes poorer as the pasty consistency of the latter increases; as a result, either the throughput becomes low or disproportionately large cooling surfaces are required. This diminishing heat transfer cannot be improved by lowering the temperature of the coolant at will, because then not only the higher-melting fatty acids but also large amounts of lower-melting fatty acids which are supposed to remain in the liquid fraction will be separated out at the excessively cooled walls of the cooler.

H. Hartmann and W. Stein; U.S. Patent 3,549,676; December 22, 1970; assigned to Henkel & Cie GmbH, Germany have found that difficulties in the process of separating mixtures of fatty acid materials can be avoided by carrying out the crystallization in two stages; i.e., if the starting fatty acid material is cooled in a first stage in the conventional manner to the extent that only a portion of the fatty acid that is to be separated in solid form crystallizes out, and if, in the second stage, the further reduction of the temperature of the fluid crystal mass formed in the first stage is brought about by forming a dispersion of this fluid crystal mass in an aqueous solution containing a wetting agent and having a temperature lower than that of the fluid crystal mass.

It has proven advantageous to carry out the separation by first chilling the fatty acid mixture in a standard cooling apparatus, such as a scraper cooler, to such an extent that 40 to 70% of the total solid fatty acid to be removed is crystallized out. When this condition has been achieved, the fluid to slurry-like liquid fatty acid containing solid fatty acid particles in a second stage is mixed with a chilled aqueous solution of wetting agent. The quantity and temperature of the aqueous solution of wetting agent is adjusted so that, after the temperature exchange has taken place between the fatty acid mixture and the wetting agent solution, the desired separating temperature is reached.

Since the aqueous solutions of wetting agent often contain electrolytes which reduce the freezing point of water, the temperature of the wetting agent solution can easily be reduced even below the freezing point of water. If necessary, crushed ice can also be stirred into the fatty acid mixture. The vessel in which the precooled fatty acid and cold wetting agent solution are mixed together should be insulated against thermal exchange with the surroundings. It is not necessary to adjust the desired final temperature in this stage of the process. The quantity of the aqueous solution of the wetting agent employed amounts to 100 to 200% of the weight of the fatty acid mixture being separated. The temperature of the wetting agent solution depends on the temperature of the fatty acid added, the desired final temperature, and the ratio of the amounts of fatty acid mixture to wetting agent solution used. The process can be combined with a process in which a wetting agent solution is used for the dispersal of the mixture of fatty acid crystals and liquid fatty acid in which the concentration of wetting agent is greater than it is to be in the final dispersion. The dispersion is then brought to the final concentration by the addition of water or a more dilute wetting agent solution. In this process, too, the dispersion of the fatty acid mixture in the wetting agent solution can be cooled down to the separating temperature if the latter has not yet been reached by mixing with the chilled wetting agent solution.

The process facilitates the cooling of the fatty acid mixture and simplifies it by eliminating a portion of the otherwise necessary scraper cooling equipment and also increases throughput. While the wetting agent solution has to be chilled before it is combined with the fatty acid mixture; this does not produce any separation of crystals, so that scraper coolers are not required for the cooling of the wetting agent solution. Furthermore, the transfer of heat from the fatty acid mixture through the wetting agent solution to the cooling brine is better than in the case of the direct cooling of the fatty acid mixture by the cooling brine. As a result, the process makes possible a highly efficient separation.

Example: The continuous cooling of a fatty acid mixture was conducted in 5 scraper coolers arranged in series and having a total cooling area of 20 m.^{2}. The first two scraper coolers were cooled with water having a temperature of 20° to 25°C., and the last three were cooled with brine having a temperature from 10° to -2°C. From the scraper coolers, the thick flowing fatty acid mixture was introduced into the first chamber of a trough which was divided by perforated partitions into five chambers arranged in tandem. In these chambers, the wetting agent solution or the wetting agent solution diluent was added to the fatty acid mixture. The material emerging from the last chamber in the trough was separated in a full jacket centrifuge into liquid fatty acid as the lighter layer, and dispersion of solid fatty acid in wetting agent solution as the heavier layer.

In a first experiment which corresponds to the procedure of the prior art, a distilled tallow fatty acid (acid number, 206; saponification number, 208; iodine number, 51.1; hardening point, 41.0°C.) was chilled from 45° to 5°C. The maximum fatty acid throughput that was possible under these conditions amounted to 1,050 kg./hr.; i.e., if the throughput was increased, the fatty acid was no longer chilled to the required end temperature of 5°C. The emerging fatty acid was thoroughly mixed in the first chamber of the trough with 5 kg./hr. of a 50% solution of sodium decyl sulfate and 400 l./hr. of 2% $MgSO_4$ solution, both at 5°C. Another

400 l./hr. of 2% MgSO4 solution at 5°C. was fed to each of the following chambers. Accordingly, approximately 2,000 l./hr. of wetting agent solution at 5°C. was consumed in the dispersing of the 1,050 kg./hr. of fatty acid mixture. The liquid fraction produced in the centrifuge had a turbidity point of 4°C., while the iodine number of the solid fraction amounted to 16.3.

In another test, the procedure was according to the process. The throughput of fatty acid was increased to 2,000 kg./hr. Since the coolant throughput and its temperature was unaltered, the fatty acid emerging from the final scraper cooler had a temperature of 19°C., at which the fatty acid flowed into the first chamber of the trough. There, 10 kg./hr. of 50% sodium decyl sulfate solution and 800 l./hr. of 2% MgSO4 solution at 0°C. were added. The remaining chambers were each supplied with 800 l/hr. of 2% MgSO4 solution at 0°C., so that the 2,000 kg./hr. of fatty acid mixture was dispersed into approximately 4,000 l./hr. of wetting agent solution.

The dispersion left the trough, which was refrigerated externally with brine at -2°C., at a temperature of 5°C. After separation in the full jacket centrifuge and removal of the solid fatty acid from the wetting agent solution, an olein having a turbidity point of 4°C. and a stearin having an iodine number of 16.8 were recovered. Thus, the fatty acid fractions obtained had substantially the same characteristics as those obtained by the prior art process; the throughput, however, had been approximately doubled in the same apparatus.

Using Crystal Modifiers

This process by D.D. Staker, R.H. Plantholt, and D.J. Kriege; U.S. Patent 3,649,657; March 14, 1972; assigned to Emery Industries, Inc. concerns crystal modifiers and method for separation by crystallization of mixtures of fatty materials of differing degrees of saturation. The fatty materials which can be separated include long chain fatty acids such as stearic acid and oleic acid and glyceride fats and oils. The method is particularly applicable to the selective crystallization of saturated fatty acids from mixtures of saturated and unsaturated fatty acids obtained from glyceride materials of animal or vegetable origin, such as tallow or other fats and oils.

These crystal modifiers are polymeric esters which are prepared by the reaction of a polybasic acid with a fatty acid ester of a polyhydric alcohol. The process involves forming a solution of the materials to be separated and the crystal modifier, and then cooling the solution to precipitate out the more saturated constituent. The polybasic acids which may be used in the preparation of the crystal modifiers are aliphatic or aromatic polybasic acids, usually dibasic acids and some tribasic acids having from 6 to 54 carbon atoms. The fatty acid esters which are used in the acidolysis reaction employed to prepare the crystal modifiers may be glycerides of either animal or vegetable origin. The fatty acid moiety may be a saturated or unsaturated aliphatic fatty acid having from 8 to 22 carbon atoms and the alcohol moiety may be a polyhydric alcohol having from 2 to 6 carbon atoms and from 2 to 6 hydroxyl groups. The preferred fatty acid esters are glycerides such as hydrogenated tallow and hydrogenated vegetable oils. The preferred polybasic acids for the acidolysis reaction are the dibasic dimer acids having 36 carbon atoms.

The amount of polybasic acid which is reacted with the fatty acid ester to produce the crystal modifiers varies over a wide range and is dependent to a large extent upon the dibasic acid employed. Usually from 5 to 50% by weight of polybasic acid, based on the total weight of the polybasic acid and fatty acid ester reactants, is used. Generally speaking, lesser amounts of the lower molecular weight dibasic acids such as adipic, azelaic, or phthalic acid are required than dimer acid or trimer acid. The preferred crystal modifiers are prepared by reacting 25 to 35% by weight dimer acid with hydrogenated tallow when tallow fatty acids are separated, the amount of dimer acid being based upon the total weight of the dimer and tallow.

The acidolysis reaction is performed by heating the polybasic acid and fatty acid ester in a reaction vessel at a temperature of 250° to 300°C., usually under reduced pressure of 1 to 5 mm. Hg. During the reaction the polybasic acid replaces some of the monobasic acids in the glyceride structure and forms the modifiers of this process. The structure of the crystal modifiers is not known although they are believed to be higher molecular weight esters containing 2 or more polyol units. The physical form of the modifier is generally a waxy amorphous solid having a higher viscosity than the original mixture.

The monobasic acids which are liberated in the reaction may be evaporated and collected by distillation. When approximately 70 to 90% by equivalent weight of the polybasic acid charged is removed in the form of monobasic acids in the distillate, the reaction is considered complete. The reaction may take place for 3 to 24 hours depending upon the temperature used and the polybasic acid and fatty acid esters which are used in the preparation of the crystal modifiers. Shorter periods generally produce a less effective modifier and longer periods than 24 hours do not enhance the quality of the modifier. In general it is desirable to use as the ester reactant, one having as the fatty acid moiety a fatty acid of the same chain length as the chain length of the fatty acid fraction being crystallized.

The separation process is conducted by first forming a solution of the fatty materials. An organic solvent, preferably a polar organic solvent, is employed as a solvent medium. The crystal forming characteristics of the resulting solutions are such that, with most fatty materials, the concentration of fatty material in the starting solution should not exceed 35 to 50% by weight of the solution. After the solution of the fatty material has been formed, the solution is chilled. The amount of crystal modifier to be employed will range from 0.5 to 1.5% based on the weight of fatty material present in the solution.

The actual separation of the fatty material into its component fractions is carried out by chilling the solution containing a crystal modifier to a temperature below the precipitation temperature of the saturated fatty material in the solvent. A sharp separation of the saturated fatty material occurs, the saturated material precipitating in the form of readily filterable crystals.

The separation can be effectively performed in a scraped surface heat exchanger such as a Votator. The solution is rapidly chilled from a temperature of as high as 35°C. to a temperature at which the more saturated fatty material precipitates in the form of crystals, usually a temperature of -10°C. The precipitated crystals are collected on a filter forming a "filter cake" and then are washed by solvent. The filter cake is collected and evaporated leaving the saturated fatty material. The unsaturated components of the fatty material mixture remain in solution and are collected as a filtrate. Evaporation of the filtrate enables recovery of the unsaturated components.

Examples 1 through 18: A number of crystal modifiers were prepared in an acidolysis reaction by reacting polybasic acids with fatty acid esters of polyhydric alcohols. The acidolysis reaction was performed by charging the polybasic acid and fatty acid ester of a polyhydric alcohol into a reaction vessel and heating the reactants for an extended period of time of 3 to 10 hours. During the reaction, monobasic acid was liberated and it was removed from the reaction and collected by distillation.

The reactions for the most part were conducted at temperatures ranging from 250° to 300°C., the lower temperature range being generally used initially with the temperature being allowed to increase as the reaction progressed. In Example 15, in which phthalic anhydride and a mixed glyceride were used to prepare the crystal modifier, a solvent toluene, was used to aid the reaction. The crystal modifier shown in Example 17 was prepared by reacting the azelaic acid and hydrogenated tallow at a temperature of 250°C. and at a pressure of 35 mm. Hg for 5 hours. The monobasic acids which were formed during the reaction were then stripped

TABLE 1: PREPARATION OF CRYSTAL MODIFIERS

Example number	Polybasic acid weight, grams	Type	Fatty acid ester of polyhydric alcohol Wt., grams	Type	Percent by wt. of polybasic acid based on total wt. of reactants	Time of reaction, hours
1	165	Dimer [1]	335	Hydrogenated tallow	35	4
2	125	Dimer	375	....do....	25	4
3	300	....do....	300	....do....	50	10
4	200	....do....	800	Hydrogenated stearic acid residue [2]	10	2.5
5	200	....do....	800	Hydrogenated stearic acid residue	20	5.5
6	100	....do....	900	....do....	10	3
7	100	....do....	900	....do....	10	6
8	100	....do....	900	....do....	10	9
9	50	....do....	950	....do....	5	5
10	200	Trimer [3]	400	Hydrogenated tallow	33	8
11	61	Trimer	345	....do....	12.5	6
12	84	....do....	309	....do....	21	6
13	100	Dimer	400	Coconut oil	20	6
14	165	....do....	335	Olive oil	33	3
15	110	Phthalic anhydride	500	Mixed glyceride [4]	18	4
16	43	Dimer	288	Ethylene glycol distearate	15	5
17	188	Azelaic	850	Hydrogenated tallow	18	5
18	66	Adipic	320	....do....	17	4

[1] Dimer acid used was Empol 1018, a polymerized tall oil fatty acid having about 83% by weight C_{36} dibasic acid and about 17% by weight C_{54} tribasic acid.
[2] Stearic acid residue is a mixture containing predominantly monoglycerides, diglycerides, triglycerides and polymerized glycerides plus small amounts of stearic acid remaining as residue after the distillation of stearic acid.
[3] The trimer acid used was Empol 1040, a polymerized tall oil fatty acid having about 80-90% by weight C_{54} tribasic acid and 10-20% by weight C_{36} dibasic acid.
[4] A mixture of 25% monoglycerides, 50% diglycerides, and 25% triglycerides.

at a pressure of 1 to 5 mm. Hg and at a temperature of 250° to 300°C. The crystal modifier shown in Example 18 was prepared by reacting the adipic acid and hydrogenated tallow for 4 hours under a carbon dioxide blanket at 240°C. The monobasic acids formed in that acidolysis reaction were stripped at the end of the 4 hour period at a pressure of 1 to 5 mm. Hg and at a temperature of 250°C.

Examples 19 through 51: A number of tests were conducted to determine the effectiveness of the crystal modifiers shown in Table 1 in the separation of fatty acid mixtures into their component fractions. The results of these tests are shown in Table 2. The crystal modifier type shown in Table 2 refers to the example number of the modifier shown in Table 1.

The tests were conducted by first forming a solution of a fatty acid mixture, the crystal modifier, and a solvent, either methanol, acetone or 2-nitropropane. The resulting solution was then cooled in a stirred, scraping crystallizer to from 0° to -20°C. depending upon the solvent and the fatty material to be removed. The resulting slurries were then filtered using a Büchner funnel while maintaining a vacuum of 5 psi until no liquid layer was visible above the crystalline layer. The resulting filter cake was then washed using 200 parts by weight of the solvent which was used to form the solution for each 100 parts of the solid cake in the funnel.

Various tests were run on the washed filter cake to determine (1) its content of solids, (2) its yield, and (3) the iodine value of the filter cake solids. The solvent was removed by heating on a steam bath followed by drying on a hot plate. A high solids content in the cake is desirable, for this indicates a correspondingly low content of solvent to be evaporated and returned to the crystallizer unit. One of the most significant features of this process is the high percentage of solids in cake which are achievable. A low iodine value is desirable because it indicates the effectiveness of the separation process, a low content of occluded unsaturated acid in the washed and dried solids fraction showing good separation. In the runs involving separation of tallow fatty acids, an iodine value of approximately 8 to 11 is regarded as satisfactory, though the values obtained in plant use might run somewhat higher (or lower), depending upon the nature of the equipment employed, and the severity of the washing step(s).

TABLE 2

Example Number	Crystal modifier from Table I	Feedstock	Solvent	Filtration temp. (°C.)	Amount of crystal modifier used in wt. percent	Percent by wt. of solids in cake	Percent by wt. fatty material in solution	Percent yield of more saturated component by wt.	Iodine value
19	1	Undistilled PFA [1]	Methanol [2]	−10	1	69.67	35		8.5
20	3	Undistilled PFA	Methanol	−10	1	51.8	35		
21	1	Hydrogenated tall oil [3]	do	−10	1	54.3	30		7.1
22	1	Undistilled PFA	do	−10	0.5	52.1	30	44.7	
23	1	do	do	−10	1.5	63.7	35	45.5	9.3
24	1	Distilled PFA	do	−10	1	44.8	35	47.8	
25	2	do	do	−10	1	41.5	35	49.7	9.5
26	None	Fleshing grease	do	−10	None	26.0	30	37.9	9.4
27	1	do	do	−10	1	61.0	30	38.7	11.4
28	(4)	do	do	−10	1	34.2	30	37.5	8.4
29	1	Undistilled PFA	Acetone	−20	1	63.6	25	45.2	7.2
30	(5)	do	do	−20	1	46.0	25	44.7	4.8
31	None	do	2-NP [6]	0	None	17.4	25	44.7	
32	1	do	2-NP	0	1	21.1	25	43.2	
33	11	Tallow	2-NP	−10	1	21.1	20	55.2	
34	3	Undistilled PFA	Methanol	−10	1	51.8	35	45.1	
35	10	do	do	−10	1	59.3	35	45.8	
36	14	Tall oil fatty acids	do	−12	1	32.0	20	29.5	100.0
37	4	Undistilled PFA	do	−10	1	57.7	35	45.5	
38	5	do	do	−10	1	69.4	35	45.7	8.2
39	(5)	do	do	−10	1	47.3	35	45.3	
40	6	do	do	−10	1	65.2	35		
41	7	do	do	−10	1	69.8	35		
42	8	do	do	−10	1	68.4	35		
43	9	do	do	−10	1	65.3	35		
44	13	do	do	−10	1	32.5	35	45.6	
45	9	do	do	−10	1	61.2	35	46.1	
46	11	do	do	−10	1	54.7	35	45.9	
47	12	do	do	−10	1	63.3	35	46.6	
48	17	do	do	−10	1	47.5	45		
49	18	do	do	−10	1	64.2	45		
50	15	do	do	−10	1	65.0	45		
51	16	do	do	−10	1	38.4	35		

[1] Pressure split fatty acids.
[2] 92.5% by weight methanol, 7.5% water.
[3] The C₁₈ fatty acid distillate recovered from polymerization of tall oil fatty acids.
[4] Hydrogenated tallow.
[5] Hydrogenated stearic acid residue.
[6] 2-nitro-propane.

From the data presented in Table 2, it may be seen that the crystal modifiers enable the use of solutions having a far greater concentration of fatty acid than would otherwise be possible, while still obtaining a solid phase which filters well, is high in solids content, has a good yield, and has a desirably low iodine value. The process can also be used in the separation of unsaturated acids such as oleic acid from more unsaturated acids such as linoleic acid or linolenic acid, and it is useful in the separation of more saturated fractions from less saturated fractions of glycerides and like materials.

SIMULTANEOUS SEPARATION AND PURIFICATION

Countercurrent Process Using NH_4OH

F.J.F. van der Plas; U.S. Patent 3,151,139; September 29, 1964; assigned to Shell Oil Company describes a process which relates to the recovery and purification of monocarboxylic acids of secondary and tertiary character obtained by the reaction of carbon monoxide and water with olefins, or by reaction of carbon monoxide and water with paraffin waxes together with hydrogen acceptors. These secondary and tertiary monocarboxylic acids are recovered in a high state of purity from these crude mixtures by a simple but highly efficient continuous selective liquid extraction procedure in which solvents and adjuvants are continuously recovered within the system.

The crude mixtures containing the aliphatic alpha-branched secondary and tertiary monocarboxylic acids in admixture with organic impurities comprising hydrocarbons and reaction products of polymeric character are subjected to liquid phase extraction with aqueous ammonium hydroxide flowing countercurrent to a water-immiscible organic solvent. This procedure separates an aqueous phase composed of ammonium salts of monocarboxylic acids from the organic phase comprising the solvent and organic impurities. The aqueous phase is then subjected to an elevated temperature which decomposes the ammonium salts liberating the monocarboxylic acids.

The strength and relative amount of the aqueous ammonium hydroxide solution will vary depending upon the specific composition of the material being extracted and the organic solvent used. The ammonium hydroxide solution is, however, always used in concentrations and amount providing a stoichiometrical excess of ammonia over that required to react with the monocarboxylic acid content of the crude organic acid charge to the system. The water-immiscible solvent used may be a substantially aromatic-free saturated hydrocarbon solvent. The extraction is carried out at substantially normal conditions of temperatures and pressures. Extraction is effected in conventional equipment for continuous countercurrent extraction.

Example: A fraction of the products obtained by thermal cracking of paraffins in the vapor phase in the presence of steam, which fraction consisted of alkenes having 8 to 10 carbon atoms was selectively hydrogenated to convert any dienes present into alkenes. After this hydrogenation the alkenes constituted 76% by weight of the mixture, viz 39% by weight of linear, 20% by weight of branched and 17% by weight of cyclic alkenes. The remainder of the mixture consisted of saturated hydrocarbons (17% by weight) and aromatics (7% by weight).

The olefinic fraction was converted to monocarboxylic acids by reaction with carbon monoxide and water at 60°C. in the presence of a catalyst consisting of H_3PO_4, BF_3 and H_2O. The reaction mixture was kept at constant volume and maintained at substantially constant composition by recycling and control of rate of feed and product removal. A monocarboxylic acid phase was separated from reactor effluence by stratification, washed at 40°C. with water and then at 20°C. with aqueous sodium bicarbonate. The resulting crude acid mixture consisted essentially of (alpha-branched) secondary and tertiary aliphatic monocarboxylic acids having 9 to 11 carbon atoms to the molecule in admixture with organic impurities which consisted essentially of hydrocarbons including unconverted charge, polymers and a lesser amount of other reaction products, the complexity of which does not permit ready determination.

The crude carboxylic acid mixture so obtained was subjected to contact with aqueous ammonium hydroxide in an extraction column of the rotary contractor type in the presence of gasoline as secondary solvent. The column was 2 meters long, had a capacity of 2 liters and was full of gasoline at the start up. The gasoline used had a boiling range of 95° to 115°C. and was introduced into the lower part of the column at the rate of 0.5 l./hr. The aqueous ammonium hydroxide, containing 6% by weight of ammonia, was introduced into the top of the column at the rate of 0.7 l./hr. The crude monocarboxylic acid was charged at 0.3 l./hr. A gasoline phase was taken continuously from the top of the column and distilled. The distillation residue consisted essentially of the organic impurities in the crude monocarboxylic acid charge and contained only 0.2 to 0.3% of the desired monocarboxylic acids.

A liquid phase, consisting essentially of aqueous solution of the ammonium salts of the monocarboxylic acids charged and ammonium hydroxide, was taken continuously from the lower part of the column and stratified. The aqueous phase comprising the ammonium salts of the monocarboxylic acids was subjected to continuous distillation at 100°C. and atmospheric pressure, thereby driving off ammonia. Distillation bottoms consisting essentially of free monocarboxylic acids were passed downwardly through a packed column maintained at 170°C. to drive off residual ammonia and water.

The yield of essentially pure alpha-branched monocarboxylic acids so obtained was 99.5% (nitrogen content 0.2 to 0.3% by weight). The monocarboxylic acids were fractionated under reduced pressure and an overhead fraction consisting of secondary and tertiary monocarboxylic acids having 9 to 11 carbon atoms to the molecule, and constituting 93% of the total acid charge to the fractional distillation, was taken overhead. This overhead fraction had an acid number of 326, a nitrogen content of 100 and a Hazen color of less than 50. Bottoms from the fractionation were found to consist predominantly of alpha-branched monocarboxylic acids having 18 to 20 carbon atoms to the molecule.

Using Acidic Clay and Boron Trifluoride Etherate

D.E. Leavens and J.M. Derfer; U.S. Patent 3,396,182; August 6, 1968; assigned to SCM Corporation describe a process for purifying and recovering crude fatty acids by recrystallization of the crude acids from liquid normal alkane solution, further purification of the recrystallized acids in liquid normal alkane solution with an acidic reagent such as boron trifluoride, removal of the acidic reagent, and recrystallization of the purified fatty acids from the liquid normal alkane solution.

Generally when the starting material is a tall oil distillation heads-cut, the crude saturated higher fatty acid fraction will consist primarily of palmitic acid. Small quantities of lauric and stearic acid and substantially larger quantities of higher unsaturated fatty acids such as oleic and linoleic acids and of an unsaponifiable material of varied and undetermined composition are also often present in the fraction. The crystalline fatty acid fraction is dissolved in a liquid nonaromatic hydrocarbon, any which is relatively inert and which is a solvent for higher saturated fatty acid may be used. Since the process involves subsequent fatty acid crystallization, liquid nonaromatic hydrocarbons boiling between 40° and 200°C. have been found to be advantageous.

The crystalline fatty acid fraction can be dissolved in the liquid aliphatic hydrocarbon by mixing one volume part of fatty acid fraction with from 2 to 4 volume parts of the liquid hydrocarbon and heating at a temperature below the boiling point of the hydrocarbon, usually between 50° to 75°C., when mineral or textile spirits are used, until solution occurs. After dissolving the fatty acid fraction in the hydrocarbon, fatty acid crystals are obtained by cooling the solution to a temperature of -10° to 10°C.

After crystallization from the liquid hydrocarbon, the saturated higher fatty acid crystals are separated from the liquid by filtration, centrifugation, decantation, etc. It is desirable to wash the crystals with cold liquid hydrocarbon and the higher fatty acid crystals will then be substantially white and will have a faint characteristic fatty acid odor. However, if crystals so treated are stored at room temperature for several weeks, they will darken and take on a more intense and rancid fatty acid odor (presumably due to the presence of unknown chromophoric and osmorphoric compounds and other impurities). Thus the crystals, while initially white and of low odor, will often undergo chemical changes, an increase in odor, and will also form color bodies upon storage.

The supernatant liquid hydrocarbon from which the fatty acid crystals are recovered is brown in color and contains unsaturated fatty acids and colored compounds which are believed to be phenolic in character. The separated crystals are then redissolved in additional liquid hydrocarbon in the concentrations and within the temperature ranges employed in forming the previously described solution.

The second solution is then treated with a small amount of acidic reagent, preferably of the Lewis acid type, which is substantially insoluble in the hydrocarbon solvent and which is also incapable of undergoing a chemical reaction with the higher fatty acid and the liquid hydrocarbon solvent. Useful acidic reagents include mineral acids, certain acidic metal salts and organic derivatives of these acidic clays and mixtures of these acidic reagents can also be employed in conjunction with a lower aliphatic aldehyde.

The amount of acidic reagent may vary depending upon the volume of solution, the concentration of fatty acid dissolved therein, the residual impurities initially present and the particular reagent employed. Generally, from 0.25 to 10% by weight, based on the weight of the fatty acid, of acidic reagent can be used.

The treatment time of the hydrocarbon solution with the acidic reagent may vary considerably depending upon the amount of impurities (e.g., chromophoric bodies and odor producing materials) in the solution as well as the (volume) of the solution employed. Generally, the time will be from 30 to 180 minutes, the longer treatment times corresponding to larger quantities of solution and more impure solutions. After completion of the treatment, the reagent phase is separated from the solution phase by filtration, centrifugation, decantation, etc.

Recrystallization of the fatty acid is then effected by cooling the liquid hydrocarbon to a temperature of -10° to 10°C. The fatty acid crystals are then conventionally separated from the liquid hydrocarbon and thoroughly washed with fresh cooled (-10° to 10°C.) liquid hydrocarbon. Then, the crystals are heated either at atmospheric pressure or in vacuo to remove residual hydrocarbon. The resulting fatty acid product (palmitic acid when the starting material is a tall oil fatty acid fraction) is of greater than 96% purity. The material has a white color and an extremely faint characteristic color, which upon storage under ambient conditions for prolonged periods of time (e.g., up to 3 months or longer) does not darken or undergo an increase in odor.

Example: Five kilograms of a tall oil heads-cut containing 63.3% of palmitic acid (as measured by vapor phase chromatography) was centrifuged to remove excess liquid. After decantation of the liquid, a crude, brown, wet crystalline solid weighing 4.2 kg. was obtained. One kilogram of the solids was dissolved in 3 kg. of textile spirits having a boiling point of 79°C. by mixing the solids with the spirits and heating the mixture to 75°C. until complete solution occurred. The resulting solution was then cooled with gentle stirring to -5°C. in an ice bath until no further crystallization occurred.

The mother liquor was filtered off and 826 grams of crystalline palmitic acid (analyzed at 96% pure by vapor phase chromatography) were obtained. The crystals were then dissolved in 2.5 liters of additional textile spirits consisting of 1 liter of mother liquor and 1.5 liters of fresh textile spirits, by heating the textile spirits and dispersed crystals to a temperature of 65°C. To the resultant solution was added, with agitation provided by a mechanical stirrer, 32.5 grams of Filtrol, a finely divided acid activated montmorillonite clay and 0.9 gram of paraformaldehyde to form a dispersion containing the solution of plamitic acid dissolved in the textile spirits in which there was dispersed a finely divided acid-activated clay and the paraformaldehyde.

The heating and agitation were continued for 150 minutes after which the dispersion was cooled to a temperature about 40°C. The clay was separated from the solution by filtration through a Büchner funnel. The solution, which was a water white color, was then cooled to -10°C. to crystallize the palmitic acid. The textile spirits were decanted from the palmitic acid crystals and the crystals were washed with cold (-5°C.) fresh textile spirits.

The excess residual textile spirits were then removed from the palmitic acid by distillation at reduced pressure (10 mm. Hg) at 40°C. A yield of 750 grams of palmitic acid, which analyzed (using vapor phase chromatography) at 98% purity was obtained. The crystals were white and had a faint characteristic fatty acid odor and an iodine value of 0.1. Upon storage for three months at 30°C., no significant change in the color and odor of the crystals was detected. When the above process was repeated using white mineral spirits in place of textile spirits substantially the same results were obtained. However, the yield of palmitic acid was reduced by 30%. The white spirits employed had a boiling point of 160°C.

COMPANY INDEX

The company names listed below are given exactly as they appear in the patents, despite name changes, mergers and acquisitions which have, at times, resulted in the revision of a company name.

Alcolac Chemical Corp. - 265
Argus Chemical Corp. - 284
Armour Industrial Chemical Co. - 116, 135, 137
BP Chemicals Ltd. - 115
Badische Anilin- & Soda-Fabrik AG - 41
Carad Corp. - 165
Celanese Corp. - 123
Commercial Solvents Corp. - 177, 216
Continental Oil Co. - 109, 153, 156, 296
Deutsche Akademie der Wissenschaften zu Berlin - 294
Diamond Alkali Co. - 181
Diamond Shamrock Corp. - 233
Distillers Co., Ltd. - 112
Du Pont - 146, 205, 301, 326
Dynamit Nobel AG - 250, 314
Eastman Kodak Co. - 273
Emery Industries, Inc. - 323, 327, 339
Esso Research & Engineering Co. - 21, 29, 32, 33, 37, 54, 91, 144, 199, 312
Ethyl Corp. - 42, 86, 94, 102, 106, 129, 251, 254, 257
Farbenfabriken Bayer AG - 186
General Electric Co. - 141
Glidden Co. - 303, 304
Th. Goldschmidt AG - 271
Gulf Research & Development Co. - 9, 169, 260, 262
Halcon International, Inc. - 245, 246
Hardman & Holden Ltd. - 239, 274
Henkel & Cie. GmbH - 337
Hoffmann-La Roche Inc. - 179
Imperial Chemical Industries Ltd. - 35, 196
Knapsack AG - 288
Kraftco Corp. - 334

Lever Brothers Co. - 70, 194, 310, 317
M & T Chemicals, Inc. - 278
Marchon Products Ltd. - 330
Minnesota Mining & Mfg. Co. - 248
Monsanto Co. - 57, 60
Morton International, Inc. - 297
National Lead Co. - 242
National Research Development Corp. - 183
Osterreichische Stickstoffwerke AG - 221
Procter & Gamble Co. - 158, 161, 209, 267
Rhone-Poulenc SA - 190, 218
Ruhrchemie AG - 65
SCM Corp. - 346
Schering AG - 73
Schuyler Development Corp. - 168
Shell Oil Co. - 2, 15, 21, 26, 80, 139, 227, 320, 344
Sinclair Refining Co. - 63
Sinclair Research, Inc. - 281
Standard Oil Co. - 5, 75, 78
Stepan Chemical Co. - 131
Studiengesellschaft Kohle mbH - 68
Teijin Ltd. - 212
Tenneco Chemicals, Inc. - 306, 309
Texaco Inc. - 23, 83
Toyo Koatsu Industries, Inc. - 97
Union Carbide Corp. - 99, 331
Union Oil Co. - 45, 50, 61
Union Oil Co. of California - 151
U.S. Secretary of Agriculture - 12, 163, 175, 193, 223, 226, 291, 311, 319
Universal Oil Products Co. - 120
Upjohn Co. - 328
Victor Wolf Ltd. - 186
Wacker-Chemie GmbH - 149

INVENTOR INDEX

Achard, R.V.J., 218
Adams, B.F., 181
Alders, L., 21
Anderson, J.E., 9
Applewhite, T.H., 291
Artman, N.R., 267
Ashworth, P.J., 35
Bagley, M.O., 175, 226
Bailey, P.S., 91
Bartlett, J.H., 144
Beal, R.E., 319
Bearden, R., Jr., 37, 54, 312
Becker, M., 245
Bennett, E.J., 326
Berry, C.B., 129
Bier, G., 250
Bittler, K., 41
Bondar, L.S., 189
Boyd, W.T., 32, 33
Bryan, T.T., 248
Bücher, K., 65
Butler, C.G., 183
Butt, W.D., 194
Callow, R.K., 183
Campbell, W.B., 333
Campen, J.P., 26
Castner, C.S., 168
Chabardes, P.J.A., 190
Chafetz, H., 23
Chao, T.S., 281
Chodsky, S.V., 265
Closson, R.D., 42
Cotton, S.M., 62
Craddock, J.H., 57, 60
Crandall, J.W., 331
Craske, J.D., 317
Cunder, J., 233
D'Addieco, A.A., 205
Davies, J.F., 70
Davis, D.D., 146
De Mott, D.N., 161
Derfer, J.M., 346
Devine, J., 70
de Vries, R., 21
Diamond, M.J., 223
Dimond, H.L., 260, 262
Douros, J.D., Jr., 199
Doyle, W.C., Jr., 309
Dubeck, M., 102, 106

Duke, R.B., Jr., 273
Eiter, K., 186
Eller, W.R., 251
Ellert, H.G., 29, 32
Ellis, A.F., 169
Elson, G.W., 196
Fanning, R.J., 257
Fenton, D.M., 50, 61, 151
Fields, E.K., 75, 78
Fishman, A.E., 254
Franke, N.W., 9
Frankenfeld, J.W., 199
Fray, G.I., 320
Freeland, J.W., 231
Friedman, B.S., 62
Furman, K.E., 2
Galefaix, R., 310
Gensike, R., 294
Geraci, J., 265
Gordon, N.D., 137
Grimm, R.C., 331
Grimme, W., 173
Haage, K., 294
Hammerberg, E.S., 135
Hampton, B.L., 303, 304
Harson, S.E., 238, 274
Hartel, H., 250
Hartmann, H., 337
Hay, A.S., 141
Hecker, A.C., 284
Heckmaier, J., 149
Hendricks, J.G., 242
Henle, W.K., 227
Hershman, A., 57, 60
Hobbs, C.C., Jr., 123
Honda, Y., 212
Howe, R., 196
Hülsmann, H.L., 314, 316
Ihrman, K.G., 42
Ishimoto, S., 212
Jacks, T.J., 193
Jaeger, R.H., 320
Jason, E.F., 75, 78
Johnston, D.L., 2
Johnston, N.C., 183
Jones, D.F., 196
Kamlet, J., 158
Keblys, K.A., 106
Kebrich, L.M., 242

Inventor Index

Kenney, H.E., 311
Kjonaas, M., 281
Klere, J., 310
Knight, H.M., 5
Koch, H., 68
Koebner, A., 330
Kollar, J., 246
Koster, R., 173
Kreuz, K.L., 83
Kriege, D.J., 339
Kunstle, G., 149
Kurhajec, G.A., 2
Lachowicz, D.R., 83
Lally, R.E., 233
Leavens, D.E., 346
Lee, R.J., 5
Leebrick, J.R., 278
LeMaster, E.J., 88
Lippincott, S.B., 144
Lohman, R.C., 29, 32, 33
Lunde, K.E., 165
Lundeen, A.J., 153
Lutz, E.F., 80, 139
MacLean, A.F., 123
Mais, A., 135
McAlister, C.G., 5
McLaughlin, H.E., 306
Merkus, H.G., 26
Mertzweiller, J.K., 37
Mihara, H., 97
Mikolajczak, K.L., 163, 175
Miller, E.J., Jr., 135
Mitchell, L.C., 94, 102
Miwa, I., 97
Möller, K.E., 68
Morel, J., 218
Morgan, E.D., 320
Morita, S., 97
Mueller, W.A., 116
Müller, W., 221
Naskar, S.S., 314, 316
Nelson, J.S., 291
Neubauer, D., 41
Newton, L.W., 99
Okunev, R.A., 189
Olivier, K.L., 45
Osbond, J.M., 179
Patterson, J.A., 23
Patton, R.A., 297
Paulik, F.E., 57, 60
Paulis, B., 26
Pawlenko, S., 73
Payne, G.R., 333
Peck, D.W., 99
Perry, M.A., 273
Philpott, P.G., 179
Pike, J.E., 328
Plantholt, R.H., 323, 339
Pollock, M.W., 284

Potts, R.H., 137
Rehberg, H., 288
Reinheckel, H., 294
Remes, N.L., 278
Renckhoff, G., 314, 316
Rinse, J., 234
Robinson, G.C., 86
Roe, E.T., 12
Roming, C., Jr., 21
Roth, J.F., 57, 60
Ruf, E., 271
Saiki, N., 212
Schmerling, L., 120
Schweighofer, J., 221
Sennewald, K., 288
Serota, S., 311
Shapiro, S.H., 137
Silverstone, G.A., 286
Simmons, T.S., 83
Smith, C.R., Jr., 226
Staker, D.D., 339
Starks, C.M., 109, 156
Stein, W., 337
Stevens, N.J., 199
Stump, J.H., Jr., 306
Sumerford, S.D., 29
Swern, D., 12
Swidler, R., 116
Szonyi, C., 317
Thompson, J.E., 209
Thornton, T., 330
Toekelt, W.G., 120
Togawa, H., 212
Trebilcock, J.W., 301
Tummes, H., 65
Turner, J.H.W., 274
Ueno, K., 97
Van de Vusse, J.G., 21
van der Plas, F.J.F., 344
von Kutepow, N., 41
Vos, J.M., 15, 21
Waale, M.J., 15
Washecheck, P.H., 109, 296
Wechsler, J.R., 131
Wehe, A.H., Jr., 32
Wehrmeister, H.L., 177, 216
Weinrotter, F., 221
Whitaker, A.C., 260, 262
White, J.O., 146
Wicke, A.F., Jr., 306
Wickens, J.C., 179
Williams, P.H., 139
Wolff, I.A., 226
Wotiz, J.H., 181
Yanick, N.S., 333
Yatsu, L.Y., 193
Yeomans, B., 112, 115
Ziegler, K., 173
Zilch, K.T., 323, 327

U.S. PATENT NUMBER INDEX

3,005,846 - 62	3,308,155 - 153	3,483,222 - 288
3,033,884 - 179	3,320,230 - 326	3.489,779 - 312
3,047,599 - 65	3,342,841 - 227	3,492,325 - 209
3,047,622 - 2	3,345,389 - 327	3,493,590 - 190
3,052,699 - 319	3,349,107 - 73	3,503,896 - 254
3,052,701 - 303	3,356,699 - 175	3,505,394 - 45
3,053,869 - 5	3,362,970 - 297	3,506,695 - 330
3,054,814 - 75	3,362,971 - 94	3,515,737 - 112
3,057,893 - 226	3,362,972 - 246	3,526,649 - 314
3,059,004 - 15	3,365,476 - 260	3,527,779 - 26
3,059,005 - 21	3,367,954 - 278	3,530,155 - 50
3,059,006 - 21	3,370,074 - 262	3,530,156 - 189
3,059,007 - 21	3,375,263 - 301	3,531,506 - 316
3,060,211 - 97	3,376,327 - 231	3,541,121 - 331
3,061,621 - 68	3,383,398 - 99	3,541,122 - 333
3,066,160 - 304	3,396,182 - 346	3,542,822 - 156
3,068,256 - 21	3,398,166 - 273	3,542,823 - 317
3,075,010 - 120	3,404,166 - 218	3,546,262 - 234
3,076,842 - 78	3,405,151 - 328	3,546,263 - 271
3,084,178 - 320	3,407,220 - 139	3,547,962 - 109
3,121,728 - 144	3,407,221 - 80	3,549,676 - 337
3,151,139 - 344	3,409,506 - 199	3,553,188 - 149
3,162,659 - 183	3,409,648 - 37	3,557,169 - 86
3,167,585 - 9	3,409,649 - 106	3,558,678 - 257
3,169,139 - 205	3,412,116 - 294	3,560,537 - 251
3,170,939 - 12	3,413,323 - 129	3,562,300 - 281
3,173,933 - 141	3,414,594 - 102	3,564,030 - 135
3,188,330 - 284	3,415,856 - 83	3,564,031 - 137
3,205,244 - 29	3,419,587 - 238	3,574,731 - 54
3,217,020 - 173	3,429,902 - 311	3,578,690 - 245
3,217,046 - 163	3,433,815 - 309	3,579,551 - 57
3,225,075 - 242	3,437,676 - 41	3,579,552 - 60
3,227,737 - 35	3,449,385 - 221	3,586,704 - 169
3,235,578 - 323	3,449,413 - 250	3,590,058 - 88
3,238,250 - 91	3,455,785 - 194	3,592,849 - 151
3,244,735 - 267	3,457,299 - 42	3,637,478 - 116
3,247,231 - 291	3,458,544 - 248	3,637,832 - 146
3,253,007 - 165	3,458,582 - 83	3,637,833 - 61
3,257,438 - 306	3,461,146 - 274	3,649,657 - 339
3,261,856 - 158	3,466,308 - 177	3,654,327 - 168
3,262,954 - 32	3,466,309 - 216	3,661,710 - 193
3,282,973 - 70	3,466,310 - 223	3,661,956 - 286
3,282,993 - 23	3,470,219 - 123	3,661,986 - 296
3,288,826 - 186	3,471,535 - 161	3,703,549 - 115
3,296,286 - 33	3,471,536 - 310	3,708,513 - 131
3,299,111 - 181	3,476,786 - 233	3,708,534 - 212
3,304,316 - 265	3,483,083 - 196	

NOTICE

Nothing contained in this Review shall be construed to constitute a permission or recommendation to practice any invention covered by any patent without a license from the patent owners. Further, neither the author nor the publisher assumes any liability with respect to the use of, or for damages resulting from the use of, any information, apparatus, method or process described in this Review.

Complete copies of the patents described in this book may be obtained at a cost of $0.50 per patent prepaid. Address order to the Commissioner of Patents, U.S. Patent Office, Washington, D.C. 20231.

LUBRICANT ADDITIVES 1973
by M. W. Ranney

Chemical Technology Review No. 2

With increasing demands being placed on lubricants and hydraulic fluids for automobiles, aircraft, and high speed machinery, many research efforts have gone toward specific improvements. Additives are now required not only for petroleum bases, but also for synthetics, such as organic esters, polyphenyl ethers, and silicone fluids.

The high level of research activity in this field of lubricant additives is nowhere more evident than in the patent literature of the last few years. This book describes the synthesis and testing of over 200 lubricant additive compounds, as reflected in the recent patent literature (since 1970). Major emphasis during this period appears to be on load carrying additives, oxidation and corrosion inhibitors, and the ashless type detergents.

A partial and condensed table of contents follows. Numbers in ( ) indicate the number of patents per topic. Chapter headings are given, followed by examples of important subtitles.

1. **ASHLESS DISPERSANTS & DETERGENTS (31)**
   Succinic Acid-Based Products
   Triazine and Phosphorous Acid
   Polyhydric Alcohols + Polycarboxylic Acids
   Modified Polyolefins
   Sulfurization and Reaction with Polyamine
   Styrene-Maleic Anhydride Copolymers

2. **ASH-FORMING DISPERSANTS & DETERGENTS (23)**
   Overbased Metal Sulfonates
   Metal Salts of Hydroxy-Aromatic Compounds
   Metal Salts of Succinic Acid Esters
   Transition Metal Aminophosphorodithioates

3. **VISCOSITY INDEX IMPROVERS AND POUR POINT DEPRESSANTS (24)**
   Hydrogenated Polyvinylcyclohexane-EPR Block Copolymers
   Succinimide-Acrylic Acid Reaction Products
   Amine-Modified Cracked Ethylene-Propylene-Diene Terpolymer
   Graft Copolymers from Degraded Ethylene-Propylene Interpolymers
   Succinamic Acid + Ethylene-Olefin Copolymers

4. **LOAD CARRYING ADDITIVES (39)**
   Mineral Oils
   Sulfurized Diels-Alder Adducts
   Sulfurized Oxymolybdenum Organophosphorodithioate
   Barium Petroleum Sulfonate + Benzotriazole
   Antimony and Bismuth Phosphorodithioate
   Chlorendic Acid-Amine Reaction Products
   Ester-P_2S_5 Reaction Products
   Halogen-Substituted Organosilicon Compounds
   Lead Naphthenate
   Molybdenum Complexes
   Cetyl Vinyl Ether and N-Vinyl Pyrrolidone Telomers
   Imido-Polyphenyl Oxides
   Di-tert.-Nonyl Polysulfide + Silicones
   Dehydrocondensed Polyorganosilicones
   Dodecenyl Succinic Acid Anhydride + Silicones
   Polyphenyl Ethers + Silicones

5. **OXIDATION AND CORROSION INHIBITORS (50)**
   N-Nitrosophenylhydroxylamine
   Metal Salts of Alkylphenolethylenamines
   Phosphinodithioic Acid-Vinyl Carboxylate Adducts
   Phosphorodithioate-Alkylene Oxide Reaction Products
   Metal Salts of Phosphorodithioic and Alkylsuccinic Acids
   Phosphorus-Containing Silane
   Lithium Salt of Substituted Succinic Acids
   Organic Esters
   α-Methyl Styrenated Aromatic Amines
   Aromatic Amines + Substituted Benzophenones
   N-Substituted Phenothiazines and Triazines
   Alkyl-Substituted Phenothiazines
   Fluorinated Aromatic Amines

6. **ADDITIVES FOR SPECIALTY LUBRICANTS (16)**
   Metal Working Oils
   Ethoxylated Fatty Amines to Prevent Corrosion
   Soluble Oils
   Inhibited Base Polyglycol Lubricant
   Inhibiting Cavitation
   Penetrating Oils

ISBN 0-8155-0471-3

336 pages

ANTIFOULING MARINE COATINGS 1973

by A. Williams

Coatings Technology Review No. 1

One of the earliest needs for performance-oriented coatings was in the marine environment. Very early formulas were designed around known toxins such as copper and mercury compounds, and the earlier patent literature is replete with hundreds of directions for using these materials in creosote and natural drying oil formulations. Later information indicated in this book involves more sophisticated materials.

The two areas of a ship requiring specialty coatings are the bottom and the boot-topping area. The boot-topping area, intermittently exposed to air, sunshine, and water, represents a surface particularly difficult to protect from the elements.

For ships' bottoms, antifouling compounds, based on copper, mercury, and tin, are incorporated into somewhat water-sensitive binders to afford gradual breakdown of the film to allow for a sustained release of the poison. This required self-erosion necessitates frequent repainting of the ship's bottom, depending on geographical location and severity of exposure. By contrast, boot-topping paints are designed to provide a high level of resistance to both salt water and weather. Typically phenolic resin-tung oil, vinyl resin combinations are used.

This book describes many patented processes which provide high performance antifouling coatings based on metal compounds as well as organic coating compositions.

A partial and abbreviated table of contents is given here. Numbers in ( ) indicate the nos. of patents or application techniques discussed under a given heading. Chapter headings are given, followed by examples of important subtitles.

1. **COPPER COMPOUNDS (22)**
   Rosin & Blown Fish Oil
   Thermosetting Resins
   Elastomeric Coating for Sonar Domes
   Cu Salts of Alkyl Mercaptans
   Oil-Soluble Organocopper Compounds
   Copper Naphthenate
   Electrolytic Copper and Chlorinated
     Coal Tar
   Silica Particles Coated with Copper
     Oxide or Borate
   Stable Cuprous Pigments

2. **MERCURY & ARSENIC COMPOUNDS (11)**
   Phenylmercury Maleates
   Arylmercury Naphthenates
   Propyl Mercuric Chloride
   Perthiocyanic Acid Salts
   Cyano & Thiosubstituted Phenarsazines
   5-Hydro-10-fluorophenarsazine

3. **TIN & ANTIMONY COMPOUNDS (14)**
   Bis(tributyltin) Sulfide
   Bis(tributyltin) Adipate
   Triphenyltin Chloride
   Alkyd Bis(organotin) Oxide
   Multiple Elastomer Coatings
   Chlorinated Methanobenzene
   Triphenyl Antimony
   Barium Carbonate + Antimony Oxide

4. **OTHER ORGANOMETAL COMPOUNDS (5)**
   Bismuth Compounds
   Terephthalic Acid Metal Salts
   2-Thiazolylbenzimidazole Complexes
   Triphenylborane-Amine Complexes

5. **NONMETAL COMPOSITIONS (18)**
   Diiodomethyl Sulfones
   2-(N,N-Dimethylthiocarbamoylthio)-5-
     nitrothiazole
   Dithiooxamide
   Pentacyclic Amides
   Thiotetrahydrophthalimide Compositions
   Chlorophenyl Methyl Carbamate
   Diacetyl Dihydrazone
   1-Bromo-3-nitrobenzene
   1,2,3-Trichloro-4,6-dinitrobenzene
   Mytilotoxin
   Polytetrafluoroethylene Sheeting
   Coal Tar-Epoxy Resin Coating
   Pitch and Tar from Cut-Back Coal
     Digestion
   Phenolics, Coal Tar Bases +
     Unsaturated Aldehydes
   Phenolics + Aldehydes Condensation
     Products
   Fluoroacetates
   Fungicidal Water-Repellent
     Concentrates

POWDER COATINGS AND FLUIDIZED BED TECHNIQUES 1971

by Dr. M. W. Ranney

It is now potentially possible to paint auto bodies and other large items in a completely automatic plant with no manual labor and no environmental pollution. This is accomplished by solventless powder coating using fluidized bed, electrostatic spray, and other techniques which can be applied to metal, glass, wood and plastic surfaces. This book describes 161 processes based on U.S. patents. Due to the actuality of the subject, most patents are of very recent date, although some older, basic patents were included to give a complete technological picture of the state of the art.

Partial contents:

I. GENERAL PROCESSES

1. FLUIDIZED BED—SPRAY— POURING TECHNIQUES
   Fluidized Bed (19 Processes)
     Basic Fluidized Bed Processes (2)
     Fluidized Bed Apparatus (2)
     Self-Supporting Bed
     Rotation of Article in Bed
     Circulating Unit
     Auxiliary Agitation
     Continuous Flow of Particles
     Two-Zone Bed with Inclined Grid
     Coating and Oven Installation
     Subambient Temperature Coating
     Air Masking Device
     Holding Devices
     Vacuum Activated Supporting Device
     General Techniques (4)
   Spray—Powder—Etc. (7)
     Laminar Flow Powder Gun
     Jet Pulverizer Unit
     Application to External Surfaces (2)
     Dust Cloud Generator
     Spray Coating
     Dispenser Unit
2. ELECTROSTATIC PROCESSES
   Fluidized Bed (4)
     Stationary Fluidized Bed
     Electrode Design
     Addition of Ba-Titanate
     PVC+TCP
   Spray Techniques (4)
     Rotary Discharge Device
     Multilayer Process
     Heated Article
     Electrostatic Powder Fixing Device

II. COATING COMPOSITIONS

3. EPOXIES
     Curing Agents—Hardeners (6)
     Modified Epoxies (8)
     Powdering Techniques (4)
       High Density Grinding Media
       Rubber Mill Blending
       Low Temp. Film Former
4. POLYOLEFINS
     Polyethylene-Peroxide Blends
     Polyethylene Powder Technique
     Addition of Lecithin
     Pretreatment with Aminophenol
     Amine-Modified Clays
     Primers & Surface Treatment (3)
     CrO_3 Surface Treatment
     Polyvinyl Acetal Primer
       Coat by Flame Spraying
     Chlorinated Polyethylene on
       Epoxy Primer
     Use of Copolymers (2)
5. VINYLS
     Vinyl Primers and Control of Film
       Thickness (2)
     Primer for Vinyl Chloride Resins (2)
     Polyesters as Fusion Aids (2)
6. OTHER RESINS (11)

III. APPLICATIONS

7. PIPE COATINGS
     Fluidized Bed (18)
     Spray and Pouring (9)
8. ELECTRICAL COMPONENTS (19)
     Electrostatic Techniques (2)
9. OTHER APPLICATIONS (24)
     Strip Coating
     Brush Roll Assembly for Metal Strip
       Coating
     Heated Mandrel for Foil
     Foam Coatings
     Interior Coating for Polyolefin Bottles
     Hot Gas Spray Unit for Construction
       Work
     Electrostatic Metal Coatings (2)
     Light Bulb Coatings
     Cathode Ray Tube Phosphor Coatings
10. INORGANIC AND
    PARTICLE COATINGS (10)

249 pages

SYNTHETIC LUBRICANTS 1972
by M. W. Ranney
Chemical Process Review No. 59

The ever increasing severity of operating conditions for industrial and military equipment has necessitated the development of high performance lubricating fluids and greases.

Polymerized olefins were produced as early as 1929 and the military demands of World War II resulted in the manufacture of ester lubricants, followed by glycols and silicones. In recent years organic phosphates, fluorocarbons, silicate esters and polyphenyl ethers have all been developed for specialty lubrication uses. Research on additives has been of prime concern, leading to lubricants with improved load-bearing characteristics as well as increased resistance to rust and oxidation.

This book presents patent-based information on 205 processes since 1966. Partial List of Contents showing process examples follows. The numbers in ( ) indicate the number of processes allocated to each topic.

I. ORGANIC ESTERS
  GENERAL SYNTHESES (16)
    Pentaerythritol and Neoalkyl Acid Esters
    Tetromethylcyclobutanediol Diesters
      of Linolenic Acid
  INHIBITED FLUID FORMULATIONS (36)
    N-Phenylnaphthylamine and Ethyl-
      diphenylazasiline
    p-Diethylaminophenylsilanes
  EXTREME PRESSURE ADDITIVES (4)
    Triphenyl Phosphorothionates and
      Chlorinated Polyaryl Compounds
    Phosphonated Dilinoleate Esters
  OTHER ADDITIVES AND
    APPLICATIONS (7)
    Polyester Thickeners contg. Glycidyl
      Ester Acid Scavengers
  GREASES (3)
    Polyfunctional Esters
II. SILICONES
  GENERAL FLUID SYNTHESES (13)
    Silphenylene-Siloxane Copolymers
    Halophenylsiloxane-Fluoroalkyl-
      siloxane Copolymers
  GREASE FORMULATIONS (22)
    Polytetrafluoroethylene as Thickener
    Siloxanylferrocenes as Stabilizers
  SOLID LUBRICANTS (4)
    Silicone-Epoxy Dry Film Lubricant
  OTHERS (3)
    Quaternary Ammonium Compounds as
      Glass Lubricants

III. POLYGLYCOLS, PHOSPHATES, AND SILICATES
  POLYGLYCOLS (8)
    Polyoxyalkylene Adducts of Phenols
    Ascorbic Acid Stabilizers
  PHOSPHATES (2)
  SILICATES (6)
IV. POLYPHENYL ETHERS
  GENERAL SYNTHESES (9)
    Diphenoxybenzenes and Diphenoxy-
      diphenyls
    Conversion of Solid Phenoxydiphenyls
      to Fluids
  ADDITIVES (6)
    Metal Acetylacetonates
    Polyalkylaminotriazines
  HALOGEN-CONTAINING ETHERS (4)
  MISCELLANEOUS (2)
V. FLUOROCARBONS
  GREASE FORMULATIONS (4)
    Tetrafluoroethylene-Thickened Greases
    Phthalocyanine Thickeners
  FLUORINATED ESTERS (4)
    Cyanoalkyl Perfluoromethylphenyl
      Phosphates
  GENERAL (8)
    Polychlorotrifluoroethylene Oils for
      Corrosion Inhibition
    Cyclic Phosphonitrile Esters for
      Corrosion Inhibition
  THREAD SEALANTS (3)
VI. PETROLEUM
  VISCOSITY INDEX IMPROVERS AND
    DISPERSANTS (11)
    Syndiotactic Alkyl Polymethacrylates
    Carbonylated Polymers
  EXTREME PRESSURE ADDITIVES (5)
    Di(organo)phosphonates plus Sulfurized
      Hydrocarbons
    Phosphorous Acid-Lanolin Reaction
      Product
  OTHER ADDITIVES (4)
    Quinizarin Dilaurate and Aminosilanes
    Diester Lubricity Additives
  GREASE FORMULATIONS (4)
  METAL WORKING FORMULAS (5)
  OTHERS (5)
    Nonspreading Lubricants
    Solid Film Lubricant
    Monomolecular Lubricant

245 pages

CATALYST MANUFACTURE, RECOVERY, AND USE 1972

by M. Sittig

Chemical Process Review No. 66

A catalyst is the modern approximation to the alchemical concept of the philosopher's stone, held to have the power of transmuting elements.

The factors that determine the effectiveness of a particular catalyst for a given chemical transformation are still obscure. Hence, simple practical knowledge must dominate any process of making and using catalysts.

In industrial practice the trend toward more and more specific catalytic processes continues. Aside from organic synthesis, the major growth area for catalyst applications lies in the field of pollution control with particular emphasis on control of automotive air pollution.

The activity of a particular catalyst frequently depends on the precise method of preparation and activation, which may greatly influence its physical and chemical properties.

This book, based on U.S. patents, describes 180 methods of manufacture and recovery in detail. A partial table of contents follows. Numbers in ( ) indicate a plurality of processes per topic. Chapter headings are given, followed by examples of important subtitles.

1. **ALKALI METAL-CONTAINING CATALYSTS (3)**
   Olefin Polymerizations
2. **COPPER-CONTAINING CATALYSTS (17)**
   Acrylonitrile Manufacture
   Automotive Exhaust Treatment
   Gasoline Treatment
   Hydration of Acetylene
   Hydrogen Manufacture
   Hydrogenation
   Oxidation-Reduction
3. **ZINC-CONTAINING CATALYSTS (3)**
   Hydrocracking-Polymerization
4. **MERCURY-CONTAINING CATALYSTS (1)**
   Vinyl Chloride Manufacture
5. **ALUMINUM-CONTAINING CATALYSTS FOR FRIEDEL-CRAFTS REACTIONS (7)**
   Catalyst Regeneration
6. **BORON FLUORIDE-CONTAINING CATALYSTS (3)**
   Polymerization-Hydrocracking
7. **ALUMINUM OXIDE CATALYSTS & SUPPORTS (13)**
   Desulfuration
   Alumina Sol Production
   Preparation of Alumina Spheres
8. **URANIUM, THORIUM & RARE EARTH CATALYSTS (6)**
9. **LEAD AND TIN-BASED CATALYSTS (5)**
   Dehydrodimerization
   Halogenation
10. **SILICA-ALUMINA CATALYSTS (21)**
    Cracking
    Transalkylation
    Catalyst Preparation
    Regeneration
    Demetallation
11. **TITANIUM-CONTAINING CATALYSTS (5)**
    Polymerization
12. **VANADIUM-CONTAINING CATALYSTS (8)**
    Oxidation-Polymerization
13. **CHROMIUM-CONTAINING CATALYSTS (7)**
14. **MOLYBDENUM-CONTAINING CATALYSTS (17)**
15. **TUNGSTEN-CONTAINING CATALYSTS (4)**
16. **MANGANESE-CONTAINING CATALYSTS (2)**
    Automotive Exhaust Treatment
17. **RHENIUM-CONTAINING CATALYSTS (3)**
18. **IRON-CONTAINING CATALYSTS (5)**
    Ammoxidation-Dehydrogenation
19. **COBALT-CONTAINING CATALYSTS (5)**
    Hydroformylation-Hydrogenation-Steam Reforming
20. **RHODIUM-CONTAINING CATALYSTS (2)**
21. **NICKEL CATALYSTS (16)**
    Hydrocracking
    Hydrogen Production
    Hydrogenation
    Olefin Isomerization
    Steam Reforming
22. **PALLADIUM CATALYSTS (8)**
    Hydrogenation-Oxidation
23. **PLATINUM CATALYSTS (19)**
    Ammoxidation
    Automotive Exhaust Treatments
    Cracking
    Dehydrogenation
    Hydrocracking
    Hydrogen Cyanide Manufacture
    Isomerization
    Reforming
24. **FUTURE TRENDS**

285 pages